SOUND & HEARING
A Conceptual Introduction

SOUND & HEARING
A Conceptual Introduction

R. Duncan Luce
University of California, Irvine

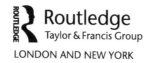

Routledge
Taylor & Francis Group

LONDON AND NEW YORK

First Published 1993 by
Lawrence Erlbaum Associates, Inc.
10 Industrial Avenue
Mahwah, New Jersey 07430

Published 2009 by Routledge
2 Park Square, Milton Park, Abingdon, Oxfordshire OX14 4RN
711 Third Avenue, New York, NY 10017

First issued in paperback 2016

Routledge is an imprint of the Taylor and Francis Group, an informa business

Library of Congress Cataloging in Publication Data

Luce, R. Duncan (Robert Duncan)
    Sound & hearing : a conceptual introduction / R. Duncan Luce.
      p. cm.
    Includes bibliographical references and index.
    ISBN 0-8058-1251-2 (hardcover)/ISBN 0-8058-1389-6 (paperback)
    1. Hearing. 2. Psychoacoustics. 3. Sound. I. Title.
II. Title: Sound and hearing.
    [DNLM: 1. Ear – physiology. 2. Hearing – physiology.
3. Psychoacoustics. 4. Sound. WV 270 L935s]
QP461.L93 1993
152.1'5 – dc20
DNLM/DLC
for Library of Congress   92–48799
                                          CIP

Publisher's Note
The publisher has gone to great lengths to ensure the quality of this reprint
but points out that some imperfections in the original may be apparent.

ISBN 13: 978-1-138-98255-0 (pbk)
ISBN 13: 978-0-8058-1251-0 (hbk)

Contents

Preface for Instructors

This text has evolved during the past decade in an attempt to convey something about scientific thinking, as evidenced in the domain of sounds and their perception, to students whose primary focus is not science. It tries to do so using a minimum of mathematics without, it is hoped, seriously compromising scientific integrity.

Its origins were in the then new Harvard University Core Curriculum. All undergraduates were required to take two semesters of science, the choices being grouped into two categories unrevealingly labeled A and B. Roughly, A courses were to correspond to scientific basics, such as particle physics and microbiology, and B courses to the more complex sciences, such as geology and biology of systems. (In practice, this partitioning was less clear-cut, which probably accounts for the fact that word labels never came to replace A and B.) David M. Green and I from the Department of Psychology and Social Relations and R. Victor Jones from the Department of Applied Physics laid out a plan for a two-semester course to fulfill both requirements: Sound and Hearing followed by Light and Seeing. The physics of the course would meet the A requirement, whereas the physiology and psychology satisfied the B requirement. Green and Jones gave the entire sequence once. Because Green did not find doing it very rewarding, he relinquished it to Jones and me. We gave Sound and Hearing the next year, but not Light and Seeing. After that I gave Sound and Hearing alone several times. As a single course it was, to my surprise, classed as A rather than B.

Since coming to the University of California, Irvine, I have given it twice to, primarily, psychology majors. As many of these students do not intend to do graduate work, and often have a decidedly limited interest in the scientific aspects of psychology, the conceptual flavor of the course has not changed greatly from its origins at Harvard.

It is safe to say that although quite a few students have taken the course— 50–75 each time it was given at Harvard and somewhat fewer at Irvine—it has never been judged a popular success. At Harvard this was due in part to the fact that the classes were full of nonscience majors who hoped it would be a relatively painless way to fulfill their Science A requirement. It was never sufficiently painless. In part this was because we made them do problems both as homework and in exams. And in part it was because many of these students were "big picture" types, and hearing, although personally important and valuable, hardly has the pizzazz of world history or cosmology or sociobiology. Yet it does serve as a neat vehicle for learning some basic physical ideas of wave motion, a bit of neurophysiology, some perception, and how these three work together. Its lack of popular acclaim was, I must acknowledge, also due to my not being a charismatic teacher.

One may ask: Why bother writing a new book on the topic? Why not just use one of the existing texts, such as Green's (1976) or Yost and Nielsen's (1985) admirable treatments? At the onset, all three of us felt that the handling of the physics in the psychology texts was insufficiently detailed and elementary for the students with whom we were dealing. So at Jones' suggestion we used Johnson, Walker, and Cutnell (1981) to cover the physics of waves, and I continued to use it until the Spring Quarter of 1991. That book, despite its being excellent and at the appropriate level, does not take up topics in my preferred order and, given its title *The Science of Hi-Fidelity,* understandably includes a great deal of material on audio equipment that is irrelevant to hearing, as such. So it seemed reasonable to incorporate the needed physics into a text whose focus is as much on hearing as on sound.

For the physiology and psychology, I have tried several of the psychology texts, the most successful proving to be Yost and Nielsen. Still, I found I had to supplement whatever book I used by various handouts. Things were patched together from various sources, something that never seems popular in elementary courses. For the physiology of the ear, the existing texts seem very satisfactory, although typically rather more detailed than I could afford to be. For the psychology, things seemed poorly organized from my perspective. One goal of the course was to make as clear as possible which phenomena can be accounted for by the physics of sine waves; then those for which the physics alone provides no explanation, but properties of the ear and the peripheral auditory nerve do; and finally those that, although well-established psychologically, have not been reduced to what we *currently* know about physics and neurons. In general, the latter phenomena are believed to be more heavily mediated by central processing than by the periphery alone. Beyond that, I wanted to segregate issues that could be studied using just single pure tones from those that necessarily involve more complex waveforms, such as harmonics and noise. In part, this was to partition a fairly substantial dose of physics into two segments separated by some physiology and psychology. To do this in the existing texts required jumping about a great deal, always bumping into inconvenient cross-references. So gradually the handouts grew in number and size, and increasingly they supplanted the text materials until in 1991 I operated solely from the notes that led to this text.

The material covered is what I covered in one semester at Harvard and in one quarter at Irvine, both of which involve 10 weeks of lectures. The course involves 28 lectures plus two 1-hour exams. The schedule that I followed, with slight adjustments for holidays, has been:

Week	Sections
1	I, II.1–4
2	II.5–10
3	II.11–12, III.1–2
4	III.3–5
5	Hour exam, IV.1–3
6	IV.4, V.1–2
7	V.3–5, VI.1–2
8	Hour exam, VI.3–4
9	VI.5–6
10	VI.7–8, review

For a course with more lectures, supplementary material will have to be added, which is certainly not hard to do because I have ignored many topics. To some degree, binaural hearing has been slighted, in part because the demonstrations, which mostly require earphones, create special classroom problems that I elected not to confront. Usually binaural phenomena are grouped together, but in this text they are separated depending on whether they are understood primarily physically, physiologically, or psychologically. Among the many topics not covered are pulsation thresholds, the dependence of pitch perception on duration, the circularity of pitch, and properties of timbre, musical scales, and various click phenomena.

The issue of classroom demonstrations is always a problem. As the course was first devised, a number were prepared and used for the physics part. I have come to abandon most of these, in part because so many of the relevant phenomena are well known to the students from their experience with water waves, ropes, pendulums, and springs. And partially because for qualitatively unfamiliar ideas, such as spectral analysis, the demonstrations seemed more confusing than illuminating. These demonstrations just did not seem to be worth the effort and time for students with little technical background.

Most of the auditory demonstrations came originally from the series of tapes prepared by David M. Green that were disseminated to professionals in the field and, no doubt, widely copied. Later, many (but unfortunately not all) of these plus some additional or modified ones were released as a compact disc by Phillips, 1126–061, which is currently available from the Acoustical Society of America. Because this disc is not very strong on some of the complex fusing and streaming phenomena, the induction of missing sounds, and various aspects of speech, I supplemented it with some of Green's tapes and with a tape prepared by A. Bregman and M. Kubovy. I am grateful to the copyright holders, A.J.M. Houtsma, T.D. Rossing, W.M. Wagenaars, Albert S. Bregman, and David M. Green, for their assistance in the preparation of the various materials for the demonstration disc, and for their permission to use those materials. The demonstrations used in this text are all on a compact disc entitled *Sound & Hearing Demonstration Disc* that is available from Lawrence Erlbaum Associates. A technical description is provided at the end of this text beginning on page 297.

My major debts are, first, to Green and Jones, with whom the initial course was developed. I have subsequently made a number of changes from that original plan; I have lost sight of just how many. And second, to Phillip Kelleher who was my head teaching assistant three times at Harvard. He was a fine source of feedback about problems in the course, an excellent instructor, and most conscientious in helping students and preparing supplementary materials. Kelleher was especially effective in preparing problems for homework and exams, and a substantial portion of the included exercises are his handiwork. In the final phase of preparation Courtney Crowther assembled the figures both from original and secondary sources and by computer generation. Dr. Bruce Berg carefully read the entire manuscript, and his comments have been extremely useful in reducing error and unclarity in the text, for which I am deeply indebted. My wife, Carolyn Scheer, has helped me in many ways, the most directly relevant being to simplify my writing.

R. Duncan Luce

Preface for Students

GOALS

The major aim of this text is to give you some idea about the ways in which scientists approach and think about a phenomenon—hearing—that intersects three quite distinct disciplines. Usually we take hearing for granted. Unless afflicted by hearing loss of one sort or another, we rarely think about it, any more than we think about how we see or talk or walk. The disciplines involved are the physics of sound sources and the propagation of sound through air and other materials, the anatomy and physiology of the transformation of the physical sound into neural activity in the brain, and the psychology of the perception that we call hearing. Physics, biology, and psychology each play a role in understanding how and what we hear.

One problem that a scientist in this area must repeatedly try to untangle is this: Given a particular phenomenon of hearing—for example, the localization of sounds—to what degree can we understand it simply in terms of the physics of sounds? Or do we need also to know something about what the ear does? Or is the phenomenon also dependent on something in the brain and psychology that lies beyond the ear and the peripheral auditory nervous system, that is, in what we refer to as the central system? We encounter examples of each.

In this text we use our gradually developing understanding of the three disciplines to try to untangle various auditory puzzles. Let it be clear at the onset that some puzzles are too complex for a text at this level to tackle and there are others that no one yet understands. Nonetheless, within our limits, there are a number of phenomena that, most likely, you do not now understand but will by the end of the text.

One aspect of these puzzles is auditory illusions. These are much like visual illusions in the sense that what one hears differs from what is physically present: something not present is heard or something that is present is not heard. The main difference is that auditory illusions typically go unnoticed by the uninitiated, whereas many visual ones are clearly paradoxical. For example, did you know that telephone communication is based in substantial part on an illusion? You hear what is in fact not physically there; more on that in Section VI.4. There is another illusion that is easier to demonstrate; yet it is one in which you, the hearer, fail to hear what is in fact there. This occurs all of the time because you are unaware of the many echos that always exist. You can hear this in Demonstration 1[1] in which various recorded sounds are played in the usual way following which they are played backward. In the backward version you will be aware of a long "shish" preceding the major sound itself. These are echos from the walls of the room in which the sounds were made, echos that one fails to hear in the forward version. In this case the listener unconsciously suppresses a sound; it is something we do all of the time unless the echos of the sound are sufficiently delayed, as in a canyon. Nevertheless, it is an auditory illusion.

PREREQUISITES

The major prerequisite is your interest in learning how science tries to provide some understanding of a basic, but nonetheless complex sensory process. The text is not intended to be the basis of a "gut" course. It involves an accumulation of knowledge and requires you to think about different ways in which that knowledge can be put together. On the other hand, the course does not presuppose that you already have a strong background in physics, biology, psychology, or mathematics.

Let me be precise about the mathematical requirements:

Elementary algebra is used freely. For example, you are expected to be able to get readily from one side of the following equation to the other:

$$1/x + 1/y = (x + y)/xy$$

Note the distinction between $1/x + 1/y$ and $1/(x + 1/y) = y/(xy + 1)$.

The only *functions* that appear as equations are:

---

[1]The demonstrations are available on the CD, *Sound & Hearing Demonstraction Disc*, from Lawrence Erlbaum Associates.

$$y = A \sin x, \ y = ax + b, \ y = ax^c, \ y = \log_{10} x.$$

The relationships represented by such equations appear often in the context of specific empirical problems. As each one is introduced, you are reminded of its basic properties.

Graphs of various types serve as effective means for summarizing a lot of information—both qualitative and quantitative. In particular, you are expected to go back and forth between the four functions listed and their corresponding graphs. (You are reminded about this as we go along.) In addition, many data are presented in graphical form. By the end of the text you will have been exposed to a least six quite different types of graphs. One goal is for you to understand and to know how to interpret data in each of these different modes of presentation, which skill is useful beyond the present subject matter.

Equipment is not much emhasized although, in fact, moderately elaborate electronic equipment is essential for carrying out original research in this area. Auditory phenomena can be demonstrated using a CD player and the demonstration disc described in footnote 1. Some of the binaural (two-ear) demonstrations on the disc can only be appreciated using earphones.

Some of the material on waves is nicely demonstrated on a computer, but I have not prepared such programs to accompany the text. In part, it seemed futile to do so given the large number of possible software packages available.

HOMEWORK

Homework problems are essential for understanding this kind of science, and a number are provided. In general, they are not multiple choice. Some involve calculations using equations you have encountered, but few can be solved by simply searching for the right formula and substituting the numbers. Rather, they require some understanding of which concepts are relevant, and only than will it be apparent what calculations to carry out.

GENERAL STRUCTURE OF THIS TEXT

Part I describes in very general terms something of the problem faced by any organism in finding out about its environment. There are similarities and differences in the several sense modalities, and some of the more important of these are cited. Part II develops the physical description of the simplest sound signals, and some important phenomena are explained. Next, Part III examines some of the anatomical, mechanical, and electromechanical properties of the inner ear. Within that framework we examine how the sound arriving at the ear is "transduced" through the inner ear and is recoded as electrical pulses on the auditory nerve. These findings play a role in Part IV, which explores some of the psychophysical (behavioral) results about these simplest sound signals. To deal with sounds of greater complexity, we examine some of the physics of more complex sounds in Part V. Finally, Part VI takes up some of the phenomena that arise with more complex signals, including several that are not really understood in terms of the physics of the signal or the physiology of the peripheral auditory neurons.

ADDITIONAL READINGS

Most of us get confused when trying to absorb a new subject, and any one presentation may confuse you to some degree. To crib a bit from Lincoln, no matter how authors try, they fail to communicate to some of the students some of the time, although presumably not all of the students all of the time. When you don't understand, often it helps to read what someone else has said about the same thing.

For the elementary physics of sound I recommend Johnson, Walker, and Cutnell (1981) as an excellent introduction. Rossing (1982) covers some of the same material plus a good deal of physiology and psychology, with a strong focus on music. Neither text uses any calculus.

For the physiology and psychology of hearing, the first reference to turn to is Yost and Nielsen (1985). Other, somewhat more advanced, alternatives are Hirsch (1952), Gluck, Gescheider, and Frisina (1989), Green (1976), Handel (1989), Moore (1982), Pickles (1988), Pierce (1983), Roederer (1975), Shiffman (1982), Stevens, Warshofsky, and Editors of *Life* (1965), Tobias (1970), or Warren (1982).

R. Duncan Luce

Greek Symbols

As in much scientific literature, there is a liberal sprinkling of Greek symbols, whose usage is deeply ingrained. They are summarized here with the section they are first introduced noted:

Symbol	Case	Name	Section	Meaning
α	lower	alpha	IV.3.3.3	exponent
β	lower	beta	IV.3.2.3	exponent
δ	lower	delta	IV.2.5	variable difference
Δ	upper	delta	II.8.3.1	fixed difference
γ	lower	gamma	IV.3.3.3	exponent
ϕ	lower	phi	II.2.1.4	phase angle
λ	lower	lambda	II.3.2.1	wavelength
μ	lower	mu	II.2.1.2	micro
ρ	lower	rho	II.7.1	density
θ	lower	theta	II.2.1	angle
τ	lower	tau	V.2.2.3	tension
ω	lower	omega	II.2.1	angular velocity

PART I

Transmission, Transduction, and Black Boxes

1. SIGNAL TRANSMISSION

For us to know about the world outside ourselves, events at some distance from us must impact one or more of the sense organs underlying the sensations known as sight, sound, taste, smell, touch, pain, and so forth. So, before information reaches the sense organ, something external must happen: A signal must be produced and that signal must be transmitted in some way to the sense organ.

What are the possible modes of transmission? Scientists know of three distinct types of transmission.

(i) A physical object can simply move from the source to the receiver — from the external site to the sense organ.

The crudest example is some form of projectile, such as a stone or a bullet, although neither is often used to transmit information in any usual sense. An informative projectile is a letter, but of course it requires some additional (visual) transmission once it is sufficiently near the intended recipient.

A more subtle example is light transmission. One of the great discoveries of the early 20th century is that light moves about in tiny packets of energy (and mass) called light quanta, which in some respects may be treated simply as projectiles. In particular, this mode of transmission does not depend on there being a physical connection — medium — between the source and the receiver. Light, for example, traverses a vacuum.

(ii) Impulses that are transmitted in a medium.

In this case, the source of a signal and the sense organ receiving it are usually bathed in the same medium,[1] and the signal moves as a pulse through the medium. Perhaps the simplest, most visible example is a surface wave on water that is generated simply by touching the surface of still water, for example, by dropping a pebble into a pond. Note that no material object is moved from the source to the receiver. For example, if a cork is floating in the pond, it will bob up and down as the impulse arising from the stone passes it, but on average it will be no closer to the receiver after the pulse has passed than it was before. Nothing but the ephemeral pulse moves through the medium.

For the purposes of this text, the key example is sound pulses that are transmitted in various materials, including air, water, and solids. Again, this is done without any particle moving from one place to another. Only the sound propagates, which may be thought of as a wave somewhat analogous to a water wave. Note that this method of transmission is not possible in a vacuum, such as outer space.

(iii) Transmission as a field, which acts somewhat like a medium, but is not.

The two most prominent examples of this form of transmission are gravity and electromagnetism. We are all very familiar with both gravitation and magnetic fields (compasses). The exact nature of fields has been the source of some controversy because, from some points of view, they act much like wave transmission, without any medium.[2] (Until the late 19th century, a medium called ether was postulated for electromagnetic transmission, until experiments established that it would have to have impossible properties.) In addition to gravity and electromagnetism, two other types of fields have been discovered called the strong and weak forces, and one of the concerns of modern physics is how these forces relate. Gravity, despite its being the first known, seems isolated from the other three. Indeed, despite major efforts to detect gravity waves, it remains unclear whether gravity exhibits a wave motion.

We focus solely on pressure impulses and waves in a medium, for it is these changes in pressure that we perceive as sound. Part II is devoted to the physics of generating and transmitting such pressure waves.

---

[1]This is not strictly necessary. For example, sounds originating in air can be rather poorly received by a person under water because, as we explore in Section II.8, some, but not a great deal, of the sound produced in air is transmitted through the air–water interface. Transmission is best when the source and receiver are in the same medium.

[2]Depending on the question asked, light, which is a special form of electromagnetism, acts either as a particle or a wave. This is known as the duality of light. Some scientists believe that gravity may ultimately be shown to exhibit the same duality.

2. SIGNAL RECEPTION

What is involved when a signal arrives at a sense organ? At the least, the person must be made aware by the sense organ that the signal has arrived. A basic generalization can be made about all such perception:

Only physical *changes* are perceived. Anything that is truly constant is never perceived.

Three examples illustrate this fact:

- Most of the time you are unaware that your entire body is under atmospheric pressure (of about 14.7 lbs/in^2). But in a rapidly moving elevator or descending airplane the external pressure can change far more rapidly than does your internal pressure, which is somewhat slower to respond, and you become (often acutely) aware of the pressure change.
- You do not notice an image that is held in a fixed location on the retina (the neural receptors at the back) of the eye. This is a difficult experiment to perform because, without any conscious awareness, the eye moves in small jumps — called saccades — several times a second. So some subtle technique and apparatus is needed to take the saccades into account in order to maintain an image at a fixed location on the retina. But when done, the fixed image rapidly disappears. (Is this assertion inconsistent with your subjective impression that you can fixate on something and it does not disappear?)
- You do not notice when there is a high level of static electricity on your body until it is rapidly discharged (preferably not into a computer), at which point you feel an electric shock. This phenomenon is very familiar to those who live in cold, dry climates; it occurs infrequently in southern California.

A corollary of this proposition states that anything perceived as a steady signal must, despite the compelling impression of steadiness, involve some change at the sense organ. Either

- **the sense organ must induce continual change, or**
- **the seeming constancy of the stimulus must be an illusion, and it really is not constant.**

As noted earlier, the eye is an example of a sense organ that induces continual change. When you gaze steadily at an unmoving object, the saccades, mentioned earlier, cause the needed change.

As an example of the second, consider a steady sound, such as a pure tone often used to test audio equipment. It sounds completely constant, but that is an illusion. A pure tone actually involves very rapid, very small changes of air pressure at the ear. They are so fast you do not notice them at a conscious level, but without them you would hear nothing.

So, each sense organ must be a device that responds to a certain class of physical changes: the eye to aspects of the light quanta impinging on it, and the ear to the changes in the pressure waves. But if they are just simple detectors of change, one can ask:

In order to understand sound and hearing (and light and seeing) why isn't it sufficient to understand the physics of the sound stimulus?

This is not a silly question. Indeed, until about 100 to 125 years ago, many scientists thought that understanding the physics of sound would be sufficient. Among those who pursued this approach were three of the most famous physicists, Newton, Fourier, and Helmholtz. They first showed how complex light and sound signals can be decomposed into a sum of very simple components: in the case of light, into the spectrum formed in a rainbow. We look into such decomposition of sound waves in Part V. Next, they postulated that if we understand how the human being responds to each of these components, then the total effect of the signal would simply be the sum of the several effects from the components. This is known as the **linear systems** approach.

Their strategy did not work because the eye and the ear do a far more complex job of processing complex signals than was realized at first. We encounter some of this processing in Part III.

Such complexity is illustrated by the existence of perceptual illusions. These were first recognized in vision, and you are no doubt familiar with some. There are auditory illusions as well, but most of us are less aware of them. The existence of illusions means that the ear and eye do a lot more than passively "transduce" the physical signal, which is discussed in some detail in the next section.

3. TRANSDUCERS

We just spoke of the ear and eye as doing more than "passively transducing" the signal. What does this term *transduce* mean?

DEFINITION: A **transducer** is any device whose (primary) function is to convert energy from one form to another while retaining information about the amount of energy involved.

The term *device* is intentionally vague, because transducers come in many guises. Some familiar examples listed in Table I.1 illustrate the breath of the concept.

TABLE I.1
Types of Transducers

Name of Device	Conversion
MICROPHONE:	sound pressure into electrical current
LOUDSPEAKER:	electrical current into sound pressure
PHOTOCELL:	light into electrical current
LIGHT BULB:	electrical current into light (+ heat)
GENERATOR:	mechanical rotation into electrical current
MOTOR:	electrical current into mechanical rotation
EAR (outer, middle, inner):	sound pressure into neural activity
VOCAL CORDS + MOUTH:	neural activity into sound
RETINA:	light into neural activity
− − −:	neural activity into light

Note that transducers mostly come in pairs, the one being, in effect, the inverse conversion of the other, except that in each case some of the energy is dissipated in the form of heat loss. Thus, for example, we use a flow of water or steam in a turbine to rotate a generator that converts some of that mechanical (flow) energy into electricity, which is then transmitted to a site, such as one's home, where some of it is used to run motors (in fans, vacuum cleaners, turntables, etc.) that once again provide mechanical power. In both conversions, heat is also generated and lost.

The major exception to such pairing is the last. Mammals simply do not generate light. Of course, some fish and some insects, such as fire flies, do.

4. BLACK AND NOT-SO-BLACK BOXES

4.1 The Black-Box Approach

In describing transducers, we speak of them in a functional way: as devices that perform a task of converting energy from one form to another. We often need to describe the exact nature (i.e., functional form) of that conversion in great detail. For example, an ideal microphone or loud-speaker has an output that is directly proportional to input, that is, if x denotes a numerical measure of the input and y a numerical measure of the output, then proportionality means that there is a positive constant c such that $y = cx$. Few microphones or loudspeakers live up to such an ideal, but usually proportionality is the goal and, roughly, it is accomplished to a degree that tends to correspond closely to the cost of the transducer. (As is pointed out later, proportionality may well not be an ideal goal for a hearing aid.) For many purposes, such a functional description may be all we need to know about the transducer. Of course, a person designing, building, or repairing a transducer needs to understand the internal structure that gives rise to the overall behavior, but few people who use transducers need to know more than the functional description.

Treating a complex device as a unitary object of known characteristics has come to be called the "black-box" approach. This image arises from the dull, usually inelegant, black casings that often housed scientific electronic devices just before and after World War II. When attention was paid only to their input–output relations, they were referred to as "black boxes." The term has been generalized. For most of us, most of the devices we encounter are treated as black boxes: TVs, computers, calculators, automobiles, locks, and so forth. Most of us usually do not care or need to know more about a device than its functional properties.

4.2 Why and When Does One Take a Black-Box Approach?

The answer to this question depends on the situation.

- The behavior of the box may be functionally much simpler than its inner mechanisms, and the external description may suffice for the purposes at hand. A good amplifier is a case in point. All it does is effect a proportional change, taking a weak electrical signal and making it strong enough to drive a transducer such as a loudspeaker. Nothing could be simpler — except that it is extremely difficult to achieve such proportionality over a wide range of inputs. To do so took years of research and development.
- We simply may not care in the slightest about how the behavior of the box is generated — unless it needs repair or it badly confuses us. The latter is often the situation facing a scientist who is trying to understand something complex, such as human behavior or earthquakes.
- Opening the black box may be infeasible (e.g., ethically), impossible (e.g., opening it destroys its function), or dangerous (e.g., opening it will release noxious substances). Obviously, there are all sorts of feasibility and ethical problems when people and their sense organs are at issue. We simply cannot take apart a human sense organ in order to learn more about how it works.
- Usually it is a good idea to have clear-cut behavioral questions before looking at the "jungle" inside a black box. Imagine trying to figure out what a computer does with neither a manual nor a wiring diagram, but just by opening it and measuring its electrical activity. That analogy is not too far

from the task facing scientists who study the relations between human behavior and neural activity.

4.3 The Black-Box Approach in Psychology

As has been hinted at in some of these examples, experimental psychology treats the person as a black box in the following sense. It tries to describe outputs, **responses,** as a function of external events (often past ones), which are usually classed into at least one of the following categories:

- **Signals** are external events of concern to the receiver.
- **Noise** is other energy in the same modality as the signal, especially energy that makes reception of the signal significantly more difficult. What is noise to one receiver may be signal to another, for example, people talking at a party.
- **Instructions** are explanations to the subject about what is to be treated as signals and how to respond to them.
- **Reinforcements** involve feedback of information about the accuracy of responses. Sometimes the feedback is accompanied by rewards, such as money or food pellets for animals, or punishments that depend on the accuracy of the responding to the signals. With animals, reinforcements are the way that instruction is communicated about what behavior the experimenter wants; it also serves to keep the animal motivated in responding differentially.
- **Social manipulations** of the subject's environment occur in some experiments, although not in many perceptual ones. One social factor that is always present and sometimes significant is the interaction between the subject and the experimenter.

There are other features of the human black box over which the experimenter has no control except by selecting subjects to meet certain criteria. These features may prove important in gaining a full understanding of the observations. Two of the most important are:

- **Cultural backgrounds** of subjects may have an impact on experimental outcomes. To the degree that this has been studied, which is not a great deal, it does not seem to be as major a factor in sensory experiments as in some others.
- **Genetic differences** may underlie some of the individual differences seen in the behavior of subjects. Of the genetic differences, the most prominent and easiest to study is sex, and studies sometimes partition the data by the sex of the subjects. This is most common when it is obvious that

it makes a big difference as, for example, in hearing loss with age (see Section IV.2.6.3).

To some extent these differences can be determined from external observation, such as sex and certain aspects of ethnic background. Other, more subtle genetic differences, such as certain chromosome patterns, can only be determined by intrusive methods. Presumably, the deep impact of culture on people is somehow stored as nearly permanent features of the brain, but at the present time we do not know what internal observations to make and we are restricted to gross external characteristics.

One example of such a black box approach that is relevant to sound and hearing is shown in Fig. I.1.

This figure, to a degree, suggests the organization of the text into the physics of the sound signal (Parts II and V), the anatomy and physiology of the ear, which is the major transducer of sound pressure into electrical activity on the neurons (Part III), and the overall stimulus–response psychology of hearing (Parts IV and VI). We follow this strategy:

We first undertake to gain some understanding of the transmission of

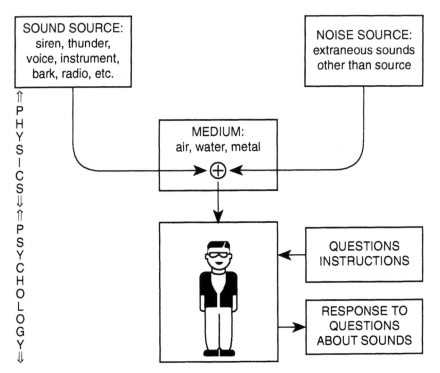

FIG. I.1 The black-box view of a person who, under instructions, is responding to a sound source in the presence of noise.

sound, and as we do so we cite examples where the physical properties of the stimulus are sufficient to account for our perceptions. For example, Part II provides an explanation for the fact that when a police car approaches with its siren blaring, the pitch of the siren changes as it passes us. And Part V explains physically why beating, which is used by piano tuners, occurs. If it cannot be explained physically, the next question is whether by opening the black box we can gain a better understanding.

4.4 Partially Opening the Black Box

Psychology, itself, does not necessarily try to open the black box to explore the internal mechanisms that lead to individuals' behavior or, in the case of sounds, to their perceptions. That is the province of neuroscience and physiology. These fields "open" (at least partially) the black box and try to understand the nature of the processes that underlie aspects of behavior — in our case, those having to do with hearing. They try to understand the mechanical, chemical, and neural-electrical activities that appear to give rise to the observed behavior.

The need to open the black box arises, in particular, when the transducer is complex in what it does. Had the ear been simply a proportionality device, like an amplifier, then the purely physical approach to hearing would have worked and there would have been little reason for psychologists to worry about what goes on in the ear. However, the ear is not much like an amplifier, although it is partially one, and so it became essential to study carefully what exactly the ear does in transducing the signal. This is taken up in Part III.

In opening the black box, one replaces it with several other black boxes at a finer level of observation. For example, we study the level of electrical activity on individual neural fibers in the auditory, or so called eighth nerve[3] coming off the inner ear, but we treat the individual neuron itself as a black box. We do not ask about the processes that go on within the nerve cell that allow electrical activity to be propagated along the nerve. Of course, there are biologists who study such matters. Each of the processes in the cell may, in turn, be taken apart further into component black boxes. This process terminates at the ultimate black box, currently thought to be a family of elementary particles and four forces (fields) among them. We stop far, far short of that.

So, for example, our first level decomposition for hearing can be diagrammed as in Fig. I.2. Further decomposition is necessary to understand the inner ear. We examine its structure in some detail, finding components that themselves will be treated as black boxes.

---

[3]In the technical literature this is usually written VIIIth nerve.

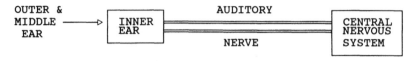

MECHANICAL   ELECTRO-CHEMICAL

FIG. I.2   A first "opening" of the overall black box into a series of component black boxes: the inner ear, the auditory nerve, and the central nervous system. Each of these can, and will, be decomposed into systems of more basic black boxes.

Having acquired some idea about the nature of the transduction effected by the ear, we then return to psychology, in Parts IV and VI. Here we describe some of the phenomena that psychologists have discovered, and we ask the degree to which we understand them either in terms of the physics of the signal or in terms of the peripheral physiology. If neither, then presumably the explanation lies in activities higher up in the brain. Although a great deal of research has and is being carried out on the neurophysiology of brain function, at the present time it does little to illuminate the psychological phenomena we encounter, and so it is not summarized here.

5. REDUCTIONISM IN SCIENCE

This, then, illustrates the *partially reductionist* strategy of the sciences.

Going between levels of analysis typically is difficult—in particular, detailed knowledge at one level does not always translate readily into predictions at an adjacent level. Probably it does not surprise you that knowledge at a higher level fails to implicate precisely the underlying processes at the next lower level, but many people seem to expect that it will be comparatively easy to pass from lower level knowledge to predictions about the higher level. Some scientists feel that when we understand enough neuroscience, then we will be able to predict the psychological processes in great detail. Perhaps that will happen in the long run, although there are sound reasons to doubt even that. But certainly matters are currently not so simple. The structure and function found at the lower level is often overwhelmingly complex, and without the behavior discovered by psychologists partially guiding the search for relevant neural processes, one simply does not have any idea what is behaviorally significant.

We turn in the next three parts to the generation and transmission of simple physical sounds, their transduction by the ear into neural activity, and to some of the basic sensory behavior that is partially illuminated by the physics and physiology.

Descriptive Physics of Pure Tones

1. PROPAGATION OF PULSES

Our first topic is the propagation of sound (or other waves) in a medium. To start, we examine a case that is simpler in two respects. First, only single pulses are propagated. Second, we consider mechanically induced pulses on a wire, which are easily demonstrated and seen.

1.1 Transverse Propagation

Consider a thin wire or string that is firmly attached to a wall at one end and held in your hand at the other end, as shown in panel a of Fig. II.1. Next, move your hand briskly upward, as shown in panel b. Then, immediately reverse direction, as in panel c. Finally, return your hand to the initial position and then simply watch the pulse that has been created. It moves along the wire from the hand toward the wall, as in panel d. This simple demonstration is easily performed. When you do it, you will find that when the pulse reaches the wall it is reflected back along the wire. We explore such reflections in Section II.5.

Such a pulse is called **transverse** because the change that is propagated is perpendicular to the direction of propagation.

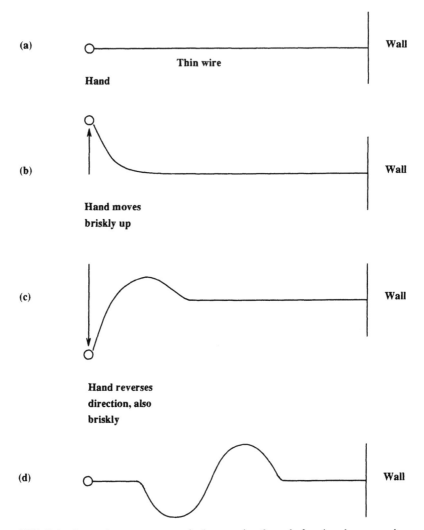

FIG. II.1   Generating a transverse pulse by snapping the end of a wire whose opposite end is firmly attached to a wall.

1.2 Longitudinal Propagation

A second, somewhat different mode of propagation is possible in some media. Consider a coiled spring, such as the children's toy called a "slinky." Again, attach one end to a fixed object such as a wall (or just have another person hold it), and hold the other end in your hand, as in panel a of Fig. II.2. Once again, move your hand briskly, but this time in the same direction as the slinky, toward the wall, as in panel b. Again, reverse direction and then immediately return your hand to the original position, as in panel c. Now, watch as the pulse propagates along the slinky. The pulse is noticeable

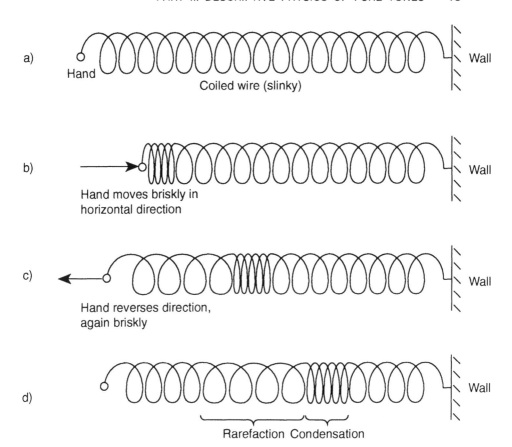

FIG. II.2 Generating a longitudinal pulse on a spring, such as a slinky, by rapid movements of the unconstrained end in the overall direction of the spring, first toward and then away from the constrained end.

because it involves a narrow region in which the spring is more tightly coiled than normal, called a **condensation,** followed by a narrow region in which it is less tightly coiled than normal, called a **rarefaction** (see panel d).

A pulse of this character is called **longitudinal** because the changes are all in the direction of the propagation.

Observe that on the slinky one can produce either a longitudinal or a transverse pulse depending on whether the hand is moved in a longitudinal or a transverse manner. Also, note that the speed of propagation of the two types of pulses differs, with the longitudinal faster than the transverse pulse; this is typical.

1.3 Propagation in a "Continuous" Medium

A continuous medium is either a gas, such as air; a liquid, such as water; or a more-or-less homogeneous solid, such as metal, stone, or wood. Any of these propagate sound pulses. Recall that in reality none of these media are really continuous, but rather are composed of many small molecules. We may idealize them as tiny billiard balls floating about in space. In a gas, the molecules are relatively independent of each other, moving around with an average velocity that depends on the temperature, and they continually collide with each other, thereby changing direction of movement irregularly. Those collisions are the source of pressure in the gas. The more densely they are packed, the more likely they are to collide, and so the pressure is higher than with less dense packing.

Now, imagine a gas trapped in a long cylinder (tube) with a moveable piston at one end. And consider moving that piston briskly to the right and then reverse it back to its original position. As with the slinky, the movement to the right forces the molecules that the piston encounters into a tight band, and when reversed it produces a region in which the molecules are sparse—a condensation followed by a rarefaction. So it is exactly analogous to propagation in a slinky, as shown in Fig. II.3.

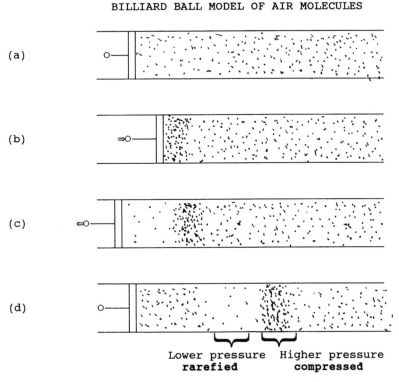

BILLIARD BALL MODEL OF AIR MOLECULES

(a)

(b)

(c)

(d)

Lower pressure   Higher pressure
    rarefied   compressed

FIG. II.3 Generating a longitudinal pulse in a gas by the rapid movement of the piston first toward and then away from the closed end of a cylinder containing the gas.

Although the pulse itself is clearly longitudinal, a graph of the local air pressure (as reflected by the density of the molecules) versus location results in a plot that looks very much like the transverse motion of a pulse on a wire, as shown in Fig. II.4.

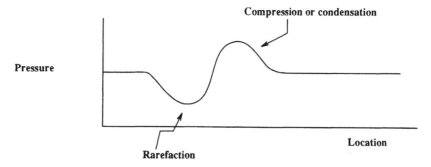

FIG. II.4 A plot of pressure versus time for a longitudinal pulse in a gas. Note that visually this plot does not differ from that of a transverse pulse on a wire.

2. GENERATION OF WAVES

A **wave** consists of a series of identical pulses, one generated immediately after another. For example, on a wire, a slinky, or a piston in a cylinder, repeat the movement of the hand over and over to produce a wave. If done with perfect repetition, it is an example of an oscillator (see Section II.2.1).

Our concern for the present is with one particularly simple class of waves, called sine waves; we investigate how sine waves may be generated and how we can describe them in terms of three numerical parameters.

2.1 Oscillators

DEFINITION: An **oscillator** is any device that repeats a pulse in time with perfect regularity.

A prototype oscillator is an idealized clock shown in Fig. II.5. Observe that the vertical height a of the radius with the arrow head is, by elementary trigonometry, given by $a = A \sin \theta,$[1] where θ denotes the angle between the radius and the horizontal, measured counterclockwise and A denotes the amplitude or length of the radius. Let us suppose that this radius is rotating at a constant rate ω, which is called the *angular velocity* of the oscillator.

---

[1]The symbol θ is often used to denote angles. There is a list of Greek symbols used in the text on p. xxiii.

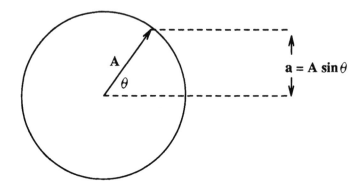

FIG. II.5   The tip of a radius A of a circle with angle θ from the horizontal has a vertical height of $a = A \sin \theta$.

Then the value of the angle θ at time t seconds after the radius was in the original horizontal location is

$$\theta = \omega t.$$

Thus, the value of the *momentary amplitude* at time t is

$$a = A \sin \omega t.$$

Figure II.6 plots the momentary amplitude as it changes with time. This function is called a **sine wave** because it is generated by the sine function. It is the wave motion generated by many natural oscillators such as a pendulum.

A sound wave in which the pressure amplitude varies as a sine wave is called a **pure tone.**

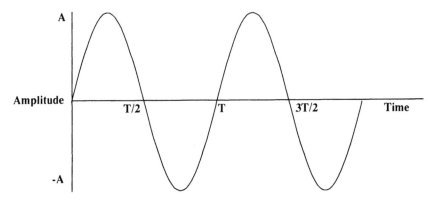

FIG. II.6   If in Fig. II.5 the angle increases in proportion to time, that is, $\theta = \omega t$, where ω is the constant called angular velocity, then plotting $a = A \sin \omega t$ versus t yields the graph shown, where T denotes the period and $1/T$ the frequency of rotation.

2.1.1 Period and Frequency.

DEFINITION. The **period** of an oscillator is the time it takes to complete one full cycle. We use the symbol T for the period. It is measured in units of time.

DEFINITION. The **frequency** of an oscillator is the number of cycles that the oscillator completes in one second. We use the symbol f for the frequency. Its units are 1/time, and one cycle per second[2] is now called Hertz, abbreviated Hz.

Thus, if time is measured in seconds, it follows from these definitions that

$$\boxed{T = 1/f \text{ and } f = 1/T.}$$ (1)

It is important to keep in mind that these relations between period and frequency hold only when T is measured in seconds. If the information about T is provided in any other units, one must first convert that unit into seconds before calculating frequency. For example, if the period is 24 hours, as it is for the Earth's daily rotation, then in seconds this is:

24 hours × (60 minutes/hour) × (60 seconds/hour) = 86,400 seconds,

and so the frequency of rotation of the Earth is approximately

$$1/86,400 = 0.00001157 \text{ Hz.}$$

2.1.2 Units of Measurement for Period and Frequency.   The most common units for *time* and their usual abbreviations are:

second (s)
minute (min) = 60 s
hour (hr) = 3,600 s
millisecond (ms) (or msec is often used) = $\frac{1}{1,000}$ s.
microsecond (μs) = $\frac{1}{1,000}$ ms = $\frac{1}{1,000,000}$ s.

The common units of *frequency* are:

Hertz (Hz) = one cycle per second
kilohertz (kHz) = 1,000 Hz
megahertz (MHz) = 1,000 kHz = 1,000,000 Hz.

Observe the following scientific conventions embodied in these terms:

---

[2]Sometimes one still sees cps, the older abbreviation of cycles per second, rather than Hz.

- A *decrease* in a measure by a factor of 1,000 is prefixed by *milli* and a decrease by a factor of 1,000,000 is prefixed by *micro*. If x is the symbol for the original unit, then milli-x is symbolized by mx and micro-x by μx.
- An *increase* by a factor of 1,000 is prefixed by *kilo* and by a factor of 1,000,000 by *mega*. The unit kilo-x is symbolized by kx, and mega-x by Mx.

Familiar examples are *micro*gram (μg), *milli*meter (mm), *milli*liter (ml), *kilo*gram (kg), *kilo*meter (km).

Some of the conversions involving various time units and frequency will arise over and over. You should become proficient in these calculations. Some examples of computations you will need to be able to do in your head are:

Period of 1 ms $= (1/1,000)$ s $\leftrightarrow f = 1/T = 1/(1/1,000) = 1,000$ Hz
Period of 5 ms $= (5/1,000)$ s $\leftrightarrow f = 1,000/5 = 200$ Hz
Period of 20 μs $= (20/1,000,000)$ s
$$\leftrightarrow f = 1,000,000/20 = 50,000 \text{ Hz}$$
$$= 50 \text{ kHz.}$$

2.1.3 Relation Between Angular Velocity and Frequency.   A very convenient unit for angle is based on the fact that a circle with a radius of 1 unit of length has a circumference of 2π units of length, where the approximate value of π is 3.1416. Thus, a complete rotation of a unit radius corresponds to the point at the end of the radius moving through the distance 2π. This suggests taking that distance divided by 2π as a natural unit, called the *radian,* for measuring angle:

DEFINITION: One cycle $= 2\pi$ **radians** $= 360°$. Thus, one radian is approximately $57.3°$.

In one full cycle, which requires T seconds to complete, the end of the radius traverses the distance 2π. *Angular velocity,* ω, is defined to be that distance divided by that time, that is,

$$\boxed{\omega = 2\pi/T = 2\pi f.} \tag{2}$$

The unit of angular velocity is *radians per second.* And the time course of the amplitude is

$$\boxed{\begin{aligned} a &= A \sin(\omega t) \\ &= A \sin(2\pi f t) \\ &= A \sin(2\pi t/T). \end{aligned}} \tag{3}$$

2.1.4 Phase Angle. Although it is quite arbitrary what instant one chooses to refer to as time 0, once an instant is selected then it serves as a reference point for other temporal events. One of these events is the oscillations that result in waves. To specify an exact wave, one must indicate the value of the amplitude of the wave at the time that has been selected to be 0. This is usually done indirectly by stating the angle ϕ, known as the **phase angle,** that corresponds to that amplitude. So, if for example one says the wave is to have the value A at time 0, then that corresponds to the value $\phi = 90°$ because $\sin 90° = 1$. Several phase angles are depicted in Fig. II.7.

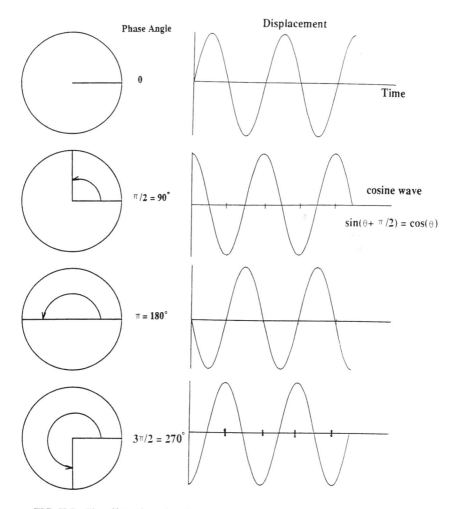

FIG. II.7 The effect of varying the phase angle ϕ on the plot of $a = A \sin(\omega t + \phi)$. The values of phase angle are equally spaced by 90°.

Given that the phase angle is ϕ, then the momentary amplitude is given by:

$$a = A \sin (2\pi ft + \phi). \tag{4}$$

2.1.5 Summary.   To sum up, any sine wave is completely characterized by knowing three numbers:

- Its phase angle ϕ, which is equivalent to stating the amplitude of the wave at time 0.
- its maximum amplitude A; and
- its frequency f.

We already know something about measuring ϕ and f, but measuring A is a more complex matter covered in Sections II.7 and 8.

2.2 Natural Oscillators

2.2.1 Pendulum.   A number of ordinary natural phenomena are sine wave oscillators. The first is the classical pendulum formed by attaching a mass m to a wire of length l, which is attached to a rigid support with a connector that introduces as little friction as possible (see Fig. II.8). Neglecting that friction and the resistance of air, its swinging motion is accurately described as a sine wave. The period T of a pendulum can be shown to have the form:

$$T = kl^{1/2},$$

where k is a constant that does not depend on either l or m and $l^{1/2} = \sqrt{l}$. Thus, in particular, we note that the period T does *not* depend on the mass m of the pendulum, but is directly proportional to the square root of the length.

Despite the fact that an ordinary pendulum, such as a child's swing, oscillates in air, it does not generate audible sound waves because the

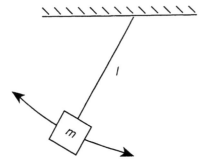

FIG. II.8   A typical pendulum of length l and mass m.

swing's natural frequency is too low—typically well below 20 Hz—to stimulate the ears.

2.2.2 Tuning Fork.   A tuning fork is a Y-shaped body of metal that vibrates at some frequency when it is struck; the exact value of its frequency depends on the shape, size, and material of the fork. It produces longitudinal sine waves in air, as depicted in panel a of Fig. II.9. If, however, a wire is attached to one tine of the fork, then the fork produces transverse sine waves in the wire, as seen in panel b.

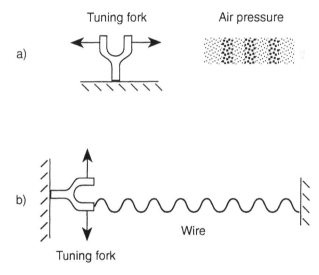

FIG. II.9   (a) A vibrating tuning fork, like the piston of Fig. II.3, compresses and then rarefies the air, thereby creating a longitudinal pressure wave in air. (b) Attaching a string or wire to one tine of the fork results in a transverse wave on the string while, at the same time, a longitudinal pressure wave of panel a is also being generated.

2.2.3 Musical Instruments.   Psychologically, sounds have at least two major aspects: pitch and loudness. Complex sounds also have an important aspect called timber,[3] which is less fully understood. This text focuses only on pitch and loudness. One obvious question is: Which physical attributes of the signal correspond to pitch and loudness? To a first approximation, pitch is governed by frequency and loudness by the amplitude of pressure wave of the signal. In some ways this is only an approximation; this is discussed later. In any event, it is clear that we need to be able to control and to measure both frequency and amplitude.

---

[3]Pronounced "tamber."

Frequency is the lesser problem. First, it is easy to measure provided that one can both count cycles and measure time, because the number of cycles in a fixed period of time provides an estimate of the period and hence of the frequency. Certainly, using a second hand on a watch, one can easily measure both for a child's swing. It is more of a chore to do with sounds, however, because the frequency is substantially higher and the counting more difficult. But it can be done. Second, it is reasonably easy to control frequency. Any natural oscillator has a natural frequency of oscillation, so it is merely a matter of selecting an appropriate oscillator in order to produce a fixed frequency.

As an example, consider a tuning fork. Pitch control in a tuning fork is exact and unchanging—it varies from fork to fork depending on the shape, size, and composition. But for any particular fork it remains the same independent of the force with which it is hit.

Thus, given a fixed set of objects that can readily be made to oscillate—strings, pipes, or tubes with holes in the side—one can produce any sequence among the available frequencies simply by selecting among them. The construction of a suitable set of oscillators is reduced to two considerations: their manufacture and some ability to make discrete choices among them when playing the instrument. True, the strings have to be adjusted to accommodate atmospheric changes and mechanical slippage, and the openings on a wind instrument or its length may well be partially affected by skill. Still, people have developed ways to tune them relatively accurately using tuning forks and the property of waves to "beat" (see Section V.1.2.3) when they differ slightly in frequency, and can learn to control variables such as openings or lengths.

In contrast, the control of loudness tends to be highly inexact because it depends on just where and how hard one does something. As a result, musicians have historically had a great deal more trouble controlling loudness than pitch. Consider some familiar examples of musical instruments shown in Table II.1.

Notice that among classical instruments, only the harpsichord has reproducible loudness, which was achieved by not allowing it to vary.

TABLE II.1
Instruments Categorized According to Types of Pitch and Loudness Controls

Loudness Control	Pitch Control		
	Mechanical	Mixed	Skill
Mechanical	Harpsichord		
Mixed			
Skill	Piano, Harp, Xylophone, Drum	Strings, Woodwinds	Horns

In the 18th- and 19th-century studies of physical acoustics, control of loudness was mechanical and very difficult to measure. In the 20th century, however, laboratory control and measurement became comparatively easy because of electronic control of electromechanical transducers. Today, it is no longer much of an issue.

We take up the measurement of sound intensity—the parameter A in Equation 4—later in Section II.8.

2.2.4 Decay of Natural Oscillators.   In the real world, decay in amplitude over time always occurs in an oscillator, and it can only be counteracted by some external source of energy (such as a parent pushing the child's swing). The major sources of decay are friction at the point of attachment and air resistance. A very long, well-designed pendulum with a tiny, massive weight has very little damping as compared, say, to an ordinary swing.

There is an important fact about the effect of damping. To state it, we need the following concept:

DEFINITION: For any function of time, its **zero crossings** are those times for which the value of the function is 0.

Observe that for a sine wave the time between successive zero crossings is simply the period of the wave.

EMPIRICAL FACT: *Despite the damping of a sine wave, the zero crossings are unaffected.*

The pattern is shown in Fig. II.10.

A commonly used measure of the decay time is the *half-life* of the oscillator, which is defined to be the time at which the amplitude has dropped to one-half of its starting value.

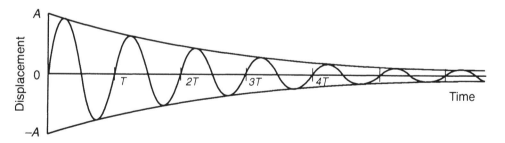

FIG. II.10 A sine wave that is subjected to (exponential) damping. In the example shown, the amount of damping is such that the amplitude is reduced to $A/2$ in about two periods of the underlying sine wave. This time is called the *half-life* of the damped wave. Note that the wave goes on indefinitely, but with an amplitude approaching 0.

3. WAVE PROPAGATION IN TIME AND SPACE

Next we examine ways to describe the propagation of a wave through both time and space. This entails understanding how the spatial and temporal aspects are in a sense the same.

3.1 Speed of Propagation

Consider the propagation of a single pulse. As it moves through a medium, one can compute its speed in the usual way as the ratio of the distance travelled to the time required, that is,

$$\textbf{speed} \text{ of pulse} = \frac{\text{distance travelled in time } t}{t}. \tag{5}$$

3.1.1 Speed of Sound.   It is fairly easy to estimate the speed of a pulse on a wire. In air we can get a good approximation as follows: If a source, such as lightening, produces both light and sound, then because light travels essentially infinitely fast (300,000 km/s) relative to sound (less than 1 km/s) we can neglect the time it takes the light to go from the source to the observer. So the time difference between the arrival of the light and the sound is an excellent estimate of the time it takes the sound to travel the distance. If we know the distance to the source, we can compute the velocity. Using such a technique, the estimated speed of a sound pulse in normal air at sea level and at 20° C is

$$\boxed{344 \text{ m/s (meters per second).}}$$

This is *roughly* 1,000 ft/s or about one mile in 5 s. You should remember these numbers. Their exact values varies somewhat with both temperature and humidity.

The speed of sound is faster in liquids and still faster in solids. Typical numbers from Weast and Astle (1980) are:

Speed of Sound in Meters per Second	
Alcohol	1,207
Water	1,497
Sea Water	1,531
Lead	2,160
Glass, pyrex	5,640
Iron	5,960
Aluminum, rolled	6,420

The value varies substantially with temperature, density, and exact composition. The figures for the liquids are at 25° C.

3.1.2 Notation for the Speed of Sound.   In order to distinguish clearly between the speed of sound in a medium and other velocities (i.e., speed together with the direction of motion), it is helpful to use a distinctive symbol. We use c for the speed of sound in whatever medium is under discussion and v for other velocities.

3.1.3 Empirical Facts About Speed of Propagation.

• If the medium of transmission is homogeneous, then the speed of propagation of a pulse of a particular type is a constant independent of exactly how that type of pulse is generated. It does not matter if the initial displacement (e.g., of the hand on the wire or piston) is small or large, the speed will be the same.
• The value of that constant for each type of wave or pulse depends only on the medium. The speed of sound is $c = (B/\rho)^{1/2}$, where B is a constant describing the elasticity and ρ the density of the medium.
• The speed of transverse and longitudinal waves in the same medium are not the same. For example, the speed of a surface pulse that is made by dropping a stone in a pond is far less than the speed of the longitudinal sound pulse made by hitting two stones together underwater.

3.2 Wavelength

3.2.1 Definition.   Consider a sine wave of period T. In other words, the amplitude of the wave is varying as a sine wave (called a sinusoidal variation) in time with the frequency $1/T$. Now, as far as the medium is concerned, each period of the wave amounts to a pulse. Like any pulse, this one propagates with some speed, c, that is a characteristic of the medium.

Now imagine the wave as existing indefinitely. Then, at any instant of time, the amplitude will form a sine wave in *space* (due to the pulse propagation) as well as one in time. This fact is familiar from surface waves in water. You can see the spatial patterns of circles, and if you fixate at a particular point you can watch the temporal change as the water rises and falls.

DEFINITION: The **wavelength** of a wave is the spatial distance between successive zero crossings of the amplitude. It is symbolized by λ (see Fig. II.11.).

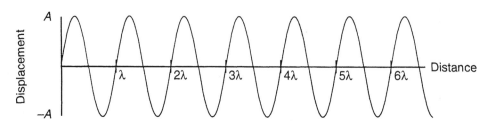

FIG. II.11   The wave in space that corresponds to a transverse sinusoid.

Observe that wavelength plays an analogous role in describing the wave in space to that of period in describing it in time.

3.2.2 Relation Among Speed, Frequency, and Wavelength.   We know the following:

- Each pulse moves through space at speed c.
- The distance between successive zero-crossings of the wave is λ.
- The time between successive zero-crossings is T.

Thus, suppose we mark an imaginary point on the wave at time 0, shown as a dot in part a of Fig. II.12. Then after time T has elapsed, one can ask where that point has gotten, as shown in part b. Because the speed of propagation is the ratio of the distance traversed by the time taken to do so, and in T seconds it travels λ units of distance, we necessarily have the important relation:

$$c = \lambda/T. \tag{6}$$

Note that the *unit* of the speed c must be the unit of distance used to measure the distance divided by the unit of time used to measure the period, T. For example, if length is measured in meters (m) and time in seconds (s), then the speed is measured in meters per second (m/s).

If we choose to measure time in seconds, then because $1/T = f$, we have

$$c = \lambda f \leftrightarrow \lambda = c/f \leftrightarrow f = c/\lambda. \tag{7}$$

Figure II.13 provides a summary of the relation between space and time of the propagation of the wave.

Table II.2 displays some values of the wavelength of sounds of different frequencies in two media. The frequencies span much of human hearing.

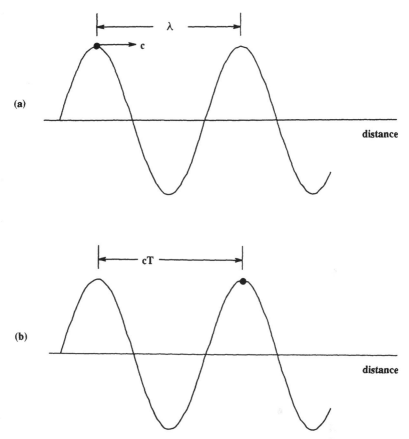

FIG. II.12 The wavelength, λ, of a transverse wave that is propagating at speed c repeats itself after the period T. Thus $\lambda = cT$, as shown.

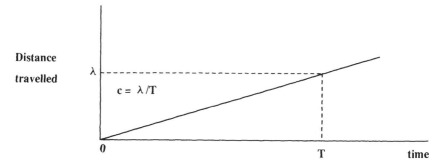

FIG. II.13 Suppose a point on a wave, such as a crest, is at the location denoted 0 on the plot at the time also denoted 0 on the plot. The distance that the point travels increases in proportion to the time elapsed, with the constant of proportionality being the speed of propagation, c. After one period, of T seconds, a new crest will be at the origin and so the point will have moved exactly one wavelength, λ. These values are shown with dotted lines. Thus, $\lambda = cT$.

TABLE II.2

Examples of the Relation Between Frequency and Wavelength in Air and Water ($\lambda = cT$ for sound source in medium)

Pitch Range	f(Hz)	T(ms)	Air (c = 344 m/s)	Water (c = 1,432 m/s)
Bottom	20	50	(344) (50)/1,000 = 17.2 m	71.6 m
Middle	256	3.9	1.34 m	5.59 m
	1,000	1	0.34 m = 34 cm	1.43 m
Upper	15 k	0.066	0.023 m = 2.3 cm	0.10 m

The 256 Hz value is included because it is the frequency of middle C, used by musicians as a standard reference frequency. The 1,000 Hz value is included because it is often used as a standard reference frequency by auditory psychologists.

Observe the enormous difference in wavelength between low and high frequencies—a factor of over 700. These differences will play a significant role in several auditory phenomena.

4. THE DOPPLER EFFECT

When a police car or ambulance passes you with its siren blaring, you hear a pronounced pitch change between its approach and its departure. The question is whether this is a perceptual illusion or whether it can be explained physically. We show it is the latter by figuring out why the frequency at the ear changes. There are several distinct cases to consider.

4.1 Source Moving Toward a Fixed Observer

Let v_s denote the velocity of source, so the situation is that shown in Fig. II.14. Let f_s denote the frequency of source signal, and let f_o be the frequency of the signal when it reaches the observer. By definition, the period in seconds of the source signal is

$$T_s = 1/f_s.$$

And the wavelength of the signal at the source is

$$\lambda_s = cT_s,$$

where c is the speed of sound in air.

During the time T_s that the wave moves the distance λ_s, the source moves the distance $v_s T_s$ toward the observer. This is diagrammed in Fig. II.15. The

Source = Siren   **Observer**

FIG. II.14 The relation between an observer and a source when the source is moving toward the observer.

actual wavelength being produced at the source is thereby reduced because the source partially catches up with the propagating wave. In fact

$$\lambda_o = \lambda_s - v_s T_s$$
$$= cT_s - v_s T_s$$
$$= (c - v_s)T_s.$$

Thus, for the observer,

$$\lambda_o = cT_o,$$

and so substituting

$$\frac{f_o}{f_s} = \frac{1/T_o}{1/T_s} = \frac{T_s}{T_o} = \frac{c}{c - v_s}. \tag{8a}$$

Thus,

$$T_o = T_s - T_s v_s/c. \tag{8b}$$

To gain some idea about the size of the effect, consider the case where f_s = 1,000 Hz, v_s = 60 miles/hr, and c = 344 m/s. First, we must put v_s and c in same units. Toward that end, recall the following conversion factors:

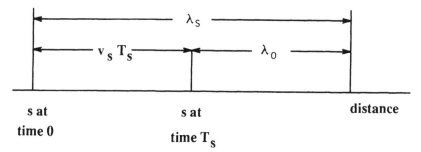

FIG. II.15 Suppose the source s of Fig. II.14 is emitting a pure tone of period T_s and wavelength λ_s. The wavelength observed by the observer is, in fact, smaller than that emitted by the source for the following reason: During any period of the wave, the wavelength of the emitted sound is λ_s; however, during that time, T_s, the source will have moved the distance $v_s T_s$ toward the observer, thereby reducing the effective wave length of the source sound to $\lambda_s - v_s T_s = \lambda_o$.

$$100 \text{ cm} = \text{m}$$
$$2.54 \text{ cm} = \text{in}$$
$$12 \text{ in} = \text{ft}$$
$$5{,}280 \text{ ft} = \text{mile}$$
$$3{,}600 \text{ s} = \text{hr.}$$

So to convert miles to meters we note:

$$(5{,}280 \text{ ft/mile}) \times (12 \text{ in/ft}) \times (2.54 \text{ cm/in}) \times (.01 \text{ m/cm}) = 1{,}609.3 \text{ m/mile},$$

and therefore

$$(60 \text{ miles/hr}) \times (1{,}609.3 \text{ m/mile}) \times (1/3{,}600 \text{ hr/s}) = 26.82 \text{ m/s}.$$

Substituting into the formula for the observer frequency

$$f_o = f_s[c/(c - v_s)]$$
$$= 1{,}000 \, [344/(344 - 26.82)]$$
$$= 1{,}084.6 \text{ Hz.}$$

So the perceived frequency is a little over 8% higher than the actual frequency of the siren. The difference occurs because, when the source moves, the wavelength of the oscillator is reduced.

Observe that something odd happens as the speed of the source approaches and then exceeds the speed of sound. As the source approaches the speed of sound, the frequency becomes larger and larger, to the point that it simply cannot be heard. At the speed of sound, the source arrives at the observer at the same time as the sound. And at speeds greater than sound, the source will pass by before the sound. The physics of sound transmission with such supersonic sources is too complex to go into here. Suffice it to say that there is great compression of the air and it is no longer a homogeneous medium.

4.2 Source Moving Away from a Fixed Observer

Once again we set up the diagram of the situation, as shown in Fig. II.16.

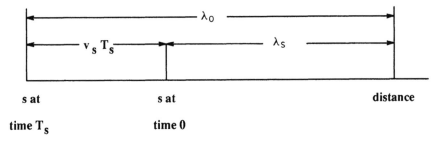

FIG. II.16 The analogue of Fig. II.15 in the case where the source is moving away from the observer. Here the effect of the movement, $v_s T_s$, is added to the wavelength of the source thereby increasing the wavelength and so reducing the frequency of the sound heard by the observer.

Following steps similar to those used in the first calculation we obtain

$$cT_o = \lambda_o = (c + v_s)T_s.$$

So

$$\frac{f_o}{f_s} = \frac{c}{c + v_s} . \qquad (9)$$

For the aforementioned example,

$$f_o = 1,000[344/(344 + 26.82)]$$
$$= 927.7 \text{ Hz.}$$

4.3 Fixed Source and a Moving Observer

Next, suppose that the source is stationary and the observer is moving at velocity, v_o. Although there appears to be a symmetry between the source moving toward a stationary observer and the observer moving toward a stationary source, it is not real. The argument as to the effective f_o is quite different because the wavelength at the observer cannot be affected by the observer's motion; it is a fact about the wave that is unaffected by the observer's motion. Therefore,

$$\lambda_o = \lambda_s = cT_s.$$

What is affected is the speed of propagation past the observer. It is no longer just the speed of the sound in air, c, because the relative motion of the wave to the observer is affected by the movement of the observer either toward or away from the source as well as by the speed of sound. Suppose that the observer's velocity is v_o, then the relative speed between observer and wave is:

$$c \pm v_o,$$

where $\pm$ means to add when o is moving toward s and to subtract when o is moving away from s. Therefore,

$$\lambda_o = (c \pm v_o)T_o.$$

But because $\lambda_o = \lambda_s$,

$$cT_s = (c \pm v_o)T_o,$$

whence,

$$f_o/f_s = \begin{cases} (c + v_o)/c \text{ for an observer moving toward the stationary source} \\ (c - v_o)/c \text{ for an observer moving away from a stationary source.} \end{cases} \qquad (10)$$

Continuing with our previous example of a 1,000 Hz siren, now suppose that $v_s = 0$ and $v_o = 60$ miles/hr toward the source. Then

$$f_o = 1,000[(344 + 26.82)/344] = 1,078.0 \text{ Hz}.$$

This is to be contrasted with the value of 1084.6 when the source is moving at the same speed toward the observer. If the observer is moving away from the source,

$$f_o = 1,000[(344 - 26.82)/344] = 922.0 \text{ Hz},$$

as contrasted with 927.7 Hz when the source is moving away from the observer.

4.4 Calculating the Doppler Effect for Light

Care must be taken in applying these Doppler formulas to the case of light transmission, which usually means to certain astronomical situations. To make the correct calculation in those cases, we must take into account a basic postulate of Albert Einstein's special theory of relativity:

No speed of a physical object exceeds the speed of light.

This has two important consequences for our calculations.

First, because it is always true that $v < c_1$ = the speed of light, the formula of Equation 8 is correct for the source moving toward the observer (Section II.4.1). The source can never arrive at the observer before the light does. In practice, this is usually not important because one is mostly concerned with sources moving away from the observer. In those cases the source frequency is decreased and the apparent wavelength is increased. This observed shift toward longer wavelengths is known as the astronomical "red shift" because the longest wavelength among visible colors is red. The empirically observed magnitude of the red shift is used, via the Doppler formula, to estimate the speed of the source away from (and indirectly the distance to) the Earth.

Second, if no speed is greater than that of light, then what happens when the observer is moving? In Section II.4.3 we said that the effective speed of propagation is $v \pm c$, which is very nearly correct when both v and c are small relative to c_1. But it cannot possibly be correct when c is the speed of light. Indeed, one can shown that "adding" v to or "subtracting" it from c_1 leads to c_1. Using this relationship in the calculation for the effect of the observer's movement we see that $f_o = f_s$. Thus, movement of the observer has no effect on the perceived frequency in the case of light sources.

5. REFLECTION AND REFRACTION OF WAVES

When a sound wave encounters a discontinuous change in medium—for example, a change between air and water—some of the sound is reflected (like light at a window) at the interface and some is transmitted (again like light at a window) into the new medium. Three major questions can be raised about the impact of such a discontinuity in the medium of propagation:

- What is the direction of propagation of the reflected wave relative to the direction of the incident wave?
- What is the direction of the transmitted wave relative to the direction of the incident wave?
- What is the magnitude (intensity) of the transmitted wave?

Knowing the answer to the last question is very important both in understanding physical acoustics, such as how to reduce sound transmission between rooms, and in understanding properties of the ear; we take this up in Section II.9. Here we deal with the first two questions.

5.1 Waves in Space

5.1.1 Spherical Waves.   Just as a stone dropped into a pond generates circular surface waves, a sound source transmits waves in a spherical fashion. A single pulse produces a compression that expands at uniform velocity in the form of an expanding sphere, as depicted in panel a of Fig. II.17.

5.1.2 Plane Waves.   If the source is very far away — idealized as being at infinity — then the spherical wave front flattens to a plane and we speak of a **plane wave,** as depicted in panel b of Fig. II.17.

In the diagrams to follow we suppose the source is sufficiently far away that the sound can be well approximated as a plane wave. We do not show the wave itself, but simply the direction of its propagation, which is perpendicular to the waves themselves.

5.2 Reflection at a Surface

Consider a plane wave that encounters a discontinuous change in medium, that is, a surface. Suppose that it approaches at an angle θ_i, called the **angle of incidence,** as measured from a perpendicular to the surface, and the reflected portion of the wave departs at an angle θ_r, called the **angle of reflection.** This situation is depicted in Fig. II.18.

The relation holding between the angle of reflected waves and the corresponding incident wave is the simplest possible:

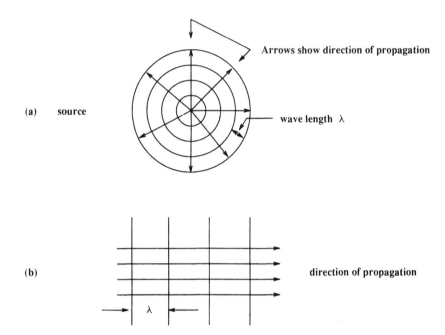

(a) source

Arrows show direction of propagation

wave length λ

(b)

direction of propagation

λ

FIG. II.17 (a) An imaginary plane is cut through the spherical expansion of a sound wave, and a "snapshot" of the places of maximum pressure are shown as solid curves, which are therefore spaced one wavelength apart. The speed of propagation is uniform in all directions, which is the reason why the pressure patterns form spheres. (b) When the source is very far away, the spheres in a bounded region are approximated by a series of planes separated by the wavelength λ. The direction, speed of propagation, and the period (or wavelength or frequency) characterize the plane wave fully. The direction of propagation is usually all that will be shown of the plane wave in diagrams.

Direction of propagation
of incident wave

Direction of propagation
of reflected wave

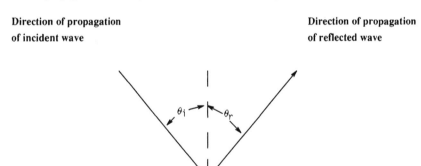

θ_i θ_r

surface

θ_i = Angle of incidence measured from the imaginary perpendicular to the surface.

θ_r = angle of reflected wave measured from same imaginary line.

FIG. II.18 A plane wave impinging on a hard, reflective surface reflects at the same angle to the perpendicular to the surface, but on the other side.

34

EMPIRICAL LAW: *The angle of reflection is identical to the angle of incidence, that is,*

$$\theta_i = \theta_r.$$ (11)

This is analogous to the way a billiard ball behaves when it strikes an edge of the table.

5.3 Refraction at a Surface

Next we consider the portion of the same wave that is transmitted through the interface or surface. At what angle does it pass into the second medium? Again, we use the symbol θ_r to denote the resultant angle, this time called the angle of refraction, as shown in Fig. II.19.

Here the empirical law is rather more complex:

EMPIRICAL LAW: *The angles of incidence and refraction are related by the speeds of sound in the two media by:*

$$\frac{\sin \theta_i}{\sin \theta_r} = \frac{c_i}{c_r}.$$ (12)

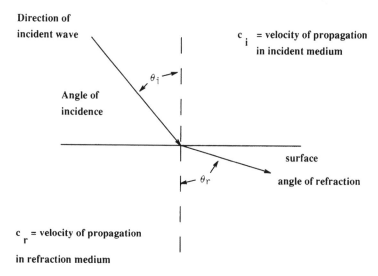

FIG. II.19 A plane wave impinging on a flat surface of a different medium being partially transmitted and refracted by the change of medium.

In optics this relationship is called Snell's law. A familiar example of the optical version is, of course, the simple fact that a stick looks as if it is bent at the point it enters water.

Because the speed of sound is greater in water than in air, in going from air to water, we have

$$c_i < c_r \text{ and so } \theta_r > \theta_i.$$

And from water to air the relations are,

$$c_i > c_r \text{ and so } \theta_r < \theta_i.$$

5.3.1 Sound Transmission During the Day and Night. A simple application of the phenomena of refraction provides understanding of how sounds carry across a lake or a valley far better at night than they do during the day. The underlying relevant facts are:

• The speed of sound in hot air exceeds that in cold air.
• During the day the reflection of sunlight from the Earth's surface causes the lower layers of air to become warmer than the higher layers.
• At night, when the source of heating is greatly reduced, the hot air rises and the cooler air comes down to replace it. This change in warmer and cooler air masses is the source of early evening winds.

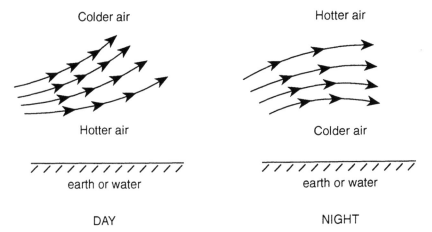

FIG. II.20   (a) A schematic showing how a sound propagating from hotter to cooler air, which is the normal daytime situation, is forced by refraction away from the surface, be it ground or water. This happens because the speed of sound increases with temperature and so, by the equation for refraction, the angle of refraction is continually decreased as one moves up from the surface. This decreasing angle means that the sound is driven away from the surface. (b) Usually at night the situation reverses, with the hot air rising and being replaced by cooler air. In this case, the speed of sound increases with the distance from the surface, and so the refraction pattern is reversed, that is, the angle of refraction increases. This means that the sound tends to be held nearer the surface, causing better transmission from one surface point to another.

Thus, if we think of air as stratified into separate layers at different temperatures, we have the refraction situations depicted in Fig. II.20.

In conclusion, it is no illusion that a stick in water looks bent or that sound transmits more clearly at night across a valley. Both have physical explanations, so neither is classified as a perceptual illusion.

5.3.2 Acoustic Tiles.   Another application of our knowledge of reflection and refraction provides some understanding of the reason for the effectiveness of acoustic tiles in reducing the amount of intelligible sound transmitted through a wall. If one looks closely at an acoustic tile, one finds that it is full of somewhat irregular holes, which in cross section look something like the diagram in Fig. II.21. Given this complex structure, it is clear that even if the incident wave is highly coherent, as in panel a of the figure, the reflected waves, as in panel b, become highly incoherent in

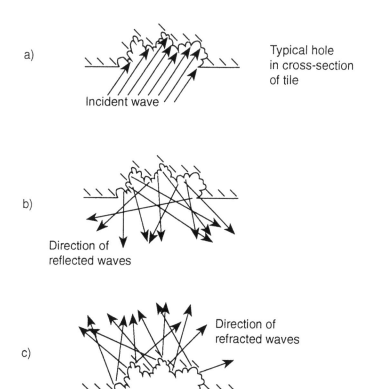

FIG. II.21   (a) A cross-sectional view of a typical hole in an acoustic tile with an incident plane wave. (b) The plane wave is reflected in random directions in different places, thereby producing an incoherent reflected wave. (c) Part of the energy of the wave is refracted, but again in random directions because of the irregularities of the surface, thereby producing an incoherent refracted wave. It is also attenuated by the change in medium, and both effects help to muffle the sound signal.

direction, thereby reducing the echos that can arise in the room. These irregularities cause the reflected sound not to have any coherent structure, and so it is much more complex than just a delayed version of the source sound.

The refracted waves, shown in panel c, are also highly incoherent in direction, thereby also reducing the intelligibility of transmitted sounds.

6. SOME FORMAL MATERIAL THAT IS USEFUL IN AUDITION

Before we can take up the measurement of sound intensity and, once we know how that is done, the calculation of the degree of loss in sound transmission across a change of medium, we need to devote some time to a useful way to write large numbers.

6.1 Powers of 10: The Scientific Notation for Very Large and Very Small Numbers

Rather than write out all of the zeros of very large or very small numbers, scientists have developed and use a system of exponential notation. The following calculation is a simple example:

$$10,000 = 100 \times 100 = 10 \times 10 \times 10 \times 10 = 10^4.$$

Note that four zeros are involved in the original number, and this is the number of times that 10 must be multiplied by itself to get that number. The symbol 10^4 is used to denote that product. More generally, 10^n denotes the product of 10 with itself n times. This pattern is further illustrated:

$$1,000 = 100 \times 10 = 10 \times 10 \times 10 = 10^3$$
$$100 = 10 \times 10 = 10^2$$
$$10 = 10^1$$
$$1 = 10^0.$$

For numbers less than 1, the rule changes slightly, as illustrated:

$$0.1 = 1/10 = 10^{-1}$$
$$0.01 = 1/100 = 1/10^2 = 10^{-2}$$
$$0.001 = 1/1000 = 1/10^3 = 10^{-3}.$$

Here the rule of thumb is to count the number of zeros after the decimal point, add one, and write it as a negative exponent.

Note the relationship we are using is:

$$10^{-m} = 1/10^m. \tag{13}$$

A major property of the exponents is:

$$10^m \times 10^n = 10^{m+n}. \tag{14}$$

These properties are very useful when multiplying large and small numbers. For example:

$$10^{-5} \times 10^8 = 100,000,000/100,000 = 1,000 = 10^3.$$

This powers-of-10 notation can also be used with ordinary numbers that are not just products of 10s. Any number can be written as the same string of numerals, but with the decimal located so it lies between 0 and 10, multiplied by the appropriate power of 10 to give the original number. Some examples are:

$$2,673 = 2.673 \times 1,000 = 2.673 \times 10^3$$

$$1,570,000 = 1.57 \times 10^6$$

$$0.085 = 8.5 \times .01 = 8.5 \times 10^{-2}.$$

6.2 Order of Magnitude of a Number

DEFINITION: A number is said to be of the **order of magnitude** 10^m if it lies between $5 \times 10^{m-1} = (1/2) \times 10^m$ and $5 \times 10^m = (1/2) \times 10^{m+1}$.

It can be helpful to carry out order of magnitude calculations (see Table II.3) in order to check approximately the reasonableness of a calculation. It is also a useful way to catch input errors when using a calculator. For example if someone says that $7,500,000 \times .0039 = 2,925$, you can point out

TABLE II.3
Some Typical Order-of-Magnitude Calculations

Number	Order of Magnitude
650,000	10^6
250,000	10^5
15	10
85	10^2

that by an order of magnitude calculation it is $10^7 \times 10^{-3} = 10^4$, which suggests an error of a factor of 10.

6.3 Logarithms

DEFINITION: The **logarithm (to the base 10)** of a number is the exponent to which you must raise 10 to get that number:

$$y = \log_{10} x \text{ if and only if } 10^y = x.$$

Thus, for example, $\log_{10} 1,000,000 = \log_{10} 10^6 = 6$.
We omit the subscript 10 of the base and write just log for $\log_{10}$.

The logarithm exhibits the following major property. It converts a multiplication of two numbers into a corresponding addition of their transformed—logarithmic—values.

This is embodied in the following formula, which you should remember:

$$\boxed{\log xy = \log x + \log y.} \tag{15}$$

This formula follows from the basic property of powers of 10. Let $a = \log x$, $b = \log y$, so by definition $x = 10^a$ and $y = 10^b$. Thus, using Equation 14, $xy = 10^a \times 10^b = 10^{a+b}$, and so $\log xy = a + b = \log x + \log y$.
The following calculation illustrates how this property may be used:

$$\begin{aligned}
\log 2,350,000 &= \log (2.35 \times 10^6) \\
&= \log 2.35 + \log 10^6 \\
&= 6 + \log 2.35.
\end{aligned}$$

Because logarithms will repeatedly play a role in the measurement of sound intensity, the values of several logarithms are worth remembering:

$$\begin{aligned}
\log 1 &= 0 \text{ (because } \log 1 = \log 10^0 = 0) \\
\log 2 &\cong .3 \\
\log 10 &= 1 \\
\log 10^m &= m.
\end{aligned}$$

The major property, Equation 15, implies all of the following properties, which we use frequently:

$$\boxed{\begin{aligned}
\log 1/x &= -\log x \\
\log x/y &= \log x - \log y \\
\log x^p &= p \log x.
\end{aligned}} \tag{16}$$

Here is the proof of log $1/x = -\log x$:

$$0 = \log 1 = \log x/x = \log x(1/x) = \log x + \log 1/x.$$

Therefore,

$$\log 1/x = -\log x.$$

In the following example some of these properties are used:

$$\begin{aligned}
\log .009 &= \log 1/(1.11 \times 10^2) \\
&= -\log (1.11 \times 10^2) \\
&= -\log 1.11 - \log 10^2 \\
&= -2 - \log 1.11.
\end{aligned}$$

7. DIMENSIONS OF PHYSICAL QUANTITIES

7.1 Basic Dimensions

Because one uses numbers to describe all sorts of qualitatively different things, such as lengths, masses, times, and so forth, one must be quite explicit about which attribute is meant. Each physical quantity is said to have a dimension as well as a magnitude. Table II.4 summarizes the four basic dimensions that play a role in audition. Temperature does not play much of a role in this text, although, as noted earlier, such things as the speed of sound increase with temperature.

The dimensions of all other quantities are expressed as products of powers of these dimensions. For example, density, ρ is defined as the ratio of the mass m of a substance occupying volume V:

$$\rho = m/V.$$

TABLE II.4
Symbols for the Four Basic Dimensions of Importance in Acoustics

Attribute	Symbol for Its Dimension
length	[L]
mass	[M]
time	[T]
temperature	[θ]

This concept captures an inherent property of substances because the following underlying physical law is true:

EMPIRICAL LAW: *In a homogeneous substance, the ratio of mass,* m, *to volume,* V, *is a constant independent of volume.*

The dimension of density is $[\rho] = [M]/[L]^3$, that is, the mass dimension to the first power and the length dimension to the minus 3 power. So, if mass is measured in grams, g, and length in centimeters, cm, then the corresponding density is measured in g/cm³.

This example is typical. The dimension of any nonbasic physical quantity depends on one or more laws relating it to other quantities — and these have to lead uniformly to dimensions of the form:

$$[L]^l[M]^m[T]^t,$$

where *l, m, t* are integers.

As another example, consider force, *F,* which according to Newton's Second Law is related to mass *m* and acceleration *a* by:

$$F = ma,$$

Then force has the dimensions

$$[F] = [M][L]/[T]^2.$$

Each expression of a physical unit in terms of others reflects some underlying physical law. Let us examine units more carefully.

7.2 Units

It is, of course, meaningless to say that the distance from point X to point Y is 300 without saying whether we are speaking of miles, kilometers, yards, meters, feet, and so on. The **magnitude** of a physical quantity is described as the ratio of the quantity in question to that of a specific standard quantity called its **unit.** For example, to say that a room is 20 m deep means that the *ratio* of the depth of the room to the length that is conventionally called *one meter* is 20. If the unit is changed, say, to cm, the ratio changes, in this case to 20 × 100 = 2,000 cm.

The most common scientific units[4] are shown in Table II.5.

---

[4]Note that some symbols receive double usage, for example, m is used both to represent an arbitrary mass, as in Newton's law, and as the symbol for the unit of length called the meter. Although such ambiguity is unfortunate, one gets used to it because the context usually makes clear what is intended.

TABLE II.5
Common Scientific Units

Unit	Dimension	Symbol	Variants
gram	mass	g	kg, mg
meter	length	m	km, cm, mm
second	time	s (sec)	ms (msec)

A number of important physical quantities arise in our discussion of sounds. These are summarized in the following table:

7.3 Summary Table: Selected Physical Units

Variable	Typical Symbol	Comments	Dimensional Notation	Units
length, distance	l, d		$[L]$	kilometer (km), meter (m), centimeter (cm), millimeter (mm) (inch, foot, etc.)
mass	m		$[M]$	kilogram (kg), gram (g), milligram (mg), microgram (μg)
time	t		$[T]$	hour (h), second (s), millisecond (ms)
area	A		$[L]^2$	km^2, m^2, etc.
volume	V		$[L]^3$	km^3, m^3, etc.
speed	c, v	rate of change of distance	$[L]/[T]$	km/h, m/s, cm/s, etc.
acceleration	a	rate of change of velocity	$[L]/[T]^2$	km/h^2, m/s^2, etc.
density	$p = m/V$	law: invariance for substance	$[M]/[L]^3$	kg/m^3, g/cm^3, etc.
force	$F = ma$	(Newton's law)	$[M][L]/[T]^2$	dyne = force to move 1 g with acceleration of 1 cm/s^2 = g - cm/s^2. Newton = 10^5 dynes
pressure	$\rho = F/A$		$[M]/[L][T]^2$	dyne/cm^2 = g/cm - s^2
energy	E	force through distance	$[M][L]^2/[T]^2$	erg = dyne - cm joule = 10^7 erg
power	P	rate of change of energy	$[M][L]^2/[T]^3$	erg/s; watt = joules/s = 10^7 erg/s
intensity	$I = P/A$		$[M]/[T]^3$	erg/cm^2 - s, watt/cm^2

The greatest complications arise in the last group of related quantities. One begins with force, and considers its application over an area, through a distance, and changing with time. Each of these leads to important new dimensions with associated units.

Pressure is defined as the amount of force being applied per unit of area. Thus, if the force is measured in dynes and the area in cm^2, then pressure is measured in dynes/cm^2. Our interest in pressure arises because sound waves are detected only when the air pressure wave impinges the ear drum causing it to move and create a series of events in the inner ear (see Sections III.1 and 2).

A second important role of force in physics is its continued application over a distance, which is called **energy.** The basic unit of energy is the **erg,** which is defined to be the exertion of a force of 1 dyne through a distance of 1 centimeter. But because this unit corresponds to an exceedingly small amount of energy, relative to ordinary human experience, it is convenient to assign a name to a far larger amount of energy, namely, 10^7 ergs, which is called the **joule.**

The rate at which energy changes in time is called **power.** With energy measured in joules, then one joule per second is called the **watt.**

The last concept, intensity, deserves a separate section.

8. MEASURING SOUND INTENSITY

8.1 Pressure and Intensity

Displacement in sound waves is a change in **air pressure,** denoted by p. Sometimes these pressures are reported or plotted as a function of time or distance, as in the lighter curve of Fig. II.22. Other times something called the **intensity** of the wave, denoted by I, is reported. I is related to p by the formula:

$$I = p^2/\rho c, \qquad (17)$$

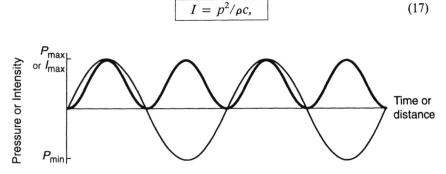

FIG. II.22 A typical sine wave (light curve): $p = P \sin 2\pi ft$; and its square (dark curve): $p^2 = P^2 (\sin 2\pi ft)^2$. Note that p^2 is definitely not a sine wave.

where

p = pressure
ρ = air density = mass/volume
c = speed of sound in the medium.

Given that p is a sine wave, and I involves squaring it, the plot of I is as shown in the darker curve of Fig. II.22. Note that I is periodic, or in other words, repeats itself, with a period that is one-half the period of the original sine wave.

The dimensions of I can be calculated by first writing the dimensions of its constituent terms:

$$[p] = [M]/[L][T]^2$$
$$[\rho] = [M]/[L]^3$$
$$[c] = [L]/[T].$$

So

$$[I] = ([M]^2/[L]^2[T]^4)([L]^3/[M])([T]/[L])$$
$$= [M]/[T]^3$$
$$= [E]/[T][A],$$

where $[E]$ is the dimension of energy and $[A]$ that of area. Because the unit of energy is the erg and the unit of power is erg/s, which is converted to watts, the units of I are:

$$\text{erg/s} - \text{cm}^2 = 10^{-7}\text{watts/cm}^2.$$

Both pressure and intensity measures are commonly used in audition.

8.2 Pressure and Intensity of Air

At sea level and 70° F, the pressure of air is about 14.7 pounds/in^2. Because 1 pound = 4.45 × 10^5 dynes, which is the usual scientific measure of force, and 1 inch = 2.54 cm, which is the usual scientific measure of length, then

14.7 pounds/in^2 = $(14.7)(4.45 \times 10^5)/(2.54)^2 = 1.0139 \times 10^6$ dynes/cm^2.

For an average young person, a change in pressure of about

$$p_0 = 2 \times 10^{-4} \text{ dynes/cm}^2 = .0002 \text{ dynes/cm}^2$$

is just detectable. As a fraction of background air pressure, this is

$$(2 \times 10^{-4})/(1.0139 \times 10^{6}) \cong 2 \times 10^{-10}.$$

This is 2 parts in 10 billion, which is the same as a bit over $600 in the U.S. national debt in early 1992 of slightly more than 3×10^{12}.

Recall that $I = p^2/\rho c$. The quantity ρc is called the *impedance* of air, and its value in still, sea level conditions is:

$$\rho c = 40 \text{ dynes/cm}^3.$$

So

$$I_0 = (2 \times 10^{-4})^2/(4 \times 10)$$
$$= 10^{-9} \text{ erg/s cm}^2$$
$$= 10^{-16} \text{ watts/cm}^2$$
$$= 10^{-12} \text{ watts/m}^2.$$

8.3 Decibels (dB)

It is usual to report pressure of sound waves as a ratio to the value of $p_0 = 0.0002$ dynes/cm^2 pressure level, and so by Equation 17 the intensity ratio is:

$$I/I_0 = (p/p_0)^2. \tag{18}$$

However, because these numbers are usually so large, they are commonly replaced by

$$10 \times \log(I/I_0).$$

This measure of intensity is called the **decibel (dB)**, that is, one tenth of a Bel, a measure named after Alexander Graham Bell who is best known for inventing the telephone. Unlike intensity itself, which has units, this quantity is dimensionless. Nevertheless, one speaks of a sound signal as having so many decibels relative to some standard intensity I_0, making it seem as if it is a unit. But it really is not a unit. It is simply a way of alerting one that the logarithmic measure of a ratio is being reported. However, given such a measure, one can convert back to an intensity ratio, and so express the intensity as its relation to I_0.

Observe that a simple factor of 2 relation holds between pressure and intensity dB measures:

$$\boxed{\begin{aligned} \text{dB} &= 10 \log I/I_0 \\ &= 10 \log (p/p_0)^2 \\ &= 20 \log (p/p_0). \end{aligned}} \tag{19}$$

When the dB is calculated relative to $p_0 = 0.0002$ dynes/cm^2, which is the usual standard, it is called **sound pressure level (dB SPL)**. So, for example, if one speaks of a sound source as having intensity 80 dB SPL, the corresponding pressure is the solution p to the equation $20 \log p/p_0 = 80$, which is equivalent to

$$p = 10^{8/2} p_0 = 10^4 p_0 = 10,000 \times 0.0002 \text{ dynes/cm}^2 = 2 \text{ dynes/cm}^2.$$

8.3.1 Facts About dB Measures.   You should memorize the following facts about dB measures because they will be repeatedly used:

$$\boxed{\begin{array}{l} I/I_0 = 2 \leftrightarrow 3 \text{ dB} \\ I/I_0 = 10 \leftrightarrow 10 \text{ dB.} \end{array}} \qquad (20)$$

These derive immediately from the fact that $\log 2 \cong .3$ and $\log 10 = 1$.

Difference in dB of the sound intensities of two sources 1 and 2 corresponds to their relative ratios:

$$\boxed{\begin{array}{l} \Delta dB = 10 \log I_1/I_2 \\ \quad = 10 \log I_1/I_0 - 10 \log I_2/I_0 \\ \quad = dB_1 - dB_2. \end{array}}$$

Here, and elsewhere Δ is used to denote a difference.

8.3.2 Summary Table: Examples of Sound Intensities.

Condition	I/I_0	dB SPL
Hearing threshold 3 kHz open field	1	0
Very quiet living room	10^4	40
Conversation, one speaker at 3 m, typical room	10^6	60
Speaker shouting	10^8	80
Subway platform arriving train (NYC, Boston)	10^9–10^{10}	90–100
30 m behind jet engine	10^{13}–10^{15}	130–150
Pain	10^{13}	130
Usual upper limit in experiments	10^{10}	100

With this material as background on how intensity is measured, we are now in a position to treat substantive matters in which intensity plays a significant role.

9. SOUND ATTENUATION THROUGH A CHANGE OF MEDIUM

In addition to making the transmitted sound incoherent (see Section II.5.3.2), acoustic tiles, like any change in medium, attenuate (reduce) the intensity of the transmitted sound. This is due to mismatches in the acoustic impedance of the two media, air and the material of the tile. **Acoustic impedance** refers to the quantity ρc, so the ratio in the two media is

$$R = (\rho c)_i/(\rho c)_r. \tag{22}$$

The subscripts refer to the media of the incident wave, i, and of the refracted wave, r. The proportion of intensity transmitted across the discontinuity of materials can be shown[5] to be given by:

$$4R/(1 + R)^2. \tag{23}$$

Note that the loss in transmission is the same in either direction because

$$\frac{4(1/R)}{(1 + 1/R)^2} = \frac{(4/R)}{(R + 1)^2/R^2} = \frac{4R}{(1 + R)^2}.$$

Let us calculate the transmission that occurs between air and seawater. The values of the acoustical impedances are:

$$(\rho c)_{air} = 40 \text{ dynes s/cm}^3$$

$$(\rho c)_{seawater} = 160{,}000 \text{ dynes s/cm}^3.$$

So,

$$R = (4 \times 10)/(16 \times 10^4) = 1/(4 \times 10^3).$$

Thus,

$$\text{Proportion transmitted} = (4 \times 4 \times 10^3)/(1 + 4 \times 10^3)^2$$
$$\cong (16 \times 10^3)/(16 \times 10^6)$$
$$= 10^{-3}.$$

That is, 1/1,000 of the intensity is transmitted and so 999/1,000 is lost. In decibels this loss is 30 dB, which is quite substantial. For example, if a person is shouting at 80 dB (see Section II.8.3.2) just above the surface of the water, then underwater it is as if the sound source is 50 dB, or at the level of whispered conversation. We are all familiar with such underwater attenuation of sounds.

The loss of 30 dB at any air–water interface plays a role in our understanding of the structure and function of the ear in Part III.

---

[5]It is beyond the scope of this text to derive this result from more basic physical principles.

10. LOCALIZING A SOUND SOURCE

This section addresses the question: What physical information exists that people can use to determine the direction from which a sound originates? We must look for some difference at the ears that varies systematically with direction. Two have been suggested: the relative time of arrival of the signal at the two ears and intensity differences of the signal at the ears. We explore both possibilities.

10.1 Time Differences

Suppose the source is fairly far away so that the spherical wave fronts are approximately planes relative to the size of the head, as is shown in Fig. II.23. Assume that the source is at angle θ to the right of straight ahead. At the instant when some portion of the wave front arrives at the right ear, R, the corresponding portion that ultimately will impact the left ear, L, is then at the point marked A. As is indicated in Fig. II.23, in order for the sound to arrive at the left ear, it must first traverse the straight distance AB to the tangent point on the head, after which it must follow the arc BL to the ear. Some elementary trigonometry leads to the following result. The excess distance the sound must travel to get to the left ear after arriving at the right is:

$$\Delta D = AB + BL = r[\sin \theta + \theta],$$

where r is the radius of the head and, as was mentioned, θ is the true angle between the sound source and the frontal direction of the head.

How long does it take sound to traverse this distance? Suppose $r = 8.75$ cm. Then because $c = 344$ m/s $= 34,400$ cm/s we see that the time difference, Δt, in seconds is given by:

$$\begin{aligned}
\Delta t &= \Delta D/c \\
&= r(\theta + \sin \theta)/c \\
&= 8.75 \ (\theta + \sin \theta)/34,400 \\
&= 254 \times 10^{-6} \times (\theta + \sin \theta).
\end{aligned}$$

Thus, Δt changes systematically with the angle θ. But observe that its value is really very small. Its maximum occurs when $\theta = \pi/2 \ (= 90°)$ in which case

$$\theta + \sin \theta = \pi/2 + 1,$$

so

$$\Delta t = 653 \times 10^{-6} s = .653 \text{ ms}.$$

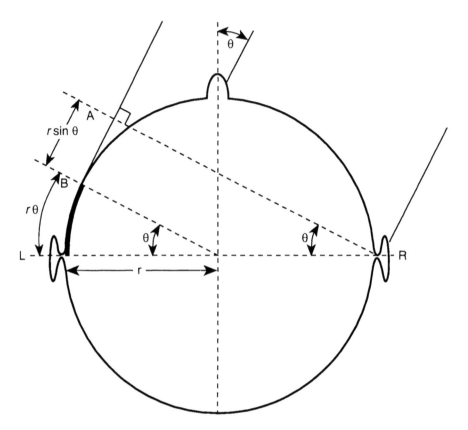

FIG. II.23 Looking down on a head with a cross-section, horizontal plane through the ears, showing an incident plane wave arriving at angle θ from straight ahead. The added route that the sound must travel to get to the left ear after it has arrived at the right ear is in two parts. The first is the straight link from A to B, which by elementary trigonometry is $r \sin \theta$. The second is the curved link around the head from B to L, which by elementary geometry is of length $r\theta$, where θ is measured in radians. Thus, the total extra distance that must be travelled is $r(\theta + \sin \theta)$.

Figure II.24 shows the exact variation of Δt with θ. Observe that for tones with a frequency in excess of 2,000 Hz, the period is less than 0.5 ms. This can result in confusion because it is not clear which of the two pressure waves at the ears is ahead of the other. This can lead to sizable errors in locating the source, as illustrated in Fig. II.25. The actual onset of the sound, of course, gives the correct result, namely that the left ear lags right by Δt. The fine structure of the rest of the wave can be interpreted either as left lags the right by Δt or the left leads the right by $T - \Delta t$. The second interpretation of what is happening, of course, shifts the estimate of the source from being to the right of straight ahead, the correct conclusion, to the left of straight ahead, which often is a rather serious error.

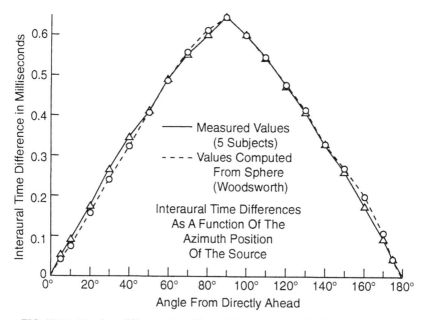

FIG. II.24 The time difference in milliseconds between the arrival at the two ears as a function of the angle of the plane wave as measured from straight ahead. From "Localization of High-frequency Tones" by W. E. Fedderson, T. T. Sandel, D. C. Teas, and L. A. Jeffress, 1957, *Journal of the Acoustical Society of America,* 29, p. 989. Copyright 1957 by American Institute of Physics. Reprinted by permission.

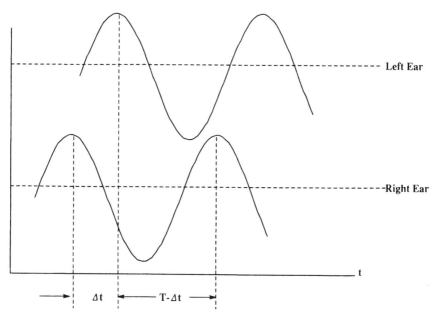

FIG. II.25 The time difference in the arrival of a sine wave shows up as an ambiguous phase difference: either the left ear lags the right by Δt or leads it by $T - \Delta t$.

10.2 Intensity Differences

The difference in intensity at the two ears is a second, independent source of information about the direction of the source. Such a difference results largely from interference introduced by the presence of the head. The amount of interference is, however, much more difficult to calculate exactly than it was to calculate the time difference. But one simple calculation is revealing.

Consider a head that is 17.5 cm in diameter. The frequency of a wave that has a wavelength of corresponding size is 34,400/17.5 = 1965.7 Hz. For frequencies lower than this, the head becomes small relative to the wavelength. And just like a small object — such as a post — in water, it has little effect on the wave pattern. For higher frequencies, however, the head is large relative to wavelength — more like an island relative to water waves. And just as the waves on the lee side of the island are much reduced in magnitude, so the head attenuates the high frequency sounds.

The data of measured dB differences as a function of f and θ are shown in Fig. II.26. Thus, there is enough information in the intensity differences to calculate the source angle for high frequency sounds.

10.3 Duplex Theory and Poor Localization
Near 2,000 Hz

In 1904, the British physicist Lord Rayleigh proposed that the brain localizes sounds by using the differences in arrival time for low frequencies and the differences in intensity for high frequencies. This hypothesis, which is referred to as **duplex theory,** appears to be correct.

Observe that according to the previous calculations, frequencies near 2,000 Hz cannot be localized very well by either mechanism. For the timing mechanism to be effective, the signals should be considerably less than 2,000 Hz, and for the intensity mechanism to be effective, they should be considerably greater than 2,000 Hz. So the region around 2,000 Hz is not well covered by either.

This prediction can be tested in the following type of two-alternative, forced-choice procedure. On each trial, the observer hears the source successively from two different angles θ and $\theta + \Delta\theta$. On a random half of the trials one temporal order is used, and on the other half it is reversed. Suppose, for example, if the angles are 30° and 40°. On a random half of the trials the observer first hears the source from 30° and then from 40°. On

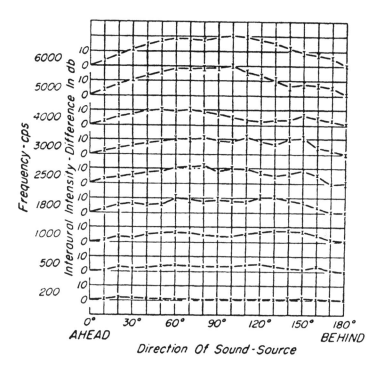

FIG. II.26 Measured values of the pressure difference in dB between the two ears as a function of the angle of the plane wave measured from straight ahead. Note that the higher the frequency the larger the difference and that the maximum difference occurs when the sound is directed at one ear, 90° from straight ahead. From "Localization of High-frequency Tones" by W. E. Fedderson, T. T. Sandel, D. C. Teas, and L. A. Jeffress, 1957, *Journal of the Acoustical Society of America*, 29, p. 989. Copyright 1957 by American Institute of Physics. Reprinted by permission.

the other half the 40° angle is heard first followed by the 30° one. The task is to identify whether the smaller angle is the first or the second member of the pair. By varying the difference $\Delta\theta$ from very small to very large, the probability of a correct response goes from a chance performance of 50% correct to a perfect performance of 100% correct. An intermediate value, say 75%, establishes a difference that can be discriminated some, but not all, of the time.

Fig. II.27 shows the contours of 75% correct performance. What is plotted here is the angular difference that yields 75% performance versus signal frequency. The several curves are for different directions—0°, 30°, 60°, and 75° from straight ahead. As predicted, the performance is distinctly poorer at frequencies in the region just below 2,000 Hz.

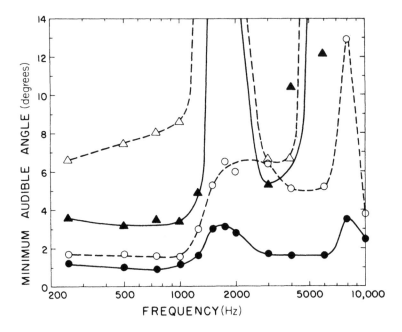

FIG. II.27 A plot of the jnd for angular discrimination as a function of signal frequency. Each curve corresponds to a different source angle, measured from straight ahead. For angles well off-center, discrimination is very poor in the region of 2,000 Hz, as predicted by the duplex theory of localization. From "Auditory Localization" in *Foundations of Modern Auditory Theory* (Vol. 2, p. 310) by A. W. Mills, 1972, New York: Academic Press. Copyright 1972 by New York: Academic Press. Reprinted by permission.

10.4 Front-Back Confusions

Most of us are familiar with front-back confusions. One hears a sound and is uncertain whether its source is in front or behind. This can happen at either low or high frequencies.

Referring back to Fig. II.24, it is evident that the same difference in time of arrival is generated whether the signal comes from the right front or the right back. Thus, for low frequencies a front-back confusion is possible.

Likewise, front-back confusions can occur at high frequencies. In these cases, the same pressure difference can arise from a source either in front or behind the observer.

One historically important case where such confusions may have occurred is in the reports of eye witnesses to the assassination of President John F. Kennedy. A number of them claimed to have heard shots originating from a location other than the one where it is known that several shots did originate. The question was whether, despite the absence of physical evidence such as spent cartridges, a second assassin had been involved. A subsequent inquiry involving acoustic experts concluded that the witnesses who reported hearing shots from the second source probably had been misled by localization confusions.

10.5 Lateralization Studies

By using earphones one can vary the parameters of stimulation in ways that cannot occur naturally. This kind of trickery is sometimes useful in attempts to figure out what information is being used by the brain.

As you probably have noticed with earphones, sounds no longer seem to arise from an external source. Rather, they seem to be located somewhere inside the head. By varying the relative intensity at the two ears, that location can be shifted from being entirely at the left ear, through the middle of the head, to entirely at the right ear. The inputs are judged equal when the resulting sound is centered.

One can use this fact to explore the trade-off between time and intensity differences, which are perfectly correlated for natural stimuli but can be uncorrelated in the earphones. So for any difference in time of arrival, one can ask the subject to adjust the relative intensities to the two ears so that the sound seems centered. The result is that for low frequencies, a small value of Δt is equivalent to a large value of ΔI (approximately 25 μs/dB), and for large frequencies, a large value of Δt is equivalent to a small value of ΔI (approximately 90 μs/dB). These effects can be heard, with earphones, on Demonstration 2. The findings are consistent with Rayleigh's duplex postulate that time differences are the primary source of localization for low frequencies, whereas intensity differences are the primary source for high frequencies.

11. RESONANCE AND FILTERS

11.1 Natural Modes of Vibration

As is true of the natural oscillators previously discussed, every physical object has a number of frequencies at which it "likes" to vibrate. These are referred to as the **natural modes of vibration.** In some cases, such as a swing, this fact is obvious. When you displace a swing, it moves with a period determined by its length—the longer the swing, the lower its frequency. Another example is a spring with a mass, as shown in Fig. II.28. And a third is a taut wire or rubber band with its ends rigidly held, as shown in Fig. II.29. This example illustrates the important fact that there usually is more than one natural frequency.

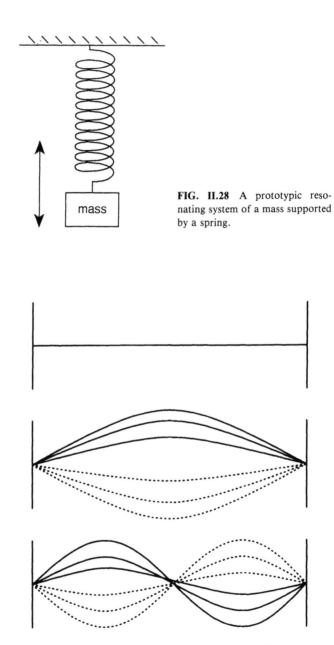

FIG. II.28 A prototypic reso-
nating system of a mass supported
by a spring.

FIG. II.29 A wire held rigidly at both ends and the envelope of its standing waves for
the fundamental and first harmonic.

11.2 Resonance

If one applies a periodic force to a body at one of its natural frequencies, then the amplitude of oscillation tends to increase. If one continues to apply the input force, however modest, the response may go out of control to the point of destroying the object. This phenomenon, called **resonance,** is familiar from swings, and it occurs with all physical bodies. It has often proved to be a serious problem in designing equipment, especially because the applied force need not be terribly large for a large and growing resonance to occur. For example, a sound wave of moderate intensity at the natural frequency of a fine crystal goblet can cause it to shatter.

Resonance can be either good or bad. The next section provides four examples of undesired resonances. On the other hand, all musical instruments as well as speech depend in large part on desirable, natural resonances. We explore that in some detail in Parts V and VI.

11.2.1 Examples of Undesirable Resonance.

• Early automobiles typically exhibited a serious vibration, called a "shimmy," at certain moderately high road speeds. Careful design has eliminated this from modern automobiles, at least at normal highway speeds.

• A somewhat similar phenomenon occurs in aircraft. Aerodynamic forces cause the wing to resonate at some natural frequency. In this case, the resonance is called "flutter," which again may be totally destructive. This was a serious problem with the Lockheed Electra from the 1950s, which are still used by the U.S. Navy for sea patrols. It was built to fly at very high speeds for propeller propulsion, but because of destructive flutter the plane has had to be restricted to substantially lower, but safe, speeds.

• Audio equipment can cause windows, plates, and so forth to rattle, and can exhibit positive feedback in which sound from the speakers can be fed through a microphone or turntable to the amplifier, thereby causing high frequency resonance.

• Resonance is a serious issue in the design of suspension bridges. A dramatic failure occurred in 1941 involving the Tacoma Narrows (Washington) bridge. As was captured on a most exciting film, very high, periodically fluctuating winds in the Narrows led the bridge to resonate with huge oscillations to the point of ripping itself apart, shown in Fig. II.30.

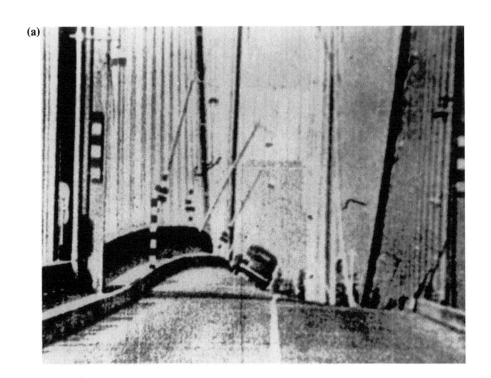

(a)

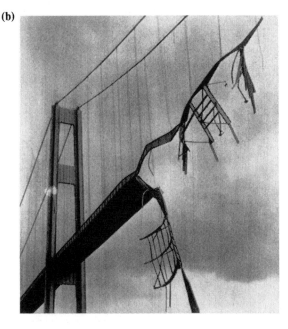

(b)

FIG. II.30 In 1940 the third longest suspension bridge in the USA was completed across the Narrows at Tacoma, Washington. On November 10, 1940 high winds caused it to writhe and twist as shown in (a), taken from a 10mm film by Prof. F.B. Farquharson of the University of Washington who was attempting to rescue a dog left in the car abandoned on the bridge. Ultimately it was torn apart and panel (b) shows the bridge after the collapse of its center span (UPI/Bettman Archive).

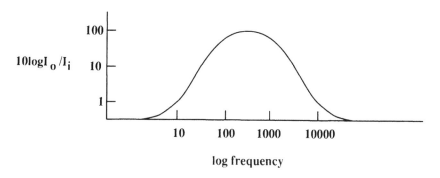

FIG. II.31   The typical response pattern of a fairly broad band filter.

11.3 Filters

11.3.1 Output–Input Ratio.   Let us begin with one way of describing the resonant response of a physical object. Let I_i denote the maximum intensity of an input sine wave applied to the body, and let I_o denote the maximum intensity of vibration output of the body when I_i is applied.[6] Consider the output–input ratio I_o/I_i as waves of different frequencies f are applied to the body in question. Typically one finds a response pattern like that shown in Fig. II.31.

Such a device is said to be a **filter** because, in analogy with mechanical filters such as a wire mesh or a coffee filter, it lets some frequencies through and attenuates others, that is, it filters them out.

11.3.2 Quality of a Filter.   A filter is said to exhibit high **quality**, which is denoted Q, if the region where it responds to the input is very narrow. The highest quality, but completely idealized, filter would have the response pattern shown in Fig. II.32 in which it responds at one frequency and not at all at any other. It is physically impossible to realize such an ideal filter, but it can be approximated with some difficulty. High quality filters play an important role in acoustic and auditory research, which we encounter in Part V.

11.3.3 A Measure of Quality.   One standard way of reporting the quality of a filter is to determine its width at the point where the response is one-half of the maximum response, as shown in Fig. II.33. Then the measure of quality, Q, is defined by the following formula:

$$Q = f/\Delta f. \qquad (24)$$

---

[6]Note that the subscripts i and o correspond to the words *input* and *output.*

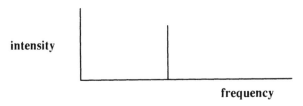

FIG. II.32   An idealized, but physically unrealizable, pure tone filter that responds at just one frequency.

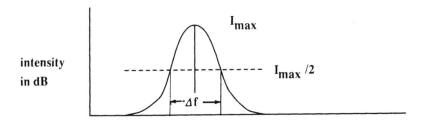

FIG. II.33   The definition of Δf used in the definition of the quality of a filter: $Q = f/\Delta f$.

Three special (and important) idealized filters can be constructed from a collection of high Q filters. Acoustic filters of the following three types are often used in experiments: low pass, high pass, and band pass filters. A **low pass filter** allows all frequencies below a cutoff to come through the filter, whereas all above the cutoff are blocked. Of course, in real filters the cutoff is not discontinuous. An idealized low pass filter is shown in panel a of Fig. II.34. A **high pass filter** does just the opposite of a low pass filter. Panel b shows an idealized case. And a **band pass filter,** panel c, allows only frequencies in an interval or a band to pass. Note that a band pass filter is equivalent to successive applications of a low pass and then a high pass filter.

A familiar example of a band pass filter — one that is also a transducer — is the telephone. Its band is roughly 300Hz to 3,000 Hz. As is discussed later, this fact together with the fact that voices do not seem greatly distorted is a bit of an auditory puzzle.

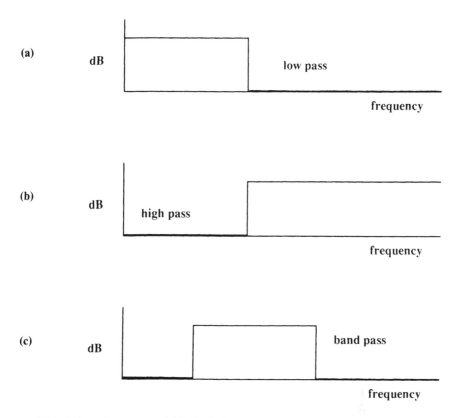

FIG. II.34 Three types of idealized filters: (a) a low pass one that passes all frequencies below the cutoff and blocks all those above; (b) a high pass one that passes the higher frequencies and blocks the lower ones; and (c) a band pass one that passes all frequencies within a band, and blocks all outside the band. Physical filters are unable to achieve a perfect cutoff, but rather exhibit a continuous change, which is referred to as a roll off and is often characterized in terms of dB per octave (i.e., a doubling of frequency).

12. SUMMARY OF THE MAIN CONCEPTS ABOUT SIMPLE WAVES

12.1 Medium of Transmission

Characteristics:

density ρ(unit: g/cm^3)
speed of propagation c (unit: m/s)
ρc is called acoustic impedance (unit: dynes-s/cm^3)

	ρ	c	ρc
Air	1.16×10^{-3}	344	40
Water	1	1,432	1.43×10^5
Seawater	1.025	1,531	1.57×10^5

12.2 Source — An Oscillator Generating a Sinusoidal Wave in Time

Characteristics of a sine wave:

period T (unit: s)
frequency $f = 1/T$ (unit: Hz when T is in seconds)
peak pressure P $=$ force/area (unit: dynes/cm^2)
phase angle ϕ (unit: radian)
pressure fluctuation $p = P \sin (2\pi ft + \phi)$

12.3 Propagation of a Wave in a Medium

Characteristic: wavelength λ (unit: m)
Physical relation: $\lambda = c/f = cT$
Doppler effect: Either the source is moving at velocity v_s or the observer is at velocity v_o. The frequency of the source is f_s and the frequency observed by the observer is f_o.

		f_o/f_s Direction of Motion	
		Toward	Away
	Source	$c/(c - v_s)$	$c/(c + v_s)$
Who is Moving			
	Observer	$(c + v_o)/c$	$(c - v_o)/c$

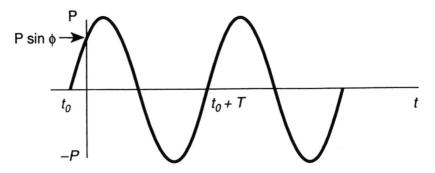

FIG. II.35 A typical sine wave of period T, amplitude P, and phase ϕ. Note: $t_o = -\phi T/2\pi$.

12.4 Intensity of Propagated Wave

Definitions: unit of force: dyne = force needed to move 1 g with acceleration of 1 cm/s^2 ≡ g-cm/s^2.

pressure = force/area; unit: dyne/cm^2.

energy = force × distance; unit: dyne-cm = erg.

power = energy/time; unit: erg/s or watt = 10^{7}erg/s.

intensity = power/area; unit: erg/s-cm^2 = 10^{-7} watt/cm^2.

Physical law: $I = p^2/\rho c$, where I is intensity, p pressure, ρ the density of the medium, and c the speed of sound in the medium.

Definition: dB = 10 $\log_{10} I/I_0$ = 10 $\log I$ − 10 $\log I_0$. This is a relative (difference) measure of intensities. For $I_0 = 10^{-9}$ erg/s-cm^2 = 10^{-12} watts/m^2, which corresponds to $P_0 = 0.0002$ dynes/cm^2 in air, the dB measure is referred to as SPL (sound pressure level).

12.5 Wave Impinging on Surface

Reflection: Fig. II.36.

Physical law: $\theta_r = \theta_i$ (angle of reflection = angle of incidence)

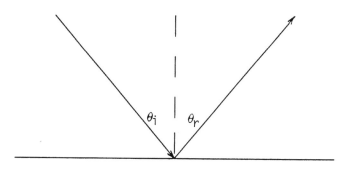

FIG. II.36   A schematic of a reflected plane wave.

Refraction: Fig. II.37.

$$\text{Physical law: } \frac{\sin \theta_i}{\sin \theta_r} = \frac{c_i}{c_r}$$

Impedance mismatch at interface:

Let $\rho_i c_i$ and $\rho_r c_r$ be the acoustic impedances of the media of the incident and refracted sound waves, respectively. Let $R = \rho_i c_i/\rho_r c_r$.

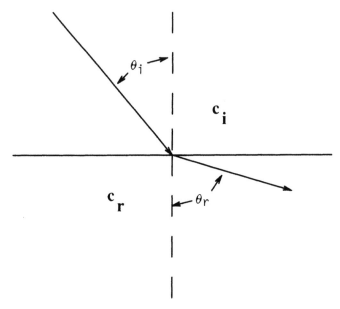

FIG. II.37   A schematic of a refracted plane wave.

Physical law: The fraction of intensity transmitted across the interface is

$$4R/(1 + R)^2.$$

From air to water, $R = 2.48 \times 10^{-4}$, so the fraction is 9.9×10^{-4} which, in dB, is a loss of 30.03 dB. The loss is the same in both directions.

13. FURTHER READING

As was noted in the preface, a good general reference, at about the same level as this text, to the physical description of sounds is Johnson, Walker, and Cutnell (1981). Rossing (1982) gives a somewhat more thorough treatment; and for those with a background of calculus, Halliday and Resnick (1978) derives the various descriptive laws from basic physical principles, although not for the attenuation of sound caused by a change of medium. Much less formal, but nonetheless sophisticated treatments, are those of Pierce (1974) and Roederer (1975). A delightful discussion of the very large and the very small in physics — powers of ten — is the book of that title by the Morrisons (1982).

PART III

Properties of the Ear

1. THE OUTER AND MIDDLE EARS

1.1 Structures

The ear is composed of three quite distinct parts called the outer, middle, and inner ears. The only part we can see is the outer ear. See Fig. III.1 for a cross-section of the entire structure.

The outer ear too can be partitioned into three parts:

Informal terms: Cup	Ear Canal	Ear Drum
↕	↕	↕
More technical: Pinna	External Auditory Meatus	Tympanic Membrane

An incoming sound wave is channeled by the pinna and external auditory meatus and, to a degree, modified by them until it reaches the tympanic membrane. At that point the middle ear comes into play.

The middle ear consists of an air-filled cavity, roughly a sphere, formed by a bony structure (see Fig. III.1). This cavity is connected to the oral cavity by the **eustachian tube.** Within the cavity are three linked bones called **ossicles,** which are suspended by means of ligaments attached to the bone forming the cavity. The first ossicle is attached to the tympanic membrane and the third to a membrane called the **oval window** that

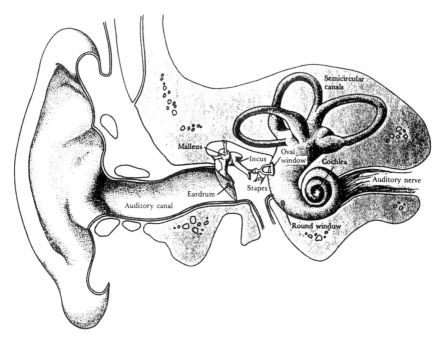

FIG. III.1 A schematic cross-section showing the major anatomical components of the ear. From *Human Information Processing: An Introduction to Psychology* (p. 221) by P. H. Lindsay and D. A. Norman, 1972, New York: Academic Press. Copyright 1972 by New York: Academic Press. Reprinted by permission.

interfaces the middle and inner ears. Basically, the ossicles simply link the outer ear to inner ear. (Their roles in hearing become clear later.)

The names of the ossicles and their linkage is as follows:

Tympanic membrane → *malleus* (also called the hammer)
  → *incus* (also called the anvil)
  → *stapes*
  → *oval window*

The part of the stapes attached to the oval window is called the **footplate.**

In addition to the suspension ligaments, muscles are located in bony tubes that connect both the malleus and the stapes to the wall of the cavity. (These are not shown in the figure.) Their role is to protect the inner ear from sounds that are so loud they can cause damage. We describe that action more fully later (Section III.1.2).

The inner ear side of the oval window consists of another bone-encased cavity, called the **cochlea,** which is filled with a fluid with a composition much like seawater. The oval window is a sealed membrane separating these two cavities; it is attached to the footplate of the stapes on the middle ear side and is hinged like a door. Movement of the tympanic membrane due to changes in air pressure is transmitted through the linkage of the ossicles to a swinging movement of the oval window. We go into detail in Section III.2 about what happens in the interior of the cochlea.

1.2 Functions

1.2.1 Overcoming the Air–Fluid Impedance Mismatch.   What functions do the outer and middle ears serve? Or put in engineering terms, what problems do they seem "designed" to solve? "Designed" is placed in quotes because for something to be designed, there must be a designer. Modern biological science treats organisms as a product of very long-term evolutionary pressures, rather than as the result of conscious design. Nonetheless, we can still ask what problem each part seems to solve, at least partially.

Given that the inner ear is filled with a liquid much like seawater, it appears very likely that the sound wave in air must be transduced (see Section I.3) into some form of water wave. That is to say, the pressure wave must be transmitted through an air–water interface. So from the physics of the situation, we know that an impedance mismatch exists that results in an intensity loss of about 30 dB (see Section II.9).

Because the pressure changes in air are already very small (recall from Section II.8.2, they are of the order of one part in 10^{10}), after a 30 dB loss (that is, another factor of $10^{3/2} \cong 32$) the task of detecting the changes is far more difficult. Amplification, not attenuation, is called for. Nevertheless, the loss can hardly be avoided because we exist and communicate in air whereas our internal biology is water based. Thus, nature faced the problem of counteracting the inherent loss of signal intensity that is involved in the change of media.

The compensation has been accomplished in three distinct ways, each being only a partial solution. It has been said, "Nature is not so much a designer as a tinkerer."

First, the outer ear is constructed so that resonances occur in the channel; in effect, the pinna serves as a frequency dependent amplifier that causes some increase in the pressure amplitude. Roughly, the resonance pattern is that shown in Fig. III.2, although there are individual differences depending on the shape of the pinna. In some of the range, the amplification is nearly two-thirds of what is needed, but overall it is much less than that. The pinna of some animals, such as rabbits and deer, is considerably more efficient than ours, especially because it can be rotated in the direction of a sound source.

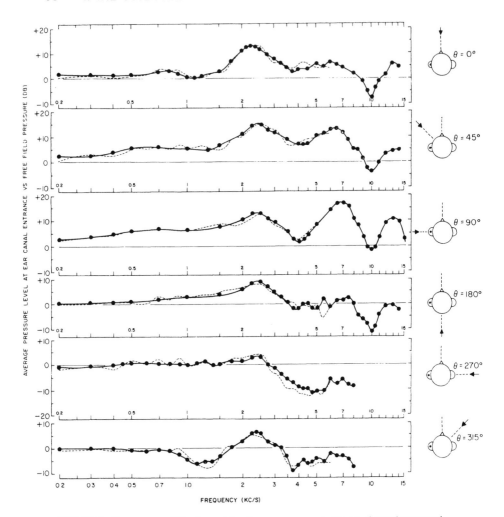

FIG. III.2 Pressure amplification arising from resonances in the ear channel presented as a function of frequency and the angle of the incident wave. This measurement is carried out by inserting a very small pressure sensor near the ear drum and an external pressure sensor near the external entrance to the outer ear. From "Earcanal Pressure Generated by a Free Sound Field" by E. A. G. Shaw, 1966, *Journal of the Acoustical Society of America, 39,* p. 469. Copyright 1966 by American Institute of Physics. Reprinted by permission.

Second, the middle ear produces mechanical leverage that amplifies the forces as follows: The effective area of the tympanic membrane is about 55 mm^2, and the area of the footplate is about 3.2 mm^2. The force input to the middle ear on the tympanic membrane must equal the force output on the oval window, which results in a pressure ratio of 55/3.2 = 17. That is about 24.6 dB.

Third, the ossicles act as a simple lever system, with a leverage factor of 1.3.

Thus, the total amplification ratio effected by the middle ear design is $17(1.3) = 22.1$. Transforming that to dB yields $10 \log(22.1)^2 = 26.9$ dB, which is reasonably close to the 30 dB loss of the impedance mismatch. This solution is hardly very elegant, but it pretty much overcomes the loss.

If this argument is correct, destruction of the ossicles or their immobilization through bone fusion should reduce hearing by about 27 dB. Observed losses in clinical cases of these types runs 20 to 30 dB, suggesting that it is roughly correct.

1.2.2 Protecting the Inner Ear from Loud Sounds.   When excess pressure is transmitted from the middle ear into the inner ear the main transducers—called "hair cells"—within the cochlea (inner ear), which convert the pressure into neural activity, can be destroyed. As discussed in Section III.3, this results in deafness. The middle ear serves the additional function of reducing this danger.

As was noted earlier, muscles are attached to the ossicles. These muscles keep the inner ear from receiving the full impact of sounds that are too loud. For sounds 80 dB or more above absolute threshold, these muscles tighten, resisting the movement of the ossicles and thereby reducing the lever action on the oval window. This decreases the transmitted intensity by about 0.6 dB for each dB of increase. Thus, for a sound of 120 dB at the tympanic membrane, the reduction is $0.6(120 - 80) = 24$ dB, thereby holding the actual exposure of the inner ear to about 96 dB.

This protective system is unsuccessful in one important way. For very loud sounds, the latency (= time elapsed) from the onset of the sound to the onset of the contraction is about 10 ms, and for less loud sounds this extends up to 150 ms. Thus, this system for attenuating loud sounds fails to provide effective protection from the initial onset of highly percussive sounds such as those of a dropped hammer, a nearby gunshot, or some rock music. Evidence that it matters comes from data on hearing loss among those continually exposed to loud percussive sounds. This is discussed further in Section III.3.3.

2. THE INNER EAR

2.1 Structure

As can be seen from the top of Fig. III.1, the cochlea looks a lot like a snail shell. It is essentially a tube coiled about two and one-half times. Its total length in the human beings is about 3.5 cm (1.38 in). Imagine that the cochlea has been unwound (which, of course, it never can be because it is made of bone) and cut lengthwise, as shown in Fig. III.3. Within this outer tube is an interior tube that is attached to the outer wall of the cochlea and to a bony shelf that extends from the inner wall of the cochlea. The inner tube (scala media) and bony shelf divides the outer tube (cochlea) into two distinct parts (called the scala vestibuli and scala tympani) that are connected only at the apical end through a small hole in the dividing membrane. This passage way is called the **helicotrema.**

At the basal end of the scala vestibuli is a second membrane, round this time, that again interfaces air. This is known as the **round window.** Its role is explained later.

In cross section, the inner tube looks somewhat triangular in shape, as shown in Fig. III.4. Its top wall is a somewhat flexible membrane known as **Reissner's membrane.** Part of the bottom wall is also a somewhat flexible membrane known as the **basilar membrane.** The basilar membrane is held rigidly in bony extensions from the wall of the cochlea, as shown in the longitudinal section in Fig. III.3. At the basal end, the membrane is narrow and stiff; at the apical end it is both wider and considerably more flaccid.

The basilar membrane is where the action is in the inner ear. Here the wave motions are transduced into neural electrical activity.

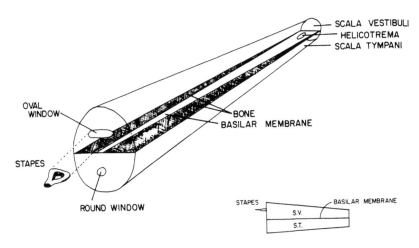

FIG. III.3   The central partition of the cochlea as it would look if one could lay it out flat. The basilar membrane is narrow at the basal end (near the round and oval windows) and wider at the apical end. The small hole in the basilar membrane at the apical end is called the helicotrema. It serves to connect the fluids on the two sides of the cochlear partition. The fluid in the region bounded by the basilar and Reissner's membrane is isolated from the other fluid. From *An Introduction to Hearing* (p. 66) by D. M. Green, 1976, Hillsdale, NJ: Lawrence Erlbaum Associates. Copyright 1976 by Lawrence Erlbaum Associates, Inc. Reprinted by permission.

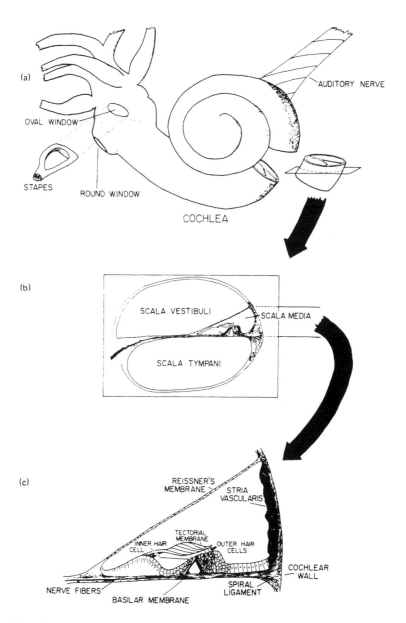

FIG. III.4 Panel a is a schematic of the cochlea showing a typical region cut out and viewed on end in panel b. Note that there are two fluid-filled regions formed by a partition down the middle of the cochlea. Panel c expands this partition and we see that it defines a third, fluid-filled region that is bounded by two somewhat flexible membranes, the basilar and Reissner's. From *An Introduction to Hearing* (p. 64) by D. M. Green, 1976, Hillsdale, NJ: Lawrence Erlbaum Associates. Copyright 1976 by Lawrence Erlbaum Associates, Inc. Reprinted by permission.

2.2 Function

Let us make clear the problem that has been solved by the cochlea. Ultimately, its output is to be electrical activity that is transmitted over neurons in the brain. Such electrical activity is how the brain has evolved to conduct rapid communications. So fluctuations in air pressure must be transduced to neural activity. Electrical activity is generated biologically by means of chemical reactions in specialized cells called **neurons.** Because such cells require a fluid environment in which to thrive, the first task of the cochlea is to convert the air pressure wave into some encoding of intensity and frequency that is transmitted through the fluid bath to these cells.

So far, we know that changes in air pressure give rise to movements of the oval window, which, in turn, introduces a pressure wave in the cochlea fluid. At the pressures involved, water is totally incompressible and the cochlea, being of bone, is totally rigid, so some way is needed to provide pressure relief, otherwise the sound waves in air will be unable to affect the basilar membrane. That relief is provided by the round window. When the internal pressure rises, the round window, being a membrane, moves slightly out into the highly compressible air of the middle ear.

One's first guess is to assume that the water wave resulting from the action of the footplate propagates down the cochlea, thereby inducing a surface wave motion along the basilar membrane. A quick calculation proves this to be impossible. In sea water, the velocity of sound is about 160,000 cm/s. So for a 1,000 Hz pressure wave, the wavelength is by Equation II.7:

$$1.6 \times 10^5/10^3 = 160 \text{ cm.}$$

However, as was remarked earlier, the basilar membrane is only 3.5 cm long. So, to a very good approximation, the pressure at any moment is the same everywhere on the basilar membrane. Thus, there is no spatial surface wave on the basilar membrane.

2.3 Traveling Waves on the Basilar Membrane

Nevertheless, over time, the pressure at any one point on the basilar membrane does indeed change quite rapidly relative to the fluid in the interior tube that is bounded by it and Reissner's membrane. Perhaps this is a situation in which resonance plays a significant role in the sense that the basilar membrane acts as a somewhat complex filter.

Suppose the basilar membrane consists, in effect, of a series of loosely coupled, fairly high Q filters (Section II.11.3). In Fig. III.3, it is as if each segment of the basilar membrane is reasonably independent of the adjacent ones. Then for each input frequency, some of the filters resonate and some do not. Each frequency is characterized by a different pattern of resonance. Of course, the amplitudes of these resonances are affected by the intensity of the input wave.

Crudely, the type of resonance motion that will occur in such a system of resonators is as shown in Fig. III.5.

This kind of resonance-induced wave is called a **traveling wave,** and its existence on the basilar membrane has been confirmed by direct observation. Such observations are technically very difficult to carry out for two reasons. First, to look inside a functioning cochlea is inherently a highly invasive procedure, one that tends inadvertently to incapacitate the system. Second, the amplitudes involved are very tiny—between 10^{-9} and 10^{-10} cm—and so measuring them at all requires great ingenuity. Of course, such measurements have only been carried out on animals.

G. von Békésy was the first to look inside a live cochlea and he made the earliest measurements of the vibratory patterns of the basilar membrane, during the 1930s and 1940s, for which research he received the Nobel Prize in 1961.

During the 1980s an increasing belief developed, initially based on neural data to be explored in Section III.4.2.4 and later confirmed by direct observations, that some considerable additional amplification of the motion occurs at the sharp rise of the resonance nearer the apical end of the traveling wave, so that the picture is something like that of Fig. III.6.

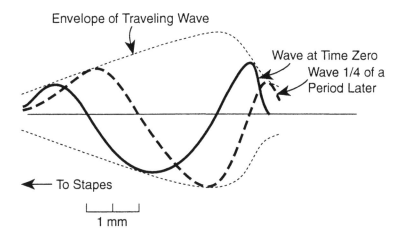

FIG. III.5 Sketch of the typical envelope of a traveling wave. To make the wave visible, the amplitude is shown in a scale many orders of magnitude larger than the distance scale. The actual displacement of the basilar membrane is tiny.

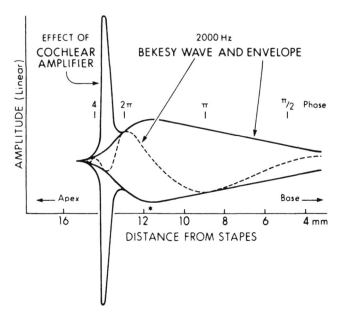

FIG. III.6 A recent modification of what the envelope of movement on the basilar membrane must be. It arises from a second source of resonance in addition to the traveling wave, one whose resonance is very peaked, that is, a high Q filter. Its existence is inferred indirectly from some aspects of neural activity discussed elsewhere, and is attributed to some ill-understood cochlear amplifier. From "An Active Process in Cochlear Mechanics" by H. Davis, 1983, *Hearing Research, 9,* p. 82. Copyright 1983 by Elsevier Science Pub., Bv. Reprinted by permission.

One may view this response pattern as arising from two independent resonance systems acting together, the one being the traveling wave of the basilar membrane itself and the other, called the **cochlear amplifier**, being of some other origin that is not well understood. The indirect evidence for its existence is described in Section III.4.2.4.

So the basilar membrane resonates in a decidedly asymmetric fashion, and the location of the sharp rise of the resonance near the basal end is determined by the frequency of the input wave (see Figs. III.7 and III.8).

The next step of the process is the conversion of that resonance into electrical, neural pulses. The key to accomplishing this are the so-called hair cells.

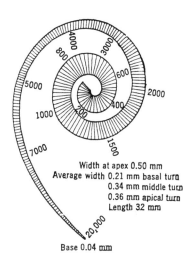

FIG. III.7 A cross-section of the cochlea indicating how the frequencies are distributed along the basilar membrane. From *An Introduction to Biophysics* (p. 286) by O. Stuhlman, 1943, New York: Wiley. Copyright 1943 by New York: John Wiley & Sons. Reprinted by permission.

Width at apex 0.50 mm
Average width 0.21 mm basal turn
0.34 mm middle turn
0.36 mm apical turn
Length 32 mm

Base 0.04 mm

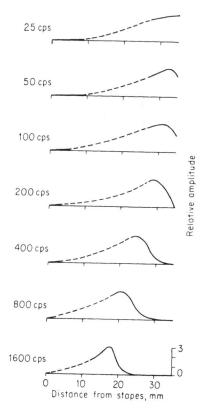

FIG. III.8 The measurements of Békésy that show how frequency corresponds to place on the basilar membrane. The solid lines were observed and the dotted ones conjectured. From *Experiments in Hearing* (p. 448) by G. von Békésy, 1960, New York: McGraw-Hill. Copyright 1960 by New York: McGraw Hill Book Company, Inc. Reprinted by permission.

3. HAIR CELLS AND THE AUDITORY NERVE

3.1 Hair Cells

The **organ of Corti** is a structure attached to the interior side of the basilar membrane. From it protrude four rows of thin cells running the length of the basilar membrane that are called **hair cells.** They are immersed in the interior fluid, called the **endolymphatic fluid,** in the tube bounded by the basilar membrane and Reissner's membrane.

The hair cells are arranged into two distinct groups. One consists of three parallel and closely spaced rows of cells called the **outer hair cells.** The remaining ones form a distinct single row of cells, parallel to but somewhat separated from the outer hair cells, called the **inner hair cells.**

On each hair cell are much smaller protuberances called **cilia.** There can be up to 100 cilia per hair cell. Because the cilia of the hair cells are just touching the **tectorial membrane,** which lies just above the organ of Corti and the hair cells, the cilia of a particular hair cell bend whenever movement occurs in the portion of the basilar membrane that underlies that hair cell.

When a cilia bends, ion molecules flow into the hair cell, which in turn releases a chemical transmitter whose action results in an electrical potential. Given the way neural fibers are constructed, this ends up as an electrical discharge that propagates along the neuron(s) connected to the hair cell. We examine something of the nature of that electrical discharge in Section III.4.

3.2 Auditory Nerve

The neurons connected to hair cells are all clustered together into a bundle, known as the **auditory (or VIIIth) nerve,** that exits the cochlea and heads toward the brain.

As shown in Fig. III.9, there are four different types of neurons that in different ways carry information to and from the hair cells. This information is shown more schematically in Fig. III.10. The neurons that send signals from the hair cells to the brain are called **afferent neurons.** They come in two major types, as shown in Fig. III.10, known as radial and outer spirals. Roughly 95% of the afferent fibers are radial, and the remaining 5% are outer spiral. Table III.1 shows some typical numbers.

The **efferent neurons** transmit signals from the brain to hair cells. In both human and cat there are from 500 to 2,500. These also come in two types, and are also shown in Fig. III.10. The acronym UCOCB is short for *uncrossed olivocochlear bundle* (also called the inner spiral). This bundle consists of 20% of the efferent neurons, and it carries signals from a part

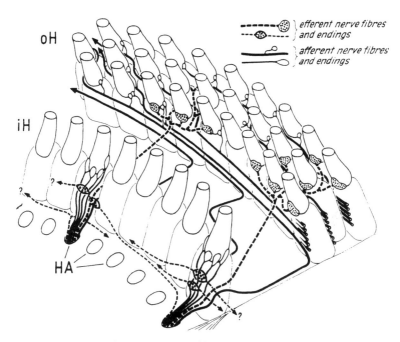

oH

iH

HA

------⊕} efferent nerve fibres
---⊛----- } and endings

⌐o} afferent nerve fibres
—— } and endings

FIG. III.9   A sketch of the anatomy of afferent and efferent nerve fiber connections to a sample of inner and outer hair cells. From "Structural Basis of Peripheral Frequency Analysis" in *Frequency Analysis and Periodicity Detection in Hearing* (p. 33) by H. Spoendlin, 1970, Leiden, The Netherlands: A. W. Sijthoff. Copyright 1970 by Kluwer Academic Publishers. Reprinted by permission.

of the brain that is on the same side as the ear in question. These fibers attach to the afferent radial fibers, but not directly to the inner hair cells. The remaining 80% of the efferent neurons, called COCB, which is short for *crossed olivocochlear bundle,* connect the side of the brain opposite to the ear sending signals to its outer hair cells.

3.3 Sources of Hearing Loss

Hearing loss can arise from problems anywhere in the auditory system. Table III.2 summarizes the major problem sources.

   One of the most important and common of these sources of hearing loss is the (partial) destruction of the hair cells. Because movement of the cilia on the hair cells results in neural activity, it is obvious that their loss is highly detrimental to the transduction from air pressure to neural activity.

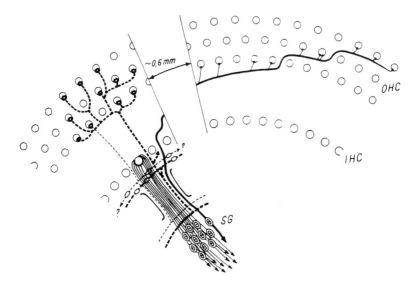

FIG. III.10 A more schematic drawing showing how the afferent and efferent nerve fibers innervate the inner and outer hair cells. The afferent fibers are of two types: the radial ones come in groups of 8 to 10 and all attach to a single inner hair cell (shown at the lower left), and the outer spiral ones (shown at upper right) each innervate about 10 outer hair cells. The efferent fibers also are of two types: those (COCB) connecting the opposite side of the brain to the outer hair cells (shown as dashed lines on the upper left), and those (UCOCB) connecting the same side of the brain to the afferent radials (but do not directly contact the inner hair cells). The latter fibers run parallel to the inner hair cells (shown on the lower left) and they are called inner spiral fibers. From "Structural Basis of Peripheral Frequency Analysis" in *Frequency Analysis and Periodicity Detection in Hearing* (p. 33) by H. Spoendlin, 1970, Leiden, The Netherlands: A. W. Sijthoff. Copyright 1970 by Kluwer Academic Publishers. Reprinted by permission.

TABLE III.1
Some Typical Numbers of Hair Cells and Afferent Neurons

| | Hair Cells | | Afferent Neurons | | |
	Inner	Outer	# Neurons per inner H.C.	# Outer H. C. per neuron	Total # neurons
Human	3,500	10,500	8–10	10	32,000
Cat	2,500	7,500	16–20	10	45,000–50,000

TABLE III.2
Some Sources of Auditory Pathology

Location	Nature	Comments
Outer ear	Blockage	Usually wax — trivial
	Scarred tympanic membrane	Must be severe to affect hearing greatly
Middle ear	Fluid	Affects movement of TM, oval, round windows
		Occurs in children and affects speech production
		Treatment: Surgical drainage
	Malfunctioning ossicles	Intensity loss up to 30 dB at all frequencies
Inner ear	Loss of hair cells	Frequency dependent hearing loss caused by loud sounds and certain drugs
	Other cochlea damage	Accidents, birth defects
Auditory nerve	Mechanical damage	Accidents, strokes
	Disease damage	Poorly understood

Observational data on the resonance occurring on the basilar membrane establishes that damage to the outer hair cells results in a marked reduction in the sharp resonance on the basilar membrane attributed in Fig. III.6 to a "cochlear amplifier." This clearly implicates the outer hair cells in an important way, but the exact mechanism remains controversial.

Such hair cell damage can occur in a number of ways, the two most important being excessive exposure to very loud, percussive sounds and exposure to certain drugs.

One very clear example of the impact of percussive sounds is the postmortem sections of the two basilar membranes of a 72-year-old hunter shown in Fig. III.11. His left ear, which was near the firing pin of his rifle when he was sighting and firing, shows a major gap in the rows of hair cells, whereas his right ear, which was shielded by the right shoulder, is more or less normal for a man of his age.

Another equally clear and sad example is found with 18- to 20-year-olds who play music very loudly through portable earphone systems. Losses of 30 dB to 40 dB in the region of 3kHz to 4kHz are common. Not only is it impossible to compensate for such losses with existing hearing aids but, as the person ages, the damage may lead to a serious ailment called *tinnitus* in which the auditory system itself generates ever-present, annoying sounds.

The following is a partial list of drugs that are known to induce hearing loss:

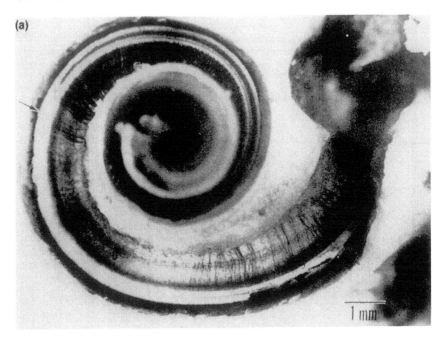

FIG. III.11 Photographs of postmortem sections of the two cochleas of a 72-year-old hunter. Note the major damage to the basilar membrane of the left cochlea. This ear was repeatedly exposed to the highly percussive sound of the rifle discharging, which inflicted the damage that led to severe hearing loss in that ear. From "Pattern of Sensorineural Degeneration in Human Ears Exposed to Noise" in *Effects of Noise on Hearing* (p. 95-96) by J. E. Hawkins and L.-G. Johnson, 1976, New York: Raven Press. Copyright 1976 by New York: Raven Press. Reprinted by permission.

Streptomycin	Used for TB. Partial destruction of hair cells.
Kanamycin	Used as a last resort for bacterial infections. Major destruction of hair cells.
Neomycin	Similar to Kanamycin.
Gentamycin	Used against staphyococcus. Major destruction of hair cells.
Viomycin	Similar to streptomycin.
Quinine	Used to treat malaria. Temporary hearing loss, but in large doses the damage becomes permanent. Very damaging to embryos.
Aspirin	Reversible hearing loss and other auditory symptoms when used in very massive doses.

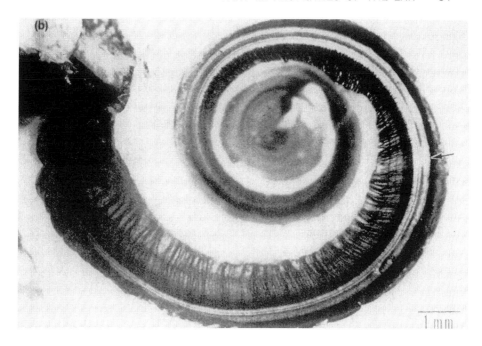

FIG. III.11 *(cont.)*

The relatively common hearing loss associated with aging, especially in men, is likely to be multifaceted — including some mix of problems with the functioning of the ossicles, changes in the characteristics of various membranes of the system, especially the basilar membrane, and loss of some hair cells, especially those at the basal end. Little is known about aging processes of central systems. Why these hearing troubles are somewhat sex linked (see Fig. IV.8) is not fully understood, although it may be partially due to be differential exposure to noise.

4. NEURAL CODING
OF AUDITORY INFORMATION

4.1 Neural Spike Trains

4.1.1 Recording Neural Activity.   During the 1960s physiological techniques developed to the point where it became possible to access the peripheral auditory (VIIIth) nerve in live animals and to penetrate individual neurons with extremely fine microelectrodes. Such research has been carried out primarily on cats and squirrel monkeys; however, because of anatomical and other physiological similarities, it is believed that substantially the same results are true for human beings (see, however, Section III.5.2).

To make electrical recordings of spikes, the microelectrode is inserted into the auditory nerve. The points of these electrodes are sufficiently small and sharp that it is possible for them to enter (see Fig. III.12) into a single auditory neuron without seriously disrupting its function, permitting measurement of electrical activity in that fiber. The potential difference between the exterior of the cell and the interior is measured and amplified so it can be seen on an oscilloscope, which is somewhat like a computer or TV monitor.

Neurons differ appreciably in diameter and most penetrations will be into those of larger diameter. Therefore, the results reported here may well be biased in that they tell us little, if anything, about the behavior of the smaller diameter neurons, which are believed to be mainly connected to the outer hair cells. What makes matters even more biased is that on a random basis the chances are 20 to 1 that the electrode will impale a radial neuron, connected to an inner hair cell. So one can hardly doubt that our knowledge is currently biased.

A second concern about any neuron that is penetrated is where it originated along the basilar membrane. Its approximate location is determined by its response pattern, which is described in the next section.

4.1.2 Neural Pulses (Spikes).   One of the earliest findings about neural activity was first observed in some very large neurons of the horseshoe crab that could be penetrated using the somewhat gross electrodes then available:

Auditory neural electrical activity is highly punctate in character.

This was later confirmed in higher mammals using much more refined microelectrodes.

Typically a neural discharge of electrical activity, as shown in Fig. III.13, does not last very long—on the order of 50 μs (microseconds)—and its electrical potential is small—on the order of 10 to 20 mv (millivolts) or less. (Sometimes these voltages are reported as microvolts, μv.) The discharge is so brief that when plotted on the more usual time scale of milliseconds, it looks like, and is often called, a **spike.**

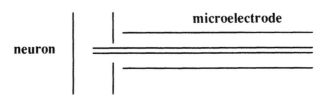

FIG. III.12   A schematic of a microelectrode penetrating an auditory nerve fiber.

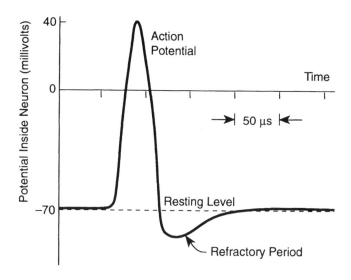

FIG. III.13   The typical voltage pattern of a neural pulse. Note that the voltage is small and measured in millivolts (mv), and the time scale is very fast and measured in microseconds (μs). When plotted on a millisecond (ms) scale it is virtually a spike.

Such a sequence of pulses over time is called a **pulse** or **spike train.** (In fact, the spikes flowing down a neuron are less like a train than like irregularly spaced cars all travelling at exactly the same velocity down a one-lane road. Nevertheless, the term *train* is used in describing their temporal sequencing.) The graph of Fig. III.14 is typical.

4.1.3 Four Important Facts About Spike Trains.

• Although the amplitude of the spikes exhibits some variability, this does not seem to encode any useful information about what is going on.[1]

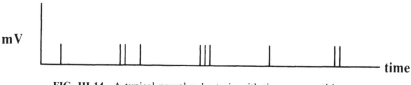

FIG. III.14   A typical neural pulse train with time measured in ms.

---

[1]A statement of this type should be viewed as highly tentative. It says what appears to be true at the time of writing, but often later work makes clear that we did not fully understand what is going on.

Apparently, the spikes are binary in character—either they occur or they don't—and this pattern of occurrences carries information into the central nervous system.[2]

• Spikes travel along the fiber at a speed characteristic of the particular neuron. The range of speeds is from 20 to 100 m/s, with the speed being roughly proportional to the diameter of the neuron.

• After a spike occurs, a second one cannot occur immediately. Once a spike has passed a given point on a neuron, a certain amount of chemical housekeeping is required within the neuron before it can transmit another pulse, and that housekeeping takes something of the order of $\frac{1}{2}$ to 1 ms to be completed on auditory neurons. The fiber is said to be **refractory** during that period. Thus, the absolute maximum firing rate is from 1,000 to 2,000 spikes per second (sps). Such high rates are never observed, but rates up to several hundred sps are possible.

• Any neuron exhibits some spiking whether or not there is any external stimulus. This is known from observations made on subjects in total silence. Of course, their breathing and blood flow are sources of some noise that cannot be controlled. This low background rate of neural firing is called the **resting** or **spontaneous rate.** It is usually between 5 and 10 sps. Thus, between the spontaneous rate and the maximum is a factor of from 100/10 = 10 to 2,000/5 = 400.

A major question confronting auditory scientists is just how intensity and frequency are encoded in these spike trains. If the neural spikes themselves do not transmit information, then what does? The only possibilities on a single fiber are the rate of firing or some temporal patterning of the spikes in the spike train. We take up firing rates first and then temporal patterns in Section III.4.3.

4.2 Coding in Terms of Neural Firing Rate

The most obvious question asks, what affects the rate of pulse generation? Because rate is the number of pulses that occur in a period of time, this amounts to asking about the reciprocal of the average time between successive pulses. Our first main empirical section is devoted just to questions about rate and how it varies with the signal.

4.2.1 Poststimulus Histograms. The three most obvious independent variables that to some degree affect neural firing rate are signal duration,

---

[2]The binary aspect of neural spikes—either they occur or they don't—has led to an analogy with digital computers. However, that particular analogy may be rather poor because synchronization as well as binariness is essential in a computer whereas in the brain synchronization seems to play a decidedly limited role. The analogy may improve with the introduction of massively parallel computers.

intensity, and frequency. This four-dimensional problem — the dependence of rate on three variables — is difficult to visualize as a whole. In such cases we try to reduce the dimensionality to two or three. One way is to hold fixed two of the three independent variables and see how rate depends on third. That is how this subsection is organized. But first, let us take up the question of estimating firing rates.

Suppose we are examining a neuron with a spontaneous rate of 10 cps and with a particular signal the rate increases to 50 sps, and suppose the signal lasts 100 ms, that is, $\frac{1}{10}$ of a second. This means that we expect, on average, five ($= 50/10$) spikes to occur while the signal is present, and, on average, one to occur in every 100 ms when the signal is not present. With such small samples, it is clear that we are not going to be able to say anything very subtle about what happens to the rate during the time the signal is on. For example, it is virtually impossible to tell from a single sample if the firing rate is the same throughout the duration of the signal or if it is decreasing or increasing.

The only way to see what is happening at that level of detail is to increase the sample with which we are working. Both the brain as well as the scientists studying the brain face the same problem of needing a much larger sample. They approach it differently. The brain has many fibers operating in parallel that provide the central system with statistically independent replicas of the same information. The scientist, with but a single electrode inserted into a single neuron, repeatedly stimulates the ear with physically identical sound signals and observes the resulting spike train arising from each stimulation. This is usually done hundreds or even thousands of times.

With such data, one can then study how the firing rate varies during the course of signal presentation as follows: Choose some small interval of time — 1, 5, and 10 ms are typical — that provides sufficiently fine temporal subdivision to enable one to see the detail desired. These time intervals are called *bin widths*. For example, partitioning a 100 ms signal, a typical duration used, into two 50 ms bins affords only the coarsest information about how the rate varies during the course of the 100 ms signal presentation. Going to 5 ms subdivides the signal duration into 20 bins, which permits one to see much more detail. One ms subdivides it into 100 bins, which is very detailed (although later we encounter bin widths another order of magnitude smaller).

Once a bin width is selected, one then enters a count in a bin each time a spike occurs in the data at a time falling within the bin. So, for example, with a 5 ms width, the bin from 21 to 25 ms will get a count every time we encounter a spike occurring 21, 22, 23, 24, or 25 ms after signal onset.

Consider, for example, the following short collection of hypothetical data of the times (measured in milliseconds) at which spikes occurred after signal onset:

5, 7, 13, 32, 33, 37, 38, 49, 62, 64, 77, 91, 94

Let us suppose that a bin width of 25 ms is used, then the classification of data leads to the following table:

Bin	1–25	26–50	51–75	76–100
Number of spikes	3	5	2	3

The bins may be identified either by their rank ordering from signal onset or, more commonly, by the average time of the bin from signal onset. When the estimated firing rate (or total number of spikes in a bin) is reported as a function of the bin location after signal onset, the plot is called a **poststimulus histogram,** usually abbreviated **PST histogram.**[3]

An aside on the reporting of data: To me, the natural way to report such data is as momentary estimates of the firing rate in spikes per second (sps), which would make it easy to compare results from different studies. That, however, is not the normal practice. Rather the plots show the total number of spikes that were observed in each bin for whatever number of signal presentations happened to be used. Both the bin width and the sample size are always reported in a technical paper, so one can estimate the actual rates, but often it cannot be done from the figures alone.

Of course, the narrower one makes each bin width, the fewer the number of spikes one expects to observe in that bin. For example, if 40 spikes is the expected number in a 5 ms width, then it is one-fifth that, or 8, when a 1 ms width is used. This necessarily means that the statistical estimate of the average rate corresponding to each bin is more variable as the bin width is made smaller. We can, of course, compensate for such increased variability by carrying out more runs. For example, if the estimate is of some acceptable quality when using 5 ms bins, then to maintain the same quality with 1 ms bins requires increasing the sample observed by a factor of five. Sometimes that will be judged too expensive or, more likely, experimentally impractical because of problems in maintaining the microelectrode in the same neuron for a long time. One has to carefully weigh the trade-off between the level of detail one needs in order to understand what is happening and the cost or practicality of getting the needed data.

4.2.2 Firing Rate as a Function of Signal Duration. Figure III.15 exhibits PST histograms from two peripheral fibers in a cat. The pattern is quite typical of what is found in the periphery. The firing rate at signal

---

[3]The term *histogram* is used whenever the data are grouped into either temporal or spatial bins, and the number of observations in each bin is represented by a bar on a graph.

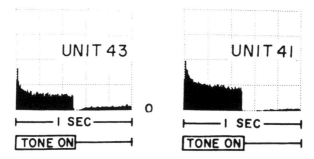

FIG. III.15 A typical poststimulus (PST) histogram for a peripheral neural fiber responding to a tone of about 500 ms duration. Note that there is an initial rate that is higher than the sustained rate for most of the duration, and that on signal offset the rate drops to zero and only recovers to the spontaneous level after about 100 ms. From *Discharge Patterns of Single Fibers in the Cat's Auditory Nerve* (p. 69) by N. Y.-S. Kiang, T. Watanabe, E. C. Thomas, and L. F. Clark, 1965, Cambridge, MA: MIT Press. Copyright 1965 by MIT Press. Reprinted by permission.

onset rises very rapidly to a peak, then decays to something like two-thirds of the peak value where it remains relatively constant until the signal is terminated. At that point the rate drops briefly to zero and then climbs back to its spontaneous rate. As far as anyone knows, this is the pattern for all peripheral neurons, although we cannot be sure what happens in those with a small diameter, which probably are rarely encountered using current microelectrodes.

Figure III.16 presents PST histograms of a neuron under several conditions. The rows are different signal intensities. The left column shows the PST histogram of a single neuron under normal conditions, and the right column is the same fiber under the same auditory stimulation but with the efferent (from the brain to the ear) fibers stimulated electrically by the experimenter.[4] Note that under such stimulation, the firing is much attenuated. This is the reason why the efferent system is said to be inhibitory, but it is not clear what else it may do. We do not really understand what role the efferent system plays in our hearing or even the conditions under which it is activated.

A certain amount of tracing of auditory neural anatomy in the brain, much of it based on dye techniques, has been carried out for both the afferent (ascending or ear-to-brain) system and for the efferent (descending or brain-to-ear) system. Many of these regions are difficult to access in order to carry out single unit recordings, and so we do not yet know what is going on in those regions in the same detail as for the auditory nerve. At

---

[4]Recall that COCB stands for *crossed olivocochlear bundle,* which means neurons that originate in the region of the brain stem, called the superior olive, on the opposite side of the brain from the cochlea to which they are connected.

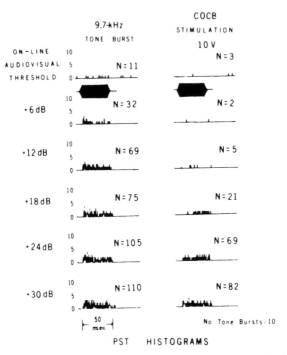

PST   HISTOGRAMS

FIG. III.16   PST histograms of a fiber to several sound intensities. The left panel is taken under normal conditions, and the right one with relevant efferent neural fibers activated electrically. The result is to inhibit the response. From "Electrophysiological Studies on the Spatial Distribution of the Crossed Olivocochlear Bundle Along the Guinea Pig Cochlea" by D. C. Teas, T. Konishi, and D. W. Nielsen, 1972, *Journal of the Acoustical Society of America, 51,* p. 1259. Copyright 1972 by American Institute of Physics. Reprinted by permission.

best, one can lay out a gross map of how the auditory nerve carries auditory information into the brain.

One major exception is the auditory cortex, which like all cortex, is located on the outer region of the upper part of the brain and so is most accessible. Single unit recordings have been made there, and the richness of activity is far greater than in the periphery. Figure III.17 presents some examples of cortical PST histograms. The fiber of the left column exhibits a burst of firing when the signal comes on, inhibition for its duration, and a return to resting level after the signal is turned off. It appears to be sensitive only to signal onset. The second neuron is more like the peripheral neurons, except that the ratio of the initial burst to the level during the rest of the presentation is quite large. The third fiber appears to be primarily one that has a constant elevated rate throughout the duration of the tone. The fiber represented by the histograms on the right clearly responds only to signal offset. Presumably, each of these patterns is derived in some fashion

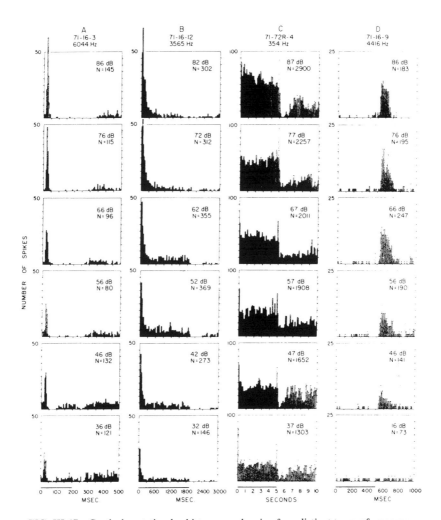

FIG. III.17 Cortical poststimulus histograms showing four distinct types of response. The neuron of A shows an initial burst of activity followed by suppression for the duration of the signal. That of B has both an initial burst and activity above the spontaneous level for the duration of the signal. This is the only one that resembles the peripheral fibers. That of C exhibits sustained activity for the duration of the signal, but without the initial spike of A or B. And that of D only shows unusual activity at signal offset. In all cases, the level of activity is dependent on the signal intensity. From "Patterns of Activity of Single Neurons of the Auditory Cortex in Monkeys" in *Basic Mechanisms in Hearing* (p. 745–766) by J. F. Brugge and M. M. Merzenich, 1973, New York: Academic Press. Copyright 1973 by Academic Press. Reprinted by permission.

from the information available from the peripheral neurons, but exactly how that is done is at present unknown.

Figure III.18 offers an idealized summary of the several patterns that have been found at the cortex. We have only a sketchy idea how these more complex units subserve hearing. For example, those that fire only at signal onset or signal offset presumably serve to alert the brain to significant changes as they occur. The steady firing pattern may well play some role in carrying out signal identification. The roles for the others are less clear, although behaviorally we know there are a number of specialized subsystems, or modules, that seem to do distinctive things in parallel. One of these modules appears to have to do with speech perception. In any event, such different firing patterns *may* reflect different roles for different modules, but at present this is speculative.

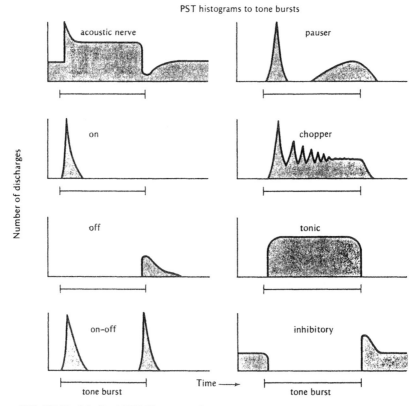

FIG. III.18   Idealized PST histograms for activity observed on cortical neurons. The exact role for all of these is unknown as is the processing that develops them from the simpler peripheral activity. From *Fundamentals of Hearing* (2nd ed., p. 103) by W. A. Yost and D. W. Nielsen, 1985, Orlando: Holt, Rinehart & Winston. Copyright 1985 by Holt, Rinehart & Winston, Inc. Reprinted by permission.

4.2.3 The Qualitative Picture of Firing Rate as a Function of Intensity and Frequency.   Given that the duration effects are relatively uniform on peripheral neurons, one can study the firing rate as a function of intensity and frequency with relatively little regard to the duration variable. One can simply lump all the data or, better, discard the initial rise immediately after signal onset and concentrate on the flat region. One then simply explores how the rate varies with intensity and frequency.

The resulting three-dimensional pattern can be described by an analogy to a butte (i.e., mountain ridge or cliff) rising from a flat valley floor to a relatively flat plateau on top, as shown in Fig. III.19. The altitude corresponds to firing rate, the north–south direction to signal intensity in dB (north being increasing intensity), and the east–west direction to the logarithm of signal frequency (east being higher frequencies). The altitude of flat valley floor corresponds to the spontaneous firing rate of the fiber; these are the intensity-frequency pairs that do not elicit any response in the

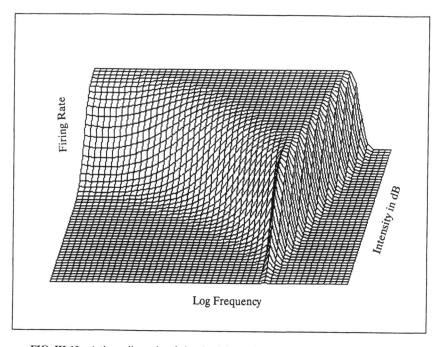

FIG. III.19   A three-dimensional sketch of the typical response pattern of a peripheral auditory neuron to a pure tone. The dependent variable is firing rate and the independent ones are intensity (in dB) and frequency (log *f*). Data are usually reported in one of the three two-dimensional plots: contours of constant firing rates, which are called tuning curves; firing rate as a function of intensity at a constant frequency, often with several curves shown for different frequencies; and firing rate as a function of frequency at constant intensity, often with several curves shown for different intensities. Examples are shown in Figs. III.20–24.

fiber beyond that which occurs with no stimulation whatsoever. The plateau on top of the ridge corresponds to the fiber firing at its maximum rate.

If one stays sufficiently far to the south—low intensities—one simply does not encounter the butte by going east or west. One remains on the valley floor. As one moves north, there is a first level at which one encounters a rise from the valley floor. This is the most southerly point of the ridge, that is, the frequency for which the neuron begins to fire with the least energy. This happens to be easy to identify because the ridge comes to a very sharp point directed toward the south. This frequency—the one for which the neuron is most sensitive—is called its **characteristic frequency** and is abbreviated CF.

We can describe this ridge of firing rates in several ways, each of which provides us with useful information that plays a role in our discussion of the perception of sounds. Each of the three descriptions involves cutting the mountain with imaginary planes and showing in a diagram just where the mountain surface intersects the planes. We discuss only planes that are easily described relative to the coordinate system we are using, which is intensity (dB), frequency (log f), and firing rate (r). So the possible planes are those of constant dB, constant f, and constant r. We deal with them in the reverse order.

4.2.4 Contours of Constant Rates of Firing: Tuning Curves. Consider the system of planes that result from constant firing rates, that is, the planes parallel to the valley floor. The resulting intersections are called contour maps in cartography, and they are considered a very useful way to sense the three-dimensional structure of mountains. It is customary in cartography to plot the contours for regularly spaced elevations, such as every 500 ft, and the comparable thing could be done for firing rates. In practice, however, only one contour is shown, usually one comparatively near the spontaneous rate of the fiber, such as the contour corresponding to a rate 10% above the spontaneous (or resting) level and 90% below the maximum firing rate. In the context of neural firing rates, such contours are called **tuning curves.** These play an important role later, so it is essential to understand them.

Several examples of such curves with different characteristic frequencies are shown in Fig. III.20. These plots make clear that the ridge does indeed have a very sharp edge directed to the south, that is, the CF is very well defined. Equally clear is the enormous asymmetry—the slope of the tuning curve for frequencies larger than the CF is very steep, whereas for lower frequencies it is far more shallow and curved.

The shape of the tuning curve has several important implications. First, a tone whose frequency is appreciably less than that of the CF of a fiber is capable of causing that fiber to fire if the signal intensity is made sufficiently large. This fact suggests that lower frequency signals of sufficient intensity are capable of interfering with the detection of weaker signals of higher frequency, whereas higher frequency signals are not nearly so likely to interfere with lower frequency ones. This, indeed, is behaviorally what happens, as we discuss in Section VI.2.1.

Second, the very sharp edge at the CF is intimately connected with the sharp resonance peak of the basilar membrane that has been attributed to some unspecified cochlear amplifier. There is evidence for this in that damage to appropriate outer hair cells attenuates both peaks markedly, that

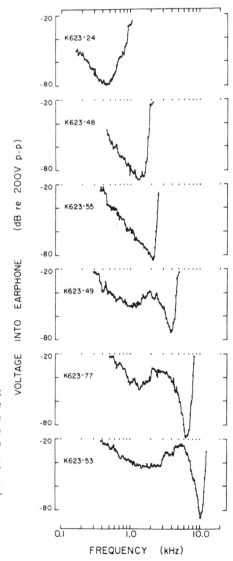

FIG. III.20 Observed tuning curves for auditory fibers whose characteristic frequency (i.e., the most sensitive frequency) range from about 400 Hz to about 10 kHz. From "Physiological Considerations in Artificial Stimulation of the Inner Ear" by N. Y.-S. Kiang and E. C. Moxon, 1972, *Annals of Otology, Rhinology and Laryngology, 81,* p. 725. Copyright 1972 by Annals Pub., Co. Reprinted by permission.

is, both the peaked motion of the basilar membrane and the corresponding sharply tuned tip of the tuning curve.

4.2.5 Firing Rate as a Function of Intensity at Fixed Frequency. The planes of constant *f* are perpendicular to the valley floor and are oriented in the north–south direction. In terms of the neural activity, the intersection of this plane with the butte shows how firing rate grows with intensity for that fixed frequency. An example of such a plane cut through at the characteristic frequency (CF) of that neuron is shown in Fig. III.21. We see that this fiber saturates at about 100 sps and has a spontaneous rate of about 5 sps. Of course, one can cut the plane through at various frequencies and plot all of the curves on the same drawing, labeling each by its frequency. This has been done for another fiber, one with CF = 1,300 Hz, in Fig. III.22. It is clear from this figure that the height of the plateau is not really constant, it falls off at frequencies substantially above and below the CF.

Note that in both figures, the range of values during which the firing rate changes from its spontaneous level to its maximum level, known as its **dynamic range,** is not terribly wide — something like 20 to 30 dB. It is evident,

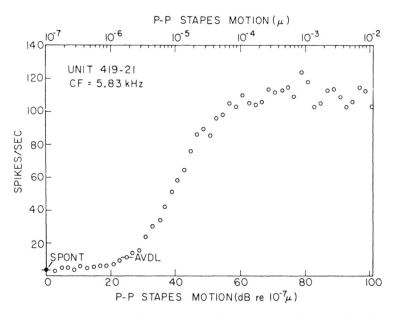

FIG. III.21 Firing rate as a function of signal intensity at the CF of the fiber. Note that the dynamic range is only about 30 dB, which means that a single fiber is incapable of coding the full dynamic range of hearing. From "A Survey of Recent Developments in the Study of Auditory Physiology" by N. Y.-S. Kiang, 1968, *Annals of Otology, Rhinology and Laryngology, 77,* p. 659. Copyright 1968 by Annals Publishing Co. Reprinted by permission.

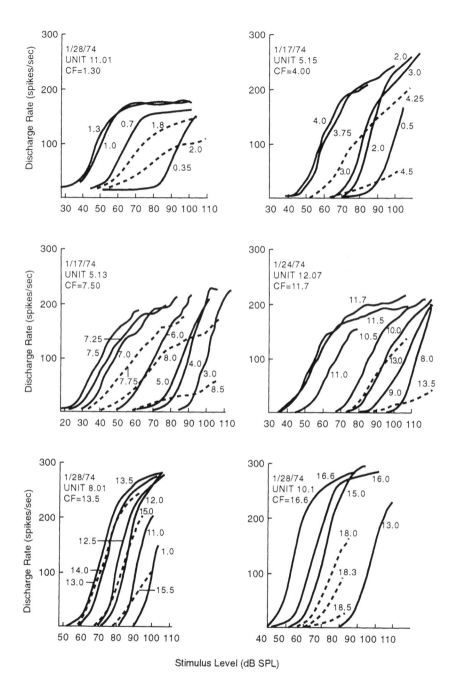

FIG. III.22 Firing rate of one neuron as a function of signal intensity at several different frequencies in addition to the CF. From "Rate Versus Level Functions for Auditory-Nerve Fibers in Cats: Tone-Burst Stimuli" by M. B. Sachs and P. J. Abbas, 1974, *Journal of the Acoustical Society of America, 56,* p. 1839. Copyright 1974 by American Institute of Physics. Reprinted by permission.

then, that a single fiber does not encode the full dynamic range of intensities that can be perceived, which is something like 150 dB. This is a problem.

The shape of the tuning curve may provide a way to understand how the whole dynamic range of intensities is handled. At low intensities, the tone will only activate fibers with CFs at or very near the frequency of the given signal. As the intensity increases, these fibers will saturate and further changes in intensity will not be reflected by any changes in their firing rates. On the other hand, the increased intensity will begin to activate some fibers with CFs larger than the signal frequency, and as the intensity increases further it will continue to recruit more fibers with larger CFs. This is one possible mechanism to explain how a wide range of intensities can be covered by neurons whose individual dynamic ranges are only 20 to 30 dB, a fraction of the total range.

There is, however, another way to encode intensity. Define the threshold of a neuron to be the lowest intensity of its tuning curve, the one corresponding to its CF. If for each frequency, there are fibers with appreciably different thresholds, then this at least partially affords a second way to cover the intensity dynamic range. Moreover, this device coupled with the other mechanism extends the range even more. Suppose one can gain as much as 70 dB from using fibers with CFs larger than the frequency in question, which from Fig. III.20 appears to be a conservative estimate, and suppose that the thresholds for a number of fibers with the same CF span a range of 60 dB. Coupled with the 20 dB range of differential activity of any fiber, we see it is possible to span a total of 70 + 60 + 20 = 150 dB, which is just what is needed.

Are there, in fact, neurons with thresholds spanning 60 dB? The answer, shown in Fig. III.23, is yes. Threshold-CF values are plotted for a number of different neurons, and we see that they span the required range of intensities. It is interesting that a correlation exists between a neuron's threshold and its spontaneous firing rate: The lower the threshold, the higher the spontaneous rate. The solid curve is the behavioral threshold for cats,[5] and we see that the fibers with the lowest threshold are very close to the behavioral ones, which is a happy agreement.

4.2.6 Firing Rate as a Function of Frequency at Fixed Intensity. The third system of planes are those at fixed intensity (oriented in the east–west direction) and perpendicular to the valley floor. Again, the several curves that are obtained for different intensities can be shown in the same drawing. Typical results for a fiber with a CF of 4,100 Hz and with planes at 10 dB intervals is shown in Fig. III.24. A considerable asymmetry is again quite

---

[5]For details on such thresholds, see Section IV.2.6.3.

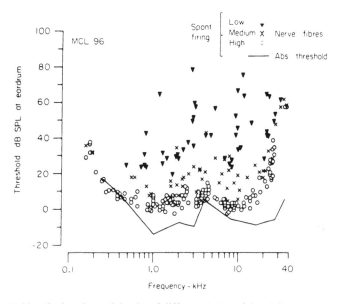

FIG. III.23 The locations of the CF of different (cat) peripheral fibers shown in the intensity-frequency plane. The behaviorally measured absolute threshold of hearing for cats is shown as the solid line. The important fact is that at each frequency there are neurons whose CF spans a wide range of intensities. From *An Introduction to the Physiology of Hearing* (p. 84) by J. O. Pickles, 1988, New York: Academic Press. Copyright 1988 by Academic Press. Reprinted by permission.

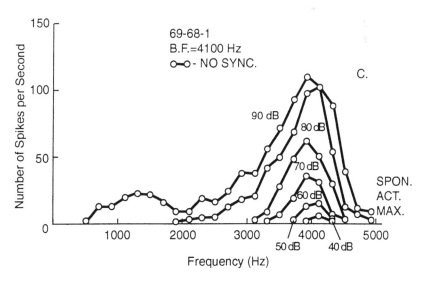

FIG. III.24 Firing rate as a function of frequency for several different levels of intensity. From "Some Effects of Stimulus Intensity on Response of Auditory Nerve Fibers in the Squirrel Monkey" by J. E. Rose, J. E. Hind, D. J. Anderson, and J. F. Brugge, 1971, *Journal of Neurophysiology, 30,* p. 687. Copyright 1971 by American Physiological Society. Reprinted by permission.

noticeable; there is relatively less spread to the right than to the left as intensity is increased. This was seen more vividly in the tuning curves.

4.2.7 Place Theory.   The previous data show that there are neurons with a CF at almost every frequency in the audible range and with a fairly wide range of thresholds. So, for each intensity-frequency combination, a sizable proportion of the 32,000 auditory neurons are active. This implies that each tone generates a characteristic pattern activity, like a mosaic to the brain, over the entire array of neurons forming the auditory nerve.

These different patterns of active neurons forming the mosaic almost certainly provide enough information to the central nervous system for it to be able to infer signal intensity and frequency. It is just a matter of its "reading" the patterns of active neurons formed across the entire 32,000 neurons forming the auditory nerve bundle. Treating a neuron as just being either "on" or "off," the number of such possible patterns is staggering:

$$2^{32,000} \cong 10^{10,000}.$$

(Recall this is the number 1 followed by 10,000 zeros.) Any theory that postulates that hearing is based on just this sort of "reading" of patterns is known as a **place theory** because the information encoded partly corresponds to location on the basilar membrane. In a sense, such theories treat the auditory nerve as quite analogous to the retina of the eye, which is an array of photosensitive cells that exhibit different patterns of activity depending on the light stimulation.

It has not proved easy in either domain to understand just how the central nervous system "reads" such arrays, and computer experts have yet to devise computer programs capable of doing the analogous thing for television arrays. In the early 1990s there is much optimism that massively parallel-computers will be able to lick this problem, but it has yet to be demonstrated. Much vision research is looking into the general question of how, without postulating an homunculus[6] to do the "reading," we are able to perceive what we do. For the auditory system, there is evidence that some of the inferences that have to be carried out may be done more simply on single fibers because the neural spike trains are tightly structured, as is pointed out in the next section.

4.3 Coding in Terms of Neural Firing Patterns

Information can be encoded by temporal patterns of binary events. That is the case for the Morse code or for that used in a computer, but these human-devised codes rely on synchronization, that is, an independent

---

[6]A hypothetical internal "person" with the very properties one is trying to explain.

means of timing, in order to tell when a spike or pulse has or has not occurred. Synchronization does not seem to be available at the periphery of the brain, so something else must be used.

Although it is conceivable that patterns involving several pulses are important, most of the work that has been done so far concentrates on the times between successive pulses. How does that time vary with different auditory inputs? For the most part the literature has focused on simple inputs such as pure tones, and that is all that is treated here.

4.3.1 Interval Histograms.   The same data that were used to generate the PST histograms can be analyzed in a different, but revealing way. Instead of referring each spike back to the onset of the signal, we can refer it back to the immediately preceding spike. Think of the spikes as cars coming along a one-way road, then one can measure the time intervals between successive cars as they pass. Thus, for the spike trains, the data to be studied are the times between successive spikes when both spikes have occurred while the signal is present. These intervals between spikes are known as **interspike intervals.** They are of interest, in part, because they afford a momentary estimate of the rate of firing, namely, 1/(interspike interval) is a (crude) estimate of the firing rate.

Now, just as we did with the intervals between signal onset and a spike, we can partition the interspike intervals into bins of varying durations and form a histogram, which in this context is known as an **interval histogram.** As an example, suppose spikes have been observed to occur at the times (in ms) after signal onset used in Section III.4.2.1, which were:

$$5, 7, 13, 32, 33, 37, 38, 49, 62, 64, 77, 91, 94.$$

The corresponding intervals between successive ones are:

$$2, 6, 19, 1, 4, 1, 11, 13, 2, 13, 14, 3.$$

If the bin widths are 5 ms, then we have:

Bin Range	*1–5*	*6–10*	*11–15*	*16–20*
# of intervals in bin	6	1	4	1

Once again a trade-off exists between the total size of the sample that we have, the bin width, and the fineness with which we wish to examine what is happening. In this case, it turns out that the fine structure is crucially important, so the bin widths have to be small and the sample size must be large. In fact, the data we will look at have bin widths of only 0.1 ms = 100 μs.

The data shown in Fig. III.25 were obtained from a single neuron of a

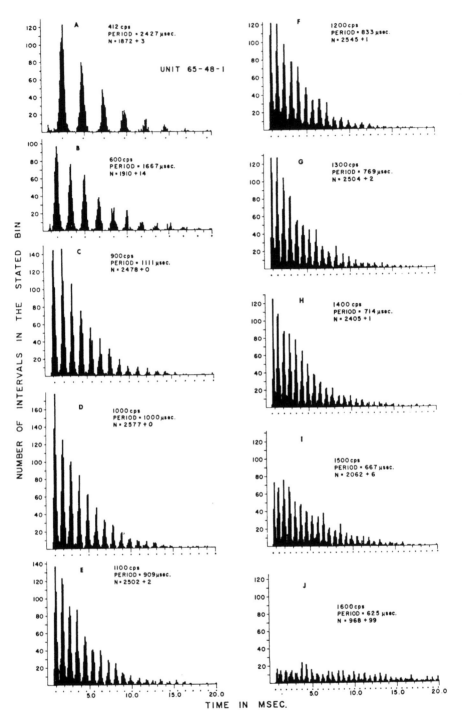

FIG. III.25 Interval histograms for a single peripheral fiber stimulated at a constant intensity and with frequencies ranging from 412 Hz to 1,600 Hz. The dots just below the abscissa are separated by the period of the stimulating pure tone. Note that the modes of the histogram are centered over these dots, showing that the firing pattern encodes frequency information. From "Phase-locked Response to Low-frequency Tones in Single Auditory Nerve Fibers of the Squirrel Monkey" by J. E. Rose, J. F. Brugge, D. J. Anderson, and J. E. Hind, 1967, *Journal of Neurophysiology, 30,* p. 772. Copyright 1967 by American Physiological Society. Reprinted by permission.

squirrel monkey when presented with tones at the same intensity, but with frequencies that varied from 412 Hz to 1,600 Hz. Except for the highest frequency, the intensity was sufficient to cause the neuron to fire above its spontaneous rate.

The most startling fact about these histograms is their extraordinarily spiky character. In order not to confuse these spikes with the spikes of the underlying neural activity, these are referred to as **modes** of the histogram.

4.3.2 Frequency Coding.   Notice that below the abscissa in each case is a row of dots. These dots are located at integral multiples of the period of the imposed tone. That is, if the frequency of the tone is f and time is measured in milliseconds, then the dots are located at $T (= 1,000/f)$, $2T$, $3T$, . . . , nT ms. If you examine the figure carefully, you will see that the highest point of each mode coincides approximately with one of the dots, and this is true for every frequency for which the neuron is active.

This means that each neuron that responds to a tone actually carries in its temporal pattern of firing information about the frequency of the tone. Thus, the central nervous system has an alternative to "reading" the pattern of activity across the entire auditory nerve in order to infer frequency. All it need do is estimate the spacing of the modes of the interval histogram, which computationally is a far simpler task than reading arrays.

How might that be done? We do not know precisely what computations a nervous system is capable of carrying out, but something equivalent to the following is sufficient: The histogram must be formed in the sense that the numbers that go into it must be accumulated. Obviously, the animal in a natural environment cannot do what the experimental scientist does and have the signal repeated over and over. Although it cannot do that, it can do something that is functionally equivalent by having each signal activate many neurons. This kind of spatial redundancy provides the needed large sample size of spike intervals; moreover, it takes no longer to accumulate the large sample than it does to collect information from a single neuron. From a computational point of view, these two ways of getting a large sample are equivalent, and as we argue later it is nature's way of solving the problem of responding both accurately and fast (see Section III.4.3.3).

Assuming much data have been collected and sorted into an interval histogram, then label each mode as follows: 1 for the one with the shortest times, 2 for the one with the group of the next shortest times, and so on. Now, the times in the first mode are each approximately T. The times in the second mode are approximately $2T$, and so dividing each of these times by 2 provides additional values that are all approximately T. In general, the times in the nth mode divided by n are each approximately of duration T. Thus, if all of these numbers are averaged, they give an estimate of T. With sample sizes in the thousands, this gives a quite accurate estimate of

T and so of f. An alternative to averaging these numbers is to find their median—that is the time such that half of the observed values are less than it and half are more. It too provides an excellent estimate of T and so of f.

Thus, in principle at least, moderately simple arithmetic calculations—those easily programmed on a computer—are sufficient to estimate signal frequency. That coupled with rate as a way of estimating intensity means that pure tones can be inferred without having to "read" an array.

4.3.3 Neural Redundancy.   This line of argument also makes it clear why there is so much redundancy in the sense of many, substantially identical, neurons all carrying statistically the same information. Consider how long an animal or person has to detect and partially identify a sound, whether soft or loud, low or high frequency. If an organism is to have any reasonable chance of surviving in a world of predators, it had better not take more than a few hundred ms. The period of a 200 Hz tone is 5 ms, so at most 20 intervals accumulate in 100 ms, and with a weak signal, it is more like 5. With a histogram based on only 5 observations, estimates of both rate and location of modes is extremely poor. One needs a much larger sample of interspike times. A minimum of 100 is needed, and 1,000 would be appreciably better. This means that the system must have from 20 to 200 neurons each carrying the same information. Thus, parallel redundancy both increases the sample size, and as a result the accuracy of identification, while simultaneously holding down the delay until the information is processed.

4.3.4 Refractoriness.   The scheme outlined earlier for estimating frequency is fine except for one thing, the refractoriness of nerve fibers. Recall that once a spike has been produced on the fiber, internal readjustments that permit the next firing to occur take something like $\frac{1}{2}$ ms. This refractoriness means that for any tone whose frequency is greater than 2,000 Hz, the first mode is actually missing because no interval can be that short. Moreover, by the same argument, for tones with frequencies over 4,000 Hz, the first two modes are missing, and so on. To deal with this, three options can be considered.

First, perhaps the estimate of refractoriness is excessive and due to inadequacies of our measurements. Although this cannot be completely ruled out, it seems unlikely, and indirect evidence is presented shortly suggesting that the $\frac{1}{2}$ ms value is not very far wrong.

Second, perhaps the auditory system uses temporal techniques for frequencies below 1 to 2 kHz and shifts to a place analysis for higher frequencies. And indeed there are some psychophysical data that make it seem as if there is some difference between the two regions, although that interpretation is far from compelling. This hypothesis has the weakness that it greatly increases the amount of neural apparatus needed beyond that required by the place theory alone, and it is not clear what purpose this would serve. However, we cannot reject the possibility that the two systems might have evolved separately in response to changing environmental pressures.

Third, perhaps the nervous system is somehow capable of examining the histogram to determine just how many modes are missing, and then it bases its inference about the frequency on just those that are available. This solution seems much simpler, and the processes involved in working out the number of missing modes might very well generate some differences in the psychophysical results found above and below the refractory boundary of 1 to 2 kHz. Moreover, in Section VI.4 we provide a vivid psychophysical demonstration in which the nervous system quite clearly infers missing modes.

4.3.5 Intensity Coding.   Figure III.26 presents interval histograms for a single fiber being activated by a tone of 1,111 Hz presented at intensities ranging from 30 dB SPL (relative to 0.0002 dynes/cm^2) to 90 dB SPL. It comes as no great surprise that the rate grows and then becomes roughly constant. This is reflected in the fact that the distribution for 30 dB is relatively flat—that is, the ratio of the proportion of short times to that of long times is modest—and it becomes progressively steeper—that is, that ratio is increased, as it must with increasing firing rate (up to about 60 or 70 dB, after which it remains roughly the same). There is no surprise here.

Is there, however, anything to be said about the overall shape of the decay in the histograms? To anyone familiar with geometric decay processes, these plots look familiar. One way to see what is going on is as follows: Let M_1 denote the number of observations in the first mode, M_2 the number in the second, M_3 in the third, and in general M_n in the nth mode. Now suppose we calculate the ratios of the sizes of successive modes: M_2/M_1, M_3/M_2, . . . , M_{n+1}/M_n, ... If we plot these ratios as a function of the index n, we find that the plot exhibits no trend. These ratios fluctuate some, but they appear to be different estimates of the same constant.

Of course, as we decrease intensity, the value of the constant decreases until it reaches a smallest value, corresponding to the spontaneous rate of the neuron.

This property that the size of each mode is a constant fraction of the size of the preceding one is characteristic of a statistical process known as the *geometric,* and it suggests a simple model for what is going on, to which we now turn.

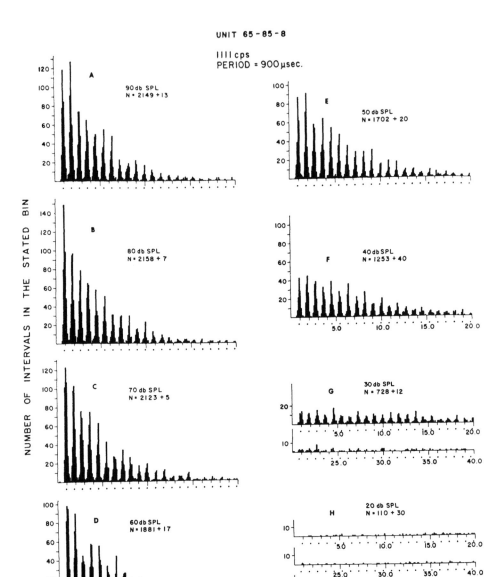

FIG. III.26 Interval histograms for a fiber stimulated at 1,111 Hz and various intensities from 30 dB to 90 dB. Note that the histogram is steeper at the higher intensities and flatter at the lower ones, which only reflects the fact that the firing rate increases over a range of intensities (see Figs. III.21–22). From "Phase-locked Response to Low-frequency Tones in Single Auditory Nerve Fibers of the Squirrel Monkey" by J. E. Rose, J. F. Brugge, D. J. Anderson, and J. E. Hind, 1967, *Journal of Neurophysiology, 30,* p. 784. Copyright 1967 by American Physiological Society. Reprinted by permission.

4.3.6 Phase-Locked Neural Firing.   Consider the intensity variations of the imposed tone:

$$p = P \sin 2\pi ft + P',$$

where P is the maximum pressure excursion, P' is the static pressure level, f is the frequency of the tone, and t is time in seconds. Consider the hypothesis that the basilar membrane and the relevant hair cells act as if they respond as follows: There is an amplitude threshold, somewhat above P' and below $P' + P$, such that when the upswing of the pressure wave passes the threshold there is some probability Q that a spike is generated. (We cannot tell if it is the upswing of pressure or the downswing that actually generates the spikes, but, as is shown later, it cannot be both.) If the threshold stays put, then as P (i.e., maximum pressure change) increases, the value of Q is assumed to increase until it reaches the maximum for that neuron.

Assume for the moment that each upswing initiates at most one neural spike—we return to this assumption shortly. Let us then calculate what happens. Suppose we start measuring time from a spike that occurred somewhere near the top of an upswing (see Fig. III.27). The next opportunity for a spike is at the next upswing, which is approximately after time T. If that fails to produce a spike, which will occur with probability $1 - Q$, then the next opportunity will be after approximately time $2T$. A spike will occur at that point with probability Q, and not occur with probability $1 - Q$. In the latter case, time again elapses for about T seconds without any spike until approximately $3T$ from signal onset, where again there is an opportunity for it to occur, and so on. Such a process is said to be (approximately) *phase-locked* to the signal.

Note that if both up- and downswings of pressure were to initiate spikes, the modes would be at multiples of $T/2$, not T. Because the data are otherwise, we know that cannot happen.

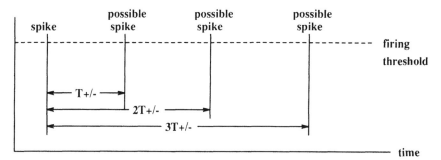

FIG. III.27   Schematic of a simple geometric model for the firing patterns that is consistent with the interval histograms.

If the total number of observations (spikes) is M, then from the previous discussion we can calculate the expected size of the modes. The first one is simply QM, the second is $(1 - Q)QM$, and the third, which entails missing the first two opportunities and then for a spike to occur on the third is $(1 - Q)(1 - Q)QM$. So, the general result is:

$$M_1 = QM$$
$$M_2 = Q(1 - Q)M$$
$$M_3 = Q(1 - Q)^2 M$$
$$\cdots$$
$$M_n = Q(1 - Q)^{n-1} M.$$

Observe that independent of n, $M_{n+1}/M_n = 1 - Q$, predicting the constant property seen in the data. It also provides a simple way to estimate Q should one want to do that.

One thing remains dangling: We assumed that no more than one spike occurs on each upswing. The entire upswing takes one-half of the period and if we assume the threshold is set sufficiently high that the relevant part is at most $T/4$, then because of refractoriness there is no conceivable way that more than one spike can occur within one upswing if $T/4 < \frac{1}{2}$ ms. Thus, for frequencies above 500 Hz the assumption is valid. However, for lower frequencies it may not be. Here the pressure may remain above the threshold for more than $\frac{1}{2}$ ms and so make it possible for two or more spikes to occur within a few milliseconds of each other. Thus, we would anticipate finding, for sufficiently low frequencies, a mode in the region of $\frac{1}{2}$ to 2 or 3 ms, one that is quite unrelated to the period of the wave. There is slight evidence for this in the 412 Hz case of Fig. III.25, and it becomes very evident in the histograms of Fig. III.28, where much lower frequencies were studied.

It is clear that the central system must somehow filter out this nonphase locked mode in inferring the signal frequency.

4.3.7 Temporal or Periodicity Theory.   Any auditory theory assuming that the temporal structure of neural spike trains is used to infer frequency by means of computations on data pooled over the fibers is called a **temporal theory** or, equally well, a **periodicity theory.** Such theories are to be contrasted strongly with the place theories that assume this information is not used; rather, the pattern of activity across all of the fibers composing the auditory nerve is the basis of both intensity and frequency inferences.

In summary, in a temporal theory the brain is assumed to accumulate interspike times, using the firing rates below the maximum rate to infer intensity and the separation of modes to infer frequencies less 500 to 1,000 Hz. At higher frequencies the pressure changes one or more times during the refractory period, and so the first few modes of the interval histogram are necessarily missing.

There are two major possibilities for dealing with the missing early

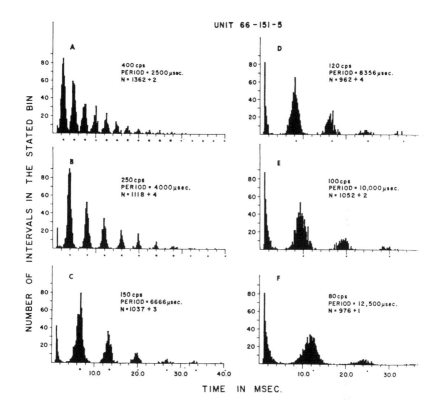

FIG. III.28 Interval histograms of low frequency signals showing a mode just a bit above the known neural refractory period as well as modes at multiples of the period of the signal. This arises because signal pressure is changing so slowly it is possible for two or more firings to occur at a single peak of the amplitude. From "Phase-locked Response to Low-frequency Tones in Single Auditory Nerve Fibers of the Squirrel Monkey" by J. E. Rose, J. F. Brugge, D. J. Anderson, J. E. Hind, 1967, *Journal of Neurophysiology, 30*, p. 776. Copyright 1967 by American Physiological Society. Reprinted by permission.

modes. One mentioned earlier suggests that a different scheme, place, is used for higher frequencies. There is a certain amount of behavioral data suggesting differences above and below 1,000 Hz. Nonetheless, if the system has a way of reading the mosaic of activity for one range of frequencies, it is unclear why it would not be used throughout. The other idea goes under the name of the **volley theory,** and is described in the next section.

4.3.8 Volley Theory.   If the activity on several fibers is combined while retaining phase information, then the refractoriness of individual fibers can be ignored. The graph of Fig. III.29 shows how adding the outputs of two fibers is able to overcome the problem.

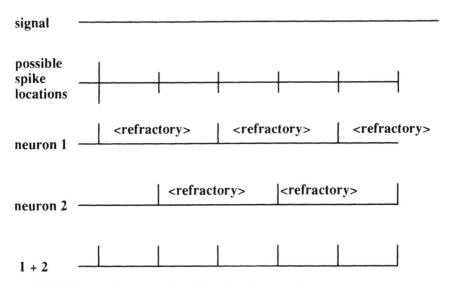

FIG. III.29 A schematic drawing of the volley theory that shows one way to overcome the effect, when the frequency is large, of neural refractoriness in eliminating the modes at low multiples of the period. If the outputs of several uncorrelated fibers can be superimposed, all of the modes will be present.

Observe that if this were possible, the only impact of refractoriness is to diminish the sample size somewhat, not to make it impossible to infer the period.

5. INTERPLAY OF BEHAVIOR
AND PHYSIOLOGY

5.1 Nonobvious Transduction

No matter whether you think the place or the temporal theory or some mix of the two is correct, one thing is very clear. The transduction carried out by the ear to the auditory nerve is far from a simple linear or nonlinear transformation of the input waveform. Stated another way, if the input is $P \sin (2\pi ft + \phi)$, there is no continuous mathematical function F of momentary pressure such that $F[P \sin (2\pi ft + \phi)]$ describes the neural spike trains that result. The ear is not remotely like many familiar, human-designed, auditory transducers — microphones, cartridges, ear phones, amplifiers, and the like — in which proportional transformations are the ideal.

One should be aware that virtually nothing said earlier about the neural coding of auditory information was or could have been inferred from purely behavioral psychological data. That is to say, using purely black-box methods, where we observe the response of the whole organism to auditory inputs, simply did not and probably could not have led one to guess at the internal transduction that underlies it. Nonetheless, the physiological results are highly consistent with much behavioral data. Indeed, a number of psychological results that, when first observed, seemed peculiar and inexplicable have become quite understandable in terms of the neural activity. One example is the masking effect of one pure tone on the detection of another pure tone of a different frequency. We find that lower frequencies can be quite effective in masking higher ones, but the reverse masking of lower frequencies by higher ones tends to be far less effective unless the frequencies are very close (Section VI.2.1). Such results are now seen as the inevitable consequences of the somewhat odd way in which the neurons encode information.

This statement does not mean there is a simple, one-way reductionism from psychological phenomena to the peripheral physiological phenomena. There are, in fact, a number of relatively simple, but striking, behavioral results that have not been explained in terms of what we know about the auditory nerves. Some are discussed and demonstrated later. Complex matters of music perception—for example, one's ability to single out individual instruments—and of speech perception are far beyond any physiological explanation at this time. To a degree, the behavioral results establish a challenge to neural scientists, telling them what to look for in the brain.

5.2 Human Behavior but Animal Physiology

One task for the psychologist is to see if our partial understanding of the transduction effected by the ear is sufficient, in itself, to account for the behavioral data, some of which are reported in Parts IV and VI. In some cases it is. In others, we have not seen how to explain the behavioral results in terms of the transducer. This may mean that we do not sufficiently understand the transducer or it may mean that the behavioral phenomenon in question is greatly mediated by central processes that are even less well understood than the peripheral ones.

Here we enter into delicate ground because much of the behavioral data come from human beings, whereas the neural and physiological data are almost entirely from animals. What of the behavioral data are unique to human beings and what relevant physiological data are being overlooked?

One can attempt to devise some behavioral studies on animal audition, but in practice this is not easy to do well and requires a well-trained, well-equipped, patient experimenter who is highly dedicated to issues of sensory perception. Moreover, some of the most interesting human auditory phenomena having to do with speech and music have no clear analogue in animals. Except for very limited observations that have been carried out during clinical surgery, the physiological and neurological data are exclusively from animals. This situation is not promising for illuminating important neurological aspects of human hearing. It will take some time to sort out which behavioral results we can reasonably expect to account for using just animal physiological results and which must await improved noninvasive techniques for studying human physiological responses. Very rapid progress is being made at present in developing computer techniques to analyze the internal sources of electrical activity that can be measured at the surface of the head, and these methods have proved informative about which (fairly gross) regions are active under various conditions of stimulation and motivation. However, such data are exceedingly crude in comparison with the detail of single unit recordings we have discussed.

6. FURTHER READING

The anatomy and general mechanical functioning of the ear is treated in every book devoted to hearing. In particular, see Gluck (1971), Green (1976), Moore (1982), Pickels (1982), Warren (1982), or Yost and Nielsen (1985). Of these, I would first consult Yost and Nielsen and then Pickels, which has by far the most comprehensive coverage. For the original observations on traveling waves on the basilar membrane, see von Békésy (1960). For data on neural pulse trains, the several papers cited in the figure captions are basic along with Kiang's (1965) monograph. The best fairly recent secondary source is Pickels (1982), and various specific topics are taken up in chapters of Tobias (1970, 1972). Discussions of place and temporal theories are found in most of the basic texts listed here. An early, important discussion is Wever (1970), which predated the modern form of the temporal theory. And, of course, the original statement of the precursor of place theory is von Helmholtz (1863/1954). For a comparison of animal and human auditory anatomy and physiology at a fairly technical level, see Dooling and Hulse (1989).

PART IV

Psychophysics of Pure Tones

1. THE ISSUES OF PSYCHOPHYSICS

As the word suggests, *psychophysics* is the field that studies the psychological (sensory) effects caused by physical stimuli. Usually the term is restricted to stimuli that are fairly simple and easily characterized. When they are more complex, such as music or speech, one speaks of *auditory perception*. Attention is restricted in this part to the simplest stimuli, the pure (sinusoidal) tones. Part VI explores some results for more complex stimuli.

For present purposes, just two major kinds of independent variables are involved:

- Physical properties of the signal such as its frequency f, intensity I, and duration t.
- Experimental procedures of various types having to do with what the observer[1] is asked to do, the information feedback to the observer about performance in the task, and instructions provided by the experimenter.

---

[1] In the psychophysical literature the term "observer" is used more commonly than "subject," which is the term of choice in most of the rest of psychology. This arises, in part, from the fact that observers are usually trained for a considerable time before the data are collected. This is almost always true for what we call local psychophysics; it may or may not be true for global psychophysics, depending on whether the data have been collected by pooling many observations from a single observer or pooling those from many subjects.

In many psychophysical studies, as the word suggests, the intervening physiology simply is ignored. In others, however, it is brought to bear, usually in an attempt to understand the origins of the observed behavior. But basically, the physiology is subservient to the relation between behavior and the physical stimuli.

Two quite distinct kinds of psychophysics exist: One, which may be characterized as being *local,* is concerned with an observer's ability to detect and to discriminate (tell apart) well-defined physical signals that are very similar to one another. They differ in either intensity or in frequency, but not by much. Local psychophysics is concerned with the lower limits of human performance—when can distinct things be told apart? The other kind of psychophysics, which can be viewed as being *global* in character, is concerned with the appreciation of sensations over large ranges of signals— what governs our appreciation of loudness or pitch?

In terms of auditory physiology, one can define two or more stimuli as forming a local cluster if they activate but do not saturate many of the same peripheral neurons; they are global if the two sets of active, nonsaturated neurons have little or no overlap.

Typical issues of local psychophysics are:

• At each frequency *f,* what is the smallest intensity that is just sufficient to detect the occurrence of the signal? This is the study of **signal detection,** and the minimum intensity that can be detected reliably is known as the **absolute threshold of hearing.** The clinically observed audiogram used to detect and measure the amount of hearing loss is a practical application (see Section IV.2.6.3).

• How far apart in intensity or in frequency must two signals be in order for an observer consistently to tell that they differ? This is the study of auditory **discrimination.** The minimum differences just sufficient to tell that they differ are known as **discrimination thresholds.**

• When one of two signals is presented at random on each trial and the subject attempts to identify which one, the design is called a **two-stimulus absolute identification experiment.** A local question is: How large must the separation in intensity or in frequency be to avoid all errors of identification?

Typical issues of global psychophysics are:

• How does the perception we call loudness grow with signal intensity and frequency? This is known as **sensory scaling.**

• How well can an observer identify one of several—say, 10—signals that are widely separated, either in intensity, in frequency, or in both? In frequency, one question is the degree to which people do or do not exhibit absolute pitch. This procedure is known as **absolute identification** and it generalizes in a natural manner the third of the local procedures.

• What combinations of intensity and frequency are perceived as equally loud, or as having equal pitch? This is the study of **equal-attribute contours** such as equal loudness or equal pitch.

Certain striking inconsistencies exist between the two kinds of results, and several approaches, both theoretical and experimental, exist to try to bridge the local and global phenomena.

2. LOCAL PSYCHOPHYSICS

2.1 Detection, Discrimination, and Identification Procedures

For the most part local psychophysical studies involve experimental designs in which, on each trial of the experiment, one or two limited time intervals are designated during which one of two distinct stimuli is presented in each interval. The observer indicates to the experimenter which interval he or she believes contained which signal. This is usually done by pressing one of two keys.

Typically the observer is seated in a sound attenuating room with earphones or, less commonly, a loudspeaker. Beginning in the 1970s, the entire procedure began to be run interactively by a computer. The observer faces a cathode ray tube (CRT), video, or computer screen and interacts with the computer via a keyboard. Typically the observer strikes the space bar or enter key when he or she is ready for a run of trials to begin, and some sort of unambiguous warning signal—a light or some symbol on the CRT—indicates the time periods during which signals may be presented. Following that, the observer responds using the keyboard in some narrowly prescribed way.

This process is repeated many times. Groups of 50 to 100 trials are typically conducted without any break; these are called **runs**. There will be several runs in a 1-hour session, and the observer may participate in from one to dozens of sessions, depending on the experimental design.

A computer-based, random procedure—equivalent to flipping a coin when there are two signals and each is equally likely to occur—usually determines which stimulus to present on each trial. In some studies, which we do not go into here, the "coin" is biased and/or the probability of presenting a stimulus depends on what happened on previous trials. The latter are known as sequential procedures, and they can become quite complex.

Have no doubt about it, these are dull, repetitive experiments, and the observer needs to be well motivated. To counteract the tedium, often some financial motivation is used to encourage the observer's attention. Sometimes this is accomplished by **information feedback** and **payoffs**. The feedback is some indication after the response as to whether it was correct or incorrect. The payoffs are some monetary function of the numbers of correct and incorrect responses.

2.2 Yes–No Detection

When one of the signals is the absence of any stimulation, we refer to that "presentation" as being the null (or no) signal case and denote it by n. The non-null signal is denoted s. The observer's task is said to be one of **detection** because he or she is attempting to detect the presence of the signal, s, against the alternative of no signal, n. In this case, the absolute identification procedure is called a **Yes–No design** because in effect the observer says on each trial either "Yes" the signal was presented or "No" it wasn't. These possible responses are abbreviated by some authors as Y and N, respectively, and by others as S and N. Often the keys to be used in responding are so marked.

The possible outcomes have been given the following descriptive names:

		RESPONSE	
		YES	NO
PRESENTATION	s	HIT	MISS
	n	FALSE ALARM	CORRECT REJECTION

A *hit* occurs when the signal is presented and the observer detects it, and a *miss* when he or she fails to detect it. A *correct rejection* occurs when the null signal is presented and the observer acknowledges that, and a *false alarm* involves saying the signal is present when in fact there is none.

The data are the numbers of observations falling in each of the four cells:

	Y	N		Numerical Example		
s	N_{sY}	N_{sN}	N_s	50	10	60
n	N_{nY}	N_{nN}	N_n	25	15	40
	N_Y	N_N	N	75	25	100

These data are usually converted into the proportion of Y and N responses for each type of trial, s and n:

TRIAL TYPE	PROPORTION		
HIT	N_{sY}/N_s		$= 50/60 = .833$
MISS	$N_{sN}/N_s = 1 - N_{sY}/N_s$		$= 10/60 = .167$
CORRECT REJECTION	N_{nN}/N_n		$= 15/40 = .375$
FALSE ALARM	$N_{nY}/N_n = 1 - N_{nN}/N_n$		$= 25/40 = .625$

The proportions are taken as estimates of underlying response probabilities.

	Y	N
s	$P(Y|s)$	$P(N|s)$
n	$P(Y|n)$	$P(N|n)$

$P(Y|s)$ denotes the probability of response Y when signal s is presented. Because

$$P(Y|s) + P(N|s) = 1 \text{ and } P(Y|n) + P(N|n) = 1,$$

there are only two independent numbers in this summary of the data, not the four suggested by the data matrix. Thus, the data from such an experiment can be summarized by a single pair of numbers for each experimental condition. The most commonly used probability pair is $\langle P(Y|s), P(Y|n) \rangle$.

Chance behavior — the observer fails to detect the signal — is the case when $P(Y|s) = P(Y|n)$. This means that a Y response gives you no information whatsoever as to whether s or n was presented.

2.3 ROC Curves

So, at first glance, it appears that we simply need to estimate these two probabilities in order to describe the observer's ability to detect the signal. It is not, however, quite so simple because of a significant phenomenon that was largely ignored until about 1950: The pair of numbers one actually obtains is markedly influenced by a number of nonsensory variables. There simply is not a unique pair that can be said to describe the detection ability of the observer; rather, there is a whole collection of such pairs, each pair being an equally valid description of sensory behavior. We consider this next.

In addition to various sensory manipulations that we can carry out — such as varying signal intensity, signal frequency, and signal duration — there are others that bear on the observer's motivations rather than on the sensory system, as such. These include such things as the instructions we give to the observer about how certain he or she should be before reporting the presence of a signal and the relative frequencies with which s and n are presented. But the easiest motivator to manipulate is the payoffs the experimenter can assign to the four kinds of outcomes that can occur. For example, the simplest symmetric payoff is:

	Y	N
s	1	−1
n	−1	1

The entries are in some monetary unit such as pennies or points that are summed over the experiment and converted into a financial bonus at the end. The symmetric case treats both correct outcomes as equally good and both errors as equally bad. Moreover, the value assigned to an error is exactly the negative of the value assigned to a correct response. So the consequence of a correct response can be wiped out by just one incorrect response, and vice versa.

It is, of course, easy to envisage detection situations in which outcomes are not all viewed as equally good or bad. For example, in some peace-time military detection situations, false alarms are deeply frowned upon. One might model that with such a payoff as:

	Y	N
s	1	−1
n	−25	1

In such a case, one anticipates that the observer will be very wary, indeed, about responding Y unless he or she is absolutely sure that a signal was presented. Equally well, the payoff matrix

	Y	N
s	25	−1
n	−1	1

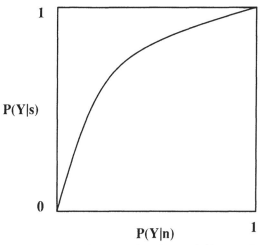

FIG. IV.1   A typical ROC (receiver operating characteristic) curve. It is the locus of possible response probability pairs ⟨P(Y|s),P(Y|n)⟩ that can be generated by varying the payoff matrix in a Yes–No experiment with a signal of fixed intensity.

is designed to incline the observer to respond Y whenever there is any indication whatsoever that the signal was presented on the trial. This payoff pattern is more likely in wartime where correct detections — hits — are crucial and commanders are usually willing to put up with a number of false alarms in an effort to avoid a miss.

These considerations suggest that by manipulating the payoff matrix, one can obtain quite a range of data pairs. Indeed, this is the case. The locus of all such pairs obtained under identical stimulus conditions is known as a Receiver Operating Characteristic,[2] usually abbreviated **ROC curve** in this literature. The typical curve looks something like that shown in Fig. IV.1.

As signal intensity is increased, the ROC curve is pushed upward and left toward the upper left corner, which point corresponds to perfect detection, that is, $P(Y|s) = 1$ and $P(Y|n) = 0$. Thus one obtains a family of curves such as shown in Fig. IV.2.

Note that chance performance, $P(Y|s) = P(Y|n)$ is the diagonal line running from $(0, 0)$ to $(1, 1)$. No behavior is expected to lie below the chance line, unless of course the observer is being either perverse and responding N when he or she detects the signal and Y otherwise or is confusing a signal with no signal, as can happen when no feedback is given.

If observers do vary their behavior with the structure of the payoff, as indeed they do, then for each payoff matrix the observed data will fall at

---

[2]This term comes from the electrical engineering literature where theories of signal detection were first formulated. They were brought into psychology in the 1950s. I made an attempt in the 1960s to introduce the somewhat more graphic term *iso-sensitivity curves,* but it failed to catch on.

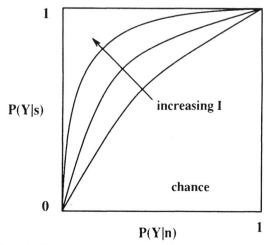

FIG. IV.2   Several ROC curves that are generated by increasing the signal intensity. Above some intensity, no errors are made and the behavior is at the point (1, 0).

one point on the curve for the signal being used. Thus, it is clear that one cannot characterize the Yes–No performance in terms of a single number, such as $P(Y|s)$, as was done for many years, or even a single pair of estimated probabilities. The entire curve must be characterized.

Two closely related ways of characterizing the detectability aspect of the curves can be found in the literature. One is to associate to each curve a number, denoted d′, that arises from a theory known as the *theory of signal detectability*. Because that rests on more mathematics than we are using, we do not go into it. The other is to use the area under the ROC curve as an overall measure of the detectability of the signal giving rise to that curve. That number is clearly $\frac{1}{2}$ when the observer is unable to detect the signal at all, and as signal strength is increased it rises smoothly from $\frac{1}{2}$ to 1, when the detection is perfect. It turns out that the area has a very simple relation to the next method of doing the detection experiment.

2.4 Two-Alternative Forced Choice

In the method called the **two-alternative forced choice** design a trial is composed of two well-defined time intervals (e.g., in an auditory discrimination experiment, visual signals, such as some mark on the CRT, are usually used to define the intervals). There are two signals, s_1 and s_2, one of which appears in the first interval and the other in the second. The subject's task is to say whether the signals were presented in the order $\langle s_1, s_2 \rangle$ or in the order $\langle s_2, s_1 \rangle$. When the signals differ only in one dimension, say intensity, then the task amounts to reporting which interval contains the more intense signal. This is called a **discrimination** design:

	1	2
$\langle s_1, s_2 \rangle$	$P(1|\langle s_1, s_2 \rangle)$	$P(2|\langle s_1, s_2 \rangle)$
$\langle s_2, s_2 \rangle$	$P(1|\langle s_2, s_1 \rangle)$	$P(2|\langle s_2, s_1 \rangle)$

Assuming that s_1 denotes the larger signal, then in analogy to the detection case, the data obtained yield estimates of two independent probabilities, for example, $P(1|\langle s_1, s_2 \rangle)$ and $P(2|\langle s_2, s_1 \rangle)$. (Note that the probabilities in each row once again sum to 1.) These two probabilities correspond to the two ways in which the observer can be correct. Their average is taken as the proportion of correct responses, which is a measure of the discriminability of the signals.

One special case of this general discrimination design is two-alternative, forced-choice detection. Here exactly one of the intervals contains the signal and the other is null. The observer's task to say which interval he or she believes contains the signal.

	1	2
$\langle s, n \rangle$	$P(1|\langle s, n \rangle)$	$P(2|\langle s, n \rangle)$
$\langle n, s \rangle$	$P(1|\langle n, s \rangle)$	$P(2|\langle n, s \rangle)$

Within the context of the theory of signal detectability, it can be shown that the area under the ROC curve of the Yes–No detection experiment is exactly equal to percent correct responding in the two-alternative, forced-choice detection experiment run under the same conditions with a perfectly symmetric payoff matrix. Thus, percent correct is usually taken to be the measure of choice, although under certain circumstances the d' measure of the Yes–No ROC curve has subtle advantages over percent correct.

2.5 Just Noticeable Differences: JNDs

The separation between two signals that is just sufficient to produce 75% correct discriminations, that is, a pair of signals s_1 and s_2 such that

$$\tfrac{1}{2}[P(1|\langle s_1, s_2 \rangle) + P(2|\langle s_2, s_1 \rangle)] = 0.75,$$

is called a **just noticeable difference**, abbreviated **jnd.** It is also called the **discrimination threshold** or, in the case of detection designs, the **absolute threshold.**[3] The choice of 75% is entirely arbitrary, and sometimes other percentages are used. The most common alternative is 71%, which arises naturally in an adaptive procedure in which one of the signals is adjusted according to the response on the preceeding trial; we do not go into such procedures here.

Suppose that two signals differ in intensity by just one jnd. Let the lower one have intensity I and the larger one, one jnd above I, have intensity I'. Then the intensity difference between them $I' - I$ is the physical equivalent of the jnd, and it is denoted by $\Delta(I)$. Thus, $I' = I + \Delta(I)$. If the signals differ in frequency by a jnd, then let f, $f + \Delta(f)$ denote the signals and so $\Delta(f)$ is the jnd of frequency.

Because we are dealing with a statistical phenomena — a probability of discriminating signals — the jnd is an estimated quantity. As is true of all estimates, the accuracy of the estimate depends on the size of the experimental sample on which it is based, in this case the number of trials run in the experiment. It is shown statistically that the error of a probability estimate improves in proportion to $1/N^{1/2}$, where N is the number of observations. This is regrettably slow — to cut the error of estimate by a factor of 10 requires the sample size be increased by a factor of 100, which is usually very expensive to do.

In practice, one typically holds I fixed and varies I'. Usually something over 100 trials are run for each pair (I, I') with 5 to 10 different values of I' spanning the region in which one expects the jnd to lie. To estimate $\Delta(I)$, we then plot, as in Fig. IV.3, the estimated probability of correctly identifying $I + \delta(I)$ as larger than I plotted as a function of $\delta(I)$. Of course, the estimate of the probability is the proportion of trials on which the correct discrimination is made. A smooth curve is then fit to the data points, as shown, and the jnd is read off from the curve. Such curves, showing a measure of accuracy, such as percentage correct, versus some measure of signal strength, are generically called **psychometric functions.**

Exactly the same procedure is followed to estimate the jnd for frequency — or for any other sensory stimulus. These methods are used for all modalities, not just sound.

---

[3]The term "threshold" dates back to earlier times when some believed that discontinuous thresholds exist, but that the data are too contaminated by measurement error to see the discontinuity. Subsequently, we have come to recognize that variability is inherent in sensory processing, and so a discontinuity is unlikely. Nonetheless, the term continues to be used, even though it is misleading. For a careful summary of this quite confusing history, see Link (1992).

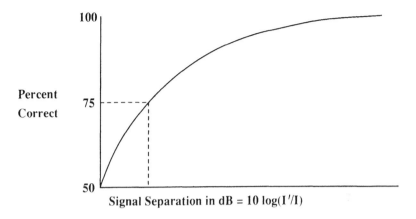

FIG. IV.3   A typical psychometric function that is generated in a two-alternative forced choice experiment by varying the intensity of one of the two signals. The independent variable is that signal difference in dB. The 75% jnd is indicated by the dotted lines.

2.6 Intensity Discrimination

2.6.1 Weber Functions.   The dimensionless quantities $\Delta(I)/I$ and $\Delta(f)/f$ are called **Weber[4] fractions.** The plot of a Weber fraction versus the stimulus level, I or f in these two cases, is called a **Weber function.** These quantities are named in honor of E. H. Weber, a German physiologist who, in the second quarter of the 19th century, first studied discrimination using procedures similar to those described. The problem in his day was not so much one of experimental design as the control over stimuli, especially over intensity.

Some scientists have argued that it is better to express the Weber fraction as:

$$I'/I = (I + \Delta I)/I = 1 + \Delta I/I,$$

in which case it can also be expressed in dB terms, as in Fig. IV.4, by writing it as:

$$10 \log[1 + \Delta(I)/I] = 10 \log (I'/I).$$

2.6.2 Weber's "Law."   As a first approximation, Weber noted that for stimulus intensity the quantity $\Delta(I)/I$ is approximately a constant, call it a, which is independent of intensity I (although it may vary with other things,

---

[4]Pronounced in the German way, Veyber.

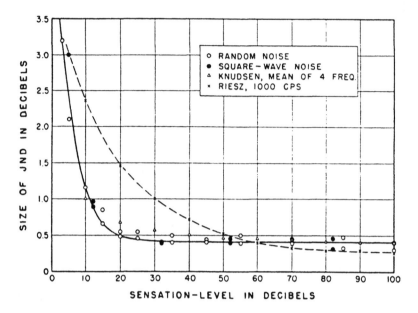

FIG. IV.4 Weber fractions, in dB, versus signal intensity, also in dB, for noise and pure tones. The smooth curves are best fitting generalized Weber's law, Equation IV.2, solid to noise and dotted to pure tones (see also Fig. IV.6). From "Sensitivity to Changes in the Intensity of White Noise and its Relation to Masking and Loudness" by G. A. Miller, 1947, *Journal of the Acoustical Society of America, 19,* p. 612. Copyright 1947 by American Institute of Physics. Reprinted by permission.

such as duration, frequency, the observer, etc.). This special relation has come to be known as **Weber's "law,"** with law in quotes because the equation

$$\Delta(I) = aI \qquad (1)$$

never really holds exactly. For example, the estimated Weber function (with the Weber fraction in dB) for noise[5] stimuli is shown in Fig. IV.4, and we see that although Weber's law is very well satisfied for sufficiently large intensities, it breaks down near threshold. These data are, however, well fit by what has been called the **generalized Weber law,**

$$\Delta(I) = aI + b, \qquad (2)$$

[5]We have not yet discussed noise in any formal sense, but do so in Section VI.3.1. It suffices to think of it as a hissing sound such as in a leaky steam pipe, that between stations on older, inexpensive FM radios, or that caused by forcing a bit too much air through a ventilation system.

where a and b are "constants" independent of I (again, they may depend on other things). This is the curve shown in Fig. IV.4. Note that the Weber fraction in this case becomes

$$\Delta(I)/I = a + b/I. \tag{3}$$

For large I (recall that at 50 dB above threshold, I is a number at least as large as 10^5) the term b/I is negligible and so in that region Equation 3 reduces to Weber's original law. But for small I (near 0) that term goes to infinity. A great deal of intensity data are well approximated by the generalized Weber law.

A major exception to this statement, however, is the discrimination of pure tones. The experiments carried out in this century (for a summary of some, see Fig. IV.5) uniformly show a Weber function that is decreasing gradually with I. Perhaps the most systematic study of pure tone discrimination is that summarized in Fig. IV.6, where $\Delta(I)/I$ is shown as a function of both I and f. There does not appear to be any significant dependence on

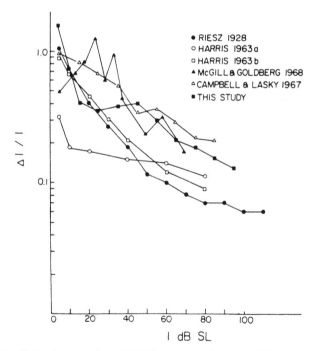

FIG. IV.5 Weber functions for a 1,000 Hz pure tone from six different experiments. The Weber fraction, shown on a logarithmic scale, is plotted as a function of signal intensity in dB. From "Neural Coding and Psychophysical Discrimination Data" by R. D. Luce and D. M. Green, 1974, *Journal of the Acoustical Society of America, 56*, p. 1559. Copyright 1974 by American Institute of Physics. Adapted by permission.

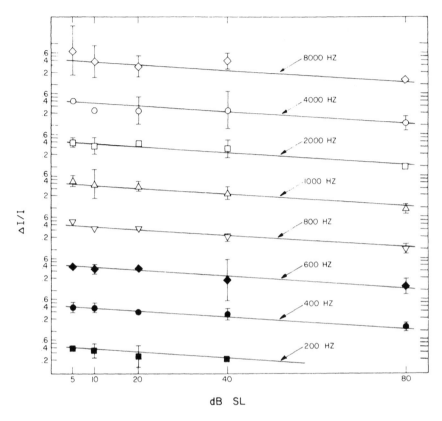

FIG. IV.6 Intensity Weber functions for pure tones of several frequencies from 200 Hz to 8 kHz. The straight lines are the best fit of the near-miss to Weber's law, Equation IV.4. The estimate of the exponent, $\mu = 0.072$, is independent of frequency. From "Intensity Discrimination as a Function of Frequency and Sensation Level" by W. Jesteadt, C. C. Wier, and D. M. Green, 1977, *Journal of the Acoustical Society of America, 61*, p. 171. Copyright 1977 by American Institute of Physics. Reprinted by permission.

f. The mathematical curve fit to the data is known as the **near-miss to Weber's law:**

$$\Delta(I)/I = aI^{-\mu}. \tag{4}$$

Note that $\log \Delta I/I = \log a - \mu \log I$. Recalling that the signal intensity in dB is given by $10 \log I$, we may rewrite Equation 4 as:

$$\log \Delta(I)/I = \log a - (\mu/10)\text{dB}.$$

Thus, the slope of the best fitting line in Fig. IV.6 is an estimate of $\mu/10$, yielding a value for μ of about 0.072.

The fact that noise satisfies the generalized Weber law whereas the individual pure tones fail to do so is viewed by many as a conundrum for the following reason. As is pointed out in Section VI.3.1, noise can be modeled as the superposition of pure tones at all frequencies but having random amplitudes. Because the Weber function for pure tones decreases with I for every frequency, it is surprising that when a large number of tones are combined to form tones, albeit with randomly varying amplitudes, the decrease disappears. Various attempts have been made to explain the conundrum, but no account has found wide acceptance as yet. Usually, the approach is to try to understand the pure tone result as some sort of artifact that vanishes in the noise case.

2.6.3 Intensity Thresholds: Audiograms.   As was noted earlier, an intensity discrimination design in which the weaker signal is null (0 intensity) is called a detection experiment, and the jnd in that case is called the **absolute threshold.** It describes the least intensity for which the observer is able to detect a signal. These data are usually collected by stepping down the signal intensity at a given frequency until the observer can no longer detect it. (Demonstration 3.)

The plot of the absolute threshold of intensity as a function of signal frequency describes the lower bound of hearing. An example is shown in Fig. IV.7 for typical young people with no known hearing defects. For a person with hearing loss, the absolute threshold function lies above this

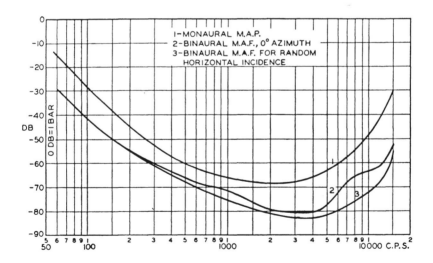

FIG. IV.7 Curves of the absolute threshold of hearing under three listening conditions. Note the appreciable dependence on frequency. From "On Minimum Audible Sound Fields" by L. J. Sivian and S. D. White, 1933, *Journal of the Acoustical Society of America, 4,* p. 313. Copyright 1933 by American Institute of Physics. Reprinted with permission.

"standard norm." Usually, and especially for older people, greater losses in detectability occur at the higher frequencies than at the lower ones, say those below 3,000 Hz.

Although most modern scientific studies report intensities in dB SPL, that is, relative to 0.0002 dynes/cm², some earlier studies reported them in dB relative to either the observer's absolute threshold or some standardized absolute threshold. These are referred to as *dB relative to sound level* and abbreviated dB SL. In reporting hearing losses, it is customary to use sound levels relative to a normal observer, that is, in terms of the difference, at each of several frequencies, between the standard normal threshold and that for the person being tested. The plot of these losses versus frequency is called an **audiogram.**

Figure IV.8 shows typical hearing loss of men and women with age for each of several frequencies. The high frequency loss with age is very widespread, as is the sharp difference between men and women.

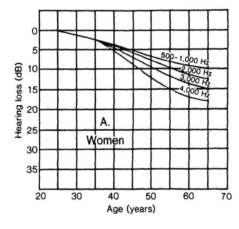

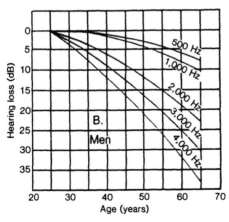

FIG. IV.8 Loss of hearing with age for men and women separately and with frequency as a parameter. The loss at each frequency and each age is reported as the amount, in dB, that the threshold level is higher on average for such a person than it is for a young person of the same sex who has no known hearing defects. Note that the loss in both sexes is more severe at the higher frequencies and that it is much more severe for men than women. For example, at age 65 the threshold at 4,000 Hz has increased, on average, less than 20 dB for women but for men, on average, it is over double that, 40 dB. From *The Science of Hi-Fidelity* (p. 129) by K. W. Johnson, W. B. Walker, and J. D. Cutnell, 1981, Dubuque, Iowa: Kendall/Hunt. Copyright 1981 by Kendall/Hunt. Reprinted by permission.

The source of the loss is not really understood. Among the possibilities are: (a) the basilar membrane, which is under considerable tension at the end near the stapes, becomes increasingly slack with age; (b) some destruction or other failure of the hair cells; (c) loss of neurons; and (d) ill-understood central problems. It may be all of these things. Exposure to very loud percussive sounds aggravates the problem through the destruction of the cilia on the hair cells or, as was the case shown in Fig. III.8, massive damage of the entire basilar membrane and its supports. The difference between men and women in Western culture is believed to be due in part to differential exposure to loud sounds and in part to other factors such as dietary differences that with age gradually affect blood flow to the ear and impair the functioning of the ear.

2.6.4 Time-Intensity Trade-off. Variables other than frequency and intensity affect the detection of signals. Perhaps the most notable is signal duration. Implicitly, we have taken for granted an experimental design in which the signals are of some arbitrary, but fixed, duration. Usually when duration is not at issue, it is set somewhere in the range from 100 to 500 ms, with different laboratories using different values. If one wishes to study the impact of duration, then a series of runs are carried out at each frequency using different durations, and the intensity is adjusted to achieve 75% correct detections. The empirical result is that durations greater than about 150 ms do not affect the jnd for intensity. But below 150 ms the intensity must be increased to compensate for shorter durations. The trade-off between duration and intensity is shown in Fig. IV.9.

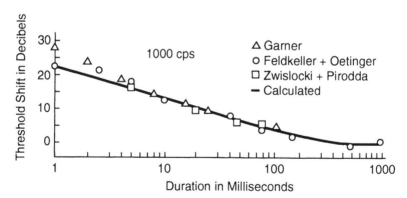

FIG. IV.9 Absolute threshold intensity for a 1,000 Hz tone as a function of signal duration. For durations below about 200 ms, there is a decided intensity-duration trade-off, but over 200 ms the threshold is largely independent of duration. From "Theory of Temporal Auditory Summation" by J. Zwislocki, 1960, *Journal of the Acoustical Society of America, 32*, p. 1053. Copyright 1960 by American Institute of Physics. Reprinted by permission.

2.7 Frequency Discrimination

Frequency discrimination is not nearly so consistent as intensity discrimination, in the sense that there are quite sizable individual differences. This can be seen in Fig. IV.10 where a number of studies are summarized in a plot of log $\Delta(f)$ versus $f^{1/2}$. (In reporting results about frequency, it is not customary to use the Weber fraction because Weber's law is not even approximately true. The use of $f^{1/2}$ rather than log f is common, although there is no strong theoretical reason for doing so.) Observe that the estimates of $\Delta(f)$ cover a considerable range—at 125 Hz the ratio between the largest and smallest estimate is about 8 to 1.

To some degree, these differences in the estimated jnd may be due to differences in experimental procedure and measurement of the stimulus, but the most likely major cause is differences among individuals. Unlike intensity discrimination, where for normal observers the individual differences are relatively minor, those for frequency are considerable. In Section IV.4.1.2 when we discuss absolute identification, we see a pronounced difference between people having "absolute pitch" and those not having it.

Perhaps the most careful study of frequency discrimination yielded the data shown in Fig. IV.11. Note that the frequency jnd depends not only on f but also on I.

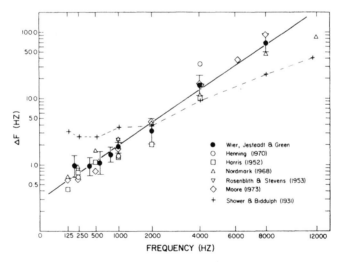

FIG. IV.10 Frequency jnd versus frequency level from several studies. The jnd, Δf, is plotted on a logarithmic scale and the frequency level is on a square root scale. Note that there are very substantial differences in the estimates, which may be due, in part, to differences in laboratories but probably is due, in substantial part, to appreciable individual differences (see also Fig. IV.26). From "Frequency Discrimination as a Function of Frequency and Sensation Level" by C. Wier, W. Jesteadt, and D. M. Green, 1977, *Journal of the Acoustical Society of America, 61,* p. 180. Copyright 1977 by American Institute of Physics. Reprinted by permission.

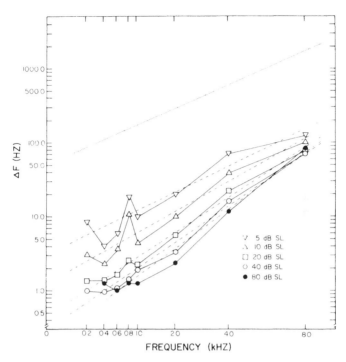

FIG. IV.11   Frequency jnd versus frequency level with intensity as a parameter. The jnd, Δf, is plotted on a logarithmic scale and the frequency level is on a square root scale. From "Frequency Discrimination as a Function of Frequency and Sensation Level" by C. Weir, W. Jesteadt, and D. M. Green, 1977, *Journal of the Acoustical Society of America, 61,* p. 180. Copyright 1977 by American Institute of Physics. Reprinted by permission.

3. GLOBAL PSYCHOPHYSICS

There is a sense in which both the plots of the Weber function and the absolute threshold as a function of frequency can be thought of as expressing something global. They show how the local performance varies over the entire frequency-intensity plane. But they are not really global in a deep sense because all they do is inform us about the discrimination of two nearby signals at any point in that plane. We turn next to more deeply global results.

3.1 A Map of Auditory Perceptual Space

3.1.1 Equal-Loudness Contours.   The curve of absolute thresholds versus frequency is, in a sense, a curve of equal loudness — it is an estimate of the point at which loudness just vanishes and the signal can no longer be detected, that is, has reached zero psychological level. Of course, because no loudness is associated with any intensity below the threshold value, there is no way that we can actually present zero loudness at one frequency and ask the observer what intensity corresponds to that signal at another frequency. In order for such an experiment to make sense, the signals must be loud enough to be heard, at least some of the time. So we use a statistical criterion, such as 75% correct responding, to determine an approximation to the upper bound of zero loudness, and we treat these "absolute thresholds" as forming the curve of equal, zero loudness.

Once we go above threshold, however, the question of equal loudness can reasonably be asked. Given a particular tone of frequency f and intensity I, then for each other frequency f', one can ask the observer to adjust the intensity to that value I' so that the tone (I', f') is perceived as having the same loudness as the tone (I, f). Denote this judgment of equal loudness by $(I', f') \sim (I, f)$. We assume, as is approximately true, that these judgments are transitive in the sense that

$$\text{if } (I, f) \sim (I', f') \text{ and } (I', f') \sim (I'', f''), \text{ then } (I, f) \sim (I'', f'').$$

Thus, by finding the equivalence for every f' (in practice, from 10 to 20 values of f'), we generate the locus (curve) of frequencies and intensities that have equal loudness. These are called *equal-loudness contours* (or curves), and some are shown in Fig. IV.12. Notice that at low intensities they exhibit much the same shape as the absolute threshold curve, and so they are a natural extension of it to the entire domain of hearing.

Note that for some values of I' it is impossible to find an f' that is equally loud as (I, f). For example, if $(I, f) = (50 \text{ dB}, 1,000 \text{ Hz})$ and I' is 30 dB, then by looking across the line corresponding to 30 dB we see that it does not intersect the equal loudness contour for (I, f).

3.1.2 Lack of Correct and Incorrect Responses. In discrimination studies the experimenter knows which signal is more intense or has higher frequency, and so it is possible to report back to the observer whether or not each response is correct. Often this is done, and such experiments are said to involve information feedback. In striking contrast, an equal-loudness study has no correct and incorrect answers. We ask the observer to make a judgment about what is heard as equally loud, and we can only accept the answer as reflecting a fact of that person's perception. Fortunately, among observers with normal hearing there is considerable consensus about what constitutes equal loudness. Nonetheless, many scientists are uncomfortable about the subjective nature of the responses in the equal-loudness experiment, and even more so about some of the designs described later. However, the experimental results are quite regular and they are widely used because they get at things we do not know how else to study.

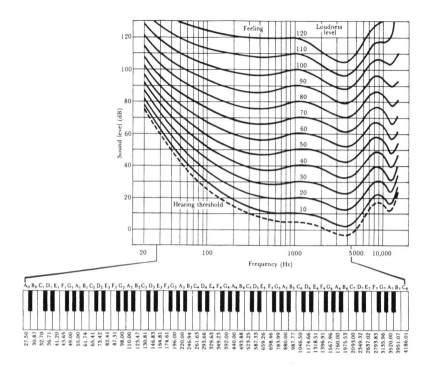

FIG. IV.12 Equal loudness contours with matches made to 1,000 Hz tones varying in intensity from 10 dB to 120 dB. From *Human Information Processing: An Introduction to Psychology* (p. 248) by P. H. Lindsay and D. A. Norman, 1972, New York: Academic Press. Copyright 1972 by Academic Press. Reprinted by permission.

3.1.3 Loudness Compensation. At low intensities the curvature of the equal loudness curves is pronounced, which is the reason that music played at very low levels of intensity (low settings of the gain control on an amplifier) sounds unbalanced, as indeed it is. One can hear neither the low nor the high frequencies as well as those in the midrange. The simplest attempt to compensate for this is called a *loudness control.* It increases the intensity of the low and high frequencies relative to the midrange ones. Many modern systems have more sophisticated *equalizers* that permit one to adjust the intensity gains at some 10 or 15 different frequencies, roughly equally spaced in log *f,* and some even have preprogrammed patterns and associate to them such names as "speech," "jazz," "rock," and "classical." If the compensation is left on when the gain control is at a middle to high setting, the music again sounds distorted because the equal loudness contour of hearing is more nearly flat but the loudness control now imposes too much intensity at the low and high frequencies relative to the middle ones.

3.1.4 Frequency and Intensity Bounds.   Another feature of Fig. IV.12 is the fairly clear impression it gives of the entire array of *(I, f)* pairs that can be heard. Roughly, hearing is bounded from below by 20 or 30 Hz and from above by 20 to 24 kHz for a young listener. By age 40 it is likely to be down to 12 kHz, and by age 70 it may be down to 8 kHz or less.

The threshold of intensity, as we have discussed, varies considerably with frequency, being lowest (i.e., best) at 2 to 4 kHz, the exact estimate depending on the study. For high intensities, the curves of equal loudness are more nearly flat and are bounded from above first by pain and then ultimately by serious damage to the inner ear. Sounds as loud as 140 dB SPL — the exposure of an unprotected aircraft handler near an accelerating jet engine or of a rock music performer in front of massive loudspeakers — should be attenuated by using earplugs or earmuffs in order to avoid damage. Laboratory studies used to go as high as 110 or 115 dB but are now mostly limited to 95 or 100 dB.

3.1.5 Indifference Curves.   As an aside, note that curves of equal values of a subjective attribute are of considerable interest not only in psychophysics but also throughout the rest of psychology and more generally in the social, biological, and physical sciences. They arise whenever two or more independent variables affect a dependent variable, and so one can ask what is the locus of values of the independent variables that yield a constant value of the dependent variable. We saw this earlier when discussing how the jnd depends on intensity and duration. In economics, when the dependent variable is a subjective value, usually called utility, such curves are called *indifference curves.* More generally, they are called *equal-X contours,* where X is the name of the dependent variable. For example, the tuning curves of Section III.4.2.4 are equal-firing-rate contours.

3.2 "Laws" to Describe Intensity Perception

Once one has equal loudness contours a natural question is: Just how loud is the loudness associated with each contour? One can debate whether or not this question is even meaningful — it is, after all, asking about the mathematical nature of something that is highly subjective. Presumably, however, the sensation we call loudness reflects something about the level of neural activity produced by the stimulus — either in terms of neural firing rates or the number of neurons that are active or, perhaps, both. It can be argued, and has been, that the answer is largely definitional, but some of the experimental results make clear that more than sheer definition is involved.

3.2.1 Fechner's "Law."   The earliest attempt to deal with the problem is probably that due to the Leipzig physicist-turned-philosopher[6] G. T. Fechner (1860/1966), and it is in a sense definitional. Fechner was quite aware that there are at least two qualitatively different types of sensory attributes: those having to do with amount, for example, loudness, brightness, weight, shock, and those having to do with quality, for example, pitch, perceived color. S. S. Stevens later termed them *prothetic* and *metathetic* attributes, respectively. The scheme Fechner proposed was limited to the prothetic, in part because Weber's law is approximately true for only the prothetic and not the metathetic.

Fechner postulated that the growth of subjective intensity – let us formulate it in terms of loudness L as a function of the intensity I of a pure tone – is such that the subjective change corresponding to a jnd has exactly the same value independent of where the jnd is evaluated, that is, independent of I. That is, if a loudness function $L(I)$ exits, then the difference $\Delta L(I) = L[I + \Delta(I)] - L(I)$ does not depend at all on I, which is to say that for some constant k that is independent of I (although as far as we know it may depend on f, signal duration, the observer, and various other things, but not intensity) such that

$$\Delta L(I) = k. \tag{5}$$

Suppose further that the generalized Weber's law, $\Delta(I) = aI + b$, Equation 3, holds. Substituting that into Fechner's postulate, Equation 5, yields:

$$L[I + aI + b] - L(I) = k. \tag{6}$$

Suppose Equation 6 holds for every statistical definition of a threshold – not only the 75% level but also for every percentage greater than 50% (chance) and less than 100%, but with the value for k depending on the criterion used. And suppose that for each value of the "threshold criterion" the generalized Weber's law holds – of course with different values for a as the criterion is varied from just above 50% to just below 100%. Then mathematicians have shown that L must be the following logarithmic function:

$$L(I) = A \log (I + b/a) + B, \tag{7}$$

where A and B are constants independent of I. In this context, the logarithmic function of Equation 7 is known as **Fechner's "law,"** once again with quotes around the word law.

---

[6]In his time psychology was not a separate discipline. Psychological studies were carried out, in part, in laboratories of physiology and in part in departments of philosophy.

It is easy to verify that L of Equation 7 has the appropriate property, Equation 6:

$$
\begin{aligned}
L[I + \Delta(I)] - L(I) &= L[I(1 + a) + b] - L(I) \\
&= A \log [I(1 + a) + b + b/a] + B \\
&\quad - A \log (I + b/a) - B \\
&= A \log [(1 + a)I + (b/a)(1 + a)] \\
&\quad - A \log (I + b/a) \\
&= A \log [(1 + a)(I + b/a)] - A \log (I + b/a) \\
&= A \log (1 + a) + A \log (I + b/a) \\
&\quad - A \log (I + b/a) \\
&= A \log (1 + a).
\end{aligned}
$$

The major mathematical difficulty is in proving that this is the only solution to Equation 6.

Of course, we know that the generalized Weber law is not precisely correct, but for noise it holds rather well and it is not far from wrong for pure tones, so the answer is approximately correct.

The exact solution to Equation 5 when Weber's law does not hold at all can be calculated approximately in the following way using the empirically known Weber function:

1. Pick any low intensity I_1, and assign it the value 1.
2. Go to the plot of $\Delta(I)/I$ vs. I, enter it at I_1 and determine $\Delta(I_1)$.
3. Let $I_2 = I_1 + \Delta(I_1)$ and assign $L(I_2) = 2$.
   Note: $L(I_2) - L(I_1) = 2 - 1 = 1$.
4. Enter the plot of the Weber function at I_2 and determine $\Delta(I_2)$.
5. Let $I_3 = I_2 + \Delta(I_2)$ and assign $L(I_3) = 3$.
   Note: $L(I_3) - L(I_2) = 3 - 2 = 1$.

And so forth. A smooth curve fitted to these discrete points is an approximate solution to Equation 5.

3.2.2 Fechner's Law and Subjective Loudness.   The most striking difficulty with Fechner's law is that it simply does not accord well with people's subjective impressions. To the extent that Weber's law is correct, Fechner's law says that loudness grows directly with dB, but most people do not agree that a change of 10 dB at low intensities generates a change in loudness that seems equivalent to a 10 dB change at high levels. This was demonstrated experimentally by E. B. Newman.

Furthermore, the use of Fechner's law led to numerous difficulties in acoustical engineering practice. In the 1920s and 1930s, sound engineers were hired to quiet work environments, for example, offices with many typewriters and mechanical calculating machines; automobiles and aircraft, and so on. In doing so, when they based design decisions on dB (= Fechner's law) their clients were dissatisfied. If in responding to a request to cut the sound transmitted by a half they cut the dB level in half, then the client found the reduction far more than half and far too expensive. If they cut the intensity in half, which is a reduction of 3 dB, the change was far too small to be called a reduction by half. For example, in Section III.7.3.1 we saw that an arriving subway train runs at 90 to 100 dB, and half of that, 45 to 50 dB, corresponds to a quiet living room. Most people feel this is a good deal quieter than 50% of the subway noise. And a 3 dB change is perceived as close to negligible. These difficulties led to the development of an alternative law and other, more direct ways of measuring loudness (and other subjective attributes of intensity).

3.2.3 Stevens' "Law." Keeping within the general framework of Fechner's approach to the problem, observe that Weber's law (not the generalized version) can be expressed in another way, namely as saying that the ratio between two signals one jnd apart is a constant independent of the intensity of the lower one:

$$[I + \Delta(I)]/I = 1 + \Delta(I)/I = 1 + a. \tag{8}$$

An a priori postulate that seems just as reasonable as Fechner's is to suppose that these ratios, not the differences corresponding to $\Delta(I)$, remain constant under the loudness function. This was suggested by J.A.F Plateau 12 years after Fechner published his work in 1860, and it has long been recognized that signal ratios are highly significant in many psychophysical results.

However, this point of view was not developed seriously until the 1950s when the psychophysicist S. S. Stevens emphasized the possibility that it may be ratios that observers hold invariant. He objected vigorously to Fechner's approach, in part, because Fechner had assumed that one could infer the overall growth of sensation from the local properties of confusions between stimuli. Stevens noted that usually in physics and engineering the connection between the quality and magnitude of observations is somewhat irregular and that in general it would be unwise to assume that knowledge of the one permits an inference about the other.

Moreover, had he known then what we know now about the representation of signals in the auditory nerve, he could have argued as follows. Discrimination between two nearby signals may very well depend on comparing changes in the firing rates on those individual neurons that are firing above their resting level but are not firing at their maximum level, whereas the overall sensation of loudness may well depend on the total number of neurons that are firing above their resting level or, perhaps, only on those that are firing at their maximum level. Fechner's idea presupposes there is a very particular relation between the number of neurons used in discriminating signals and those that underlie the sensation of loudness.

Rather than work with a conjectured relation between magnitude and discriminability, Stevens said that the important property of the subjective function is its preservation of ratios, of which Equation 8 is only a special case.

Assuming that stimulus ratios are preserved by the loudness function, then a straightforward mathematical question must be solved. What loudness function L is such that physical intensity ratios are all preserved, that is, what increasing functions L has the property:

$$\text{if } I'/I = c, \text{ then } L(I')/L(I) = k(c), \tag{9}$$

where c is any positive constant and k is some function of c. It turns out that the only solution to this problem for which $L(I)$ is an increasing function of I is:

$$L(I) = AI^{\beta}, \tag{10}$$

where A and β are both positive constants independent of I. (As an exercise, verify that Equation 10 does in fact satisfy the condition stated in Equation 9; it is rather more difficult to show that it is the only increasing function that does so, but that is also true.) In mathematics, such functions are called **power functions,** and they abound in physics. In this context, as a "law" describing subjective growth of intensity, it has come to be called **Stevens' (power) "law."**

No a priori way exists to choose with any confidence between Fechner's and Stevens' hypotheses (and possibly others of a similar sort); it seems to be a matter of trying to find experiments that bear on their descriptive accuracy. This is what Stevens did, and in the process introduced new experimental procedures to which we now turn.

3.3 Magnitude Methods

3.3.1 The Three Procedures.   Stevens' new approach can be caricatured: Just ask clients to tell you what their numerical loudnesses are. It all began in Fechner's time when Plateau asked a number of painters to mix greys half-way between a dark and a light grey. He pointed out that when the physical intensity was measured, "half-way" was not where it should be on a dB scale. Stevens generalized this to a method of fractionization and to three related methods. In all of these, we assume signals that vary in just the intensity dimension.

The first, called **magnitude estimation,** presents signals one at a time to the observer. Usually the signals are spaced equally in dB and they are presented in irregular order among the intensities. The observer is instructed to assign a positive number to each presentation, selecting these numbers so that their ratios reflect the subjective intensity—for example, loudness—ratios among the signals.

The second method, called **magnitude production**, has the experimenter present positive numbers and the observer adjusts the signal intensity so that, again, the ratios of the numbers reflect the subjective ratios of the chosen signal intensities.

And the third is **cross-modal matching** in which stimuli from one modality, such as sounds, are presented and the observer is required "to match" attribute values, such as intensity, on a different modality, such as light, to the presented stimulus. Presumably one is matching brightness to loudness. One can view magnitude estimation and production as special cases of cross-modal matching in which one attribute is the real numbers together with the operation of multiplication.

At first encounter, such instructions may seem peculiar, if not actually perverse, and almost impossible to carry out. But people do not find the tasks difficult and, whatever it is that they do, their behavior is surprisingly regular.

3.3.2 Magnitude Estimation and Production Data.   The major empirical finding is that both magnitude methods do establish relations that are reasonably well described by Stevens' law. Note that if Stevens' law is true, then by taking the logarithm of it we obtain

$$\log L(I) = \beta \log I + \log A$$
$$= (\beta/10)\text{dB} + B, \tag{11}$$

which says that when the logarithm of the magnitude estimates are plotted against the signal intensity in dB, the resulting function is a straight line with the slope of $\beta/10$. So, the data from these experiments are plotted in what are called log-log coordinates for the variables $L(I)$ and I. For $L(I)$ versus dB, only the ordinate need be logarithmic and the dB are plotted linearly. Plotting paper ruled in these coordinates is known as semi-log paper.

For the most part, Stevens collected only a few data from each of several subjects.[7] Often he used 10 to 30 subjects, 5 to 10 stimuli, and obtained only 2 observations per stimulus from each subject. The reported data are then either the median or the geometric mean response to each signal.[8]

---

[7]Here the term "subject" seems more appropriate than "observer."

[8]The *median* response is the one such that half of the responses are larger than it and half are smaller than it. The *arithmetic mean,* often just called the *mean* or the *average,* is the sum of all n observations divided by n. The *geometric mean* of n observations is the nth root of the product of all the responses. It is equivalent to computing the arithmetic mean of the logarithm of each response and then taking the inverse of the logarithm, the exponential, of that mean. For example, suppose the observations are 5, 6, 7, 8, and 10. Then the median is 7, the arithmetic mean is 7.2, and the geometric mean is 6.999.

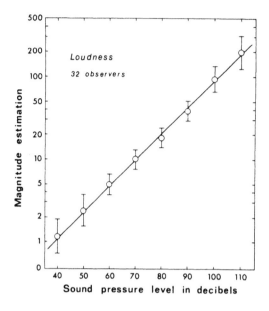

FIG. IV.13 Magnitude estimates of loudness versus signal intensity. Both scales are logarithmic. The data points are geometric means of two observations from each of 32 observers, and one standard deviation error bar is shown. The straight line represents the best fitting version of Stevens' law, Equation IV.10. From *Psychophysics* (p. 28) by S. S. Stevens, 1975, New York: Wiley. Copyright 1975 by John Wiley & Sons. Reprinted by permission.

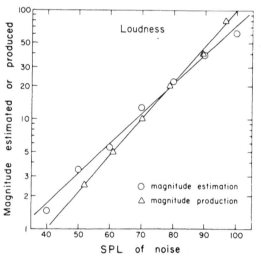

FIG. IV.14 A comparison of magnitude estimates and magnitude productions of loudness showing some lack of agreement, which has been called a "regression effect." From "Regression Effect in Psychophysiological Judgment" by S. S. Stevens and H. B. Greenbaum, 1966, *Perception & Psychophysics, 1,* p. 441. Copyright 1966 by The Psychonomic Society of America. Reprinted by permission.

Figure IV.13 shows the magnitude estimation of loudness and Fig. IV.14 compares magnitude estimation and magnitude production for sound intensity. Both curves conform to the prediction of Equation 11 quite well. The most peculiar thing about these plots is seen in Fig. IV.14, where we observe that the slope of the magnitude estimation line is less than that of the magnitude production one. This discrepancy almost always occurs and Stevens called it a "regression effect" (although, for various reasons, that term is not particularly felicitous, especially given its specialized meaning in statistics). Whatever it is called, we do not really understood why it happens.

3.3.3 Loudness Magnitudes of Some Deaf People.   Although there is not much sign of it in Figs. IV.13 and IV.14, the magnitude curves often droop at low intensities, producing much larger slopes than at higher intensities. Such a droop can be induced to occur at higher intensities by adding noise to the signal. Figures IV.15 and IV.16 are examples of this phenomenon. Such a low-intensity droop is quite characteristic of deafness due to neural loss. This fact makes clear why such people either fail to hear what is being said or, when voices are raised slightly, they grumpily complain that one is shouting. The reason is not simple perversity, but rather that the band of intensities over which the loudness function goes from zero to normal, but high level, loudness is much, much narrower for such deaf people than it is for those with normal hearing. Speakers have difficulty in maintaining speech within a sufficiently narrow range both to be heard and not to become excessively loud.

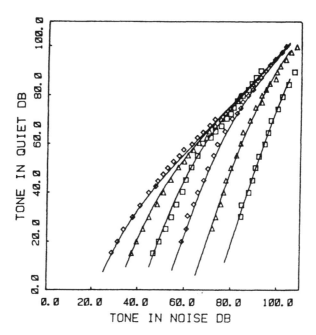

FIG. IV.15   Loudness matches of a pure tone of several intensities in quiet to the same tone in noise. Each curve corresponds to a different level of noise. The smooth curves are the best fit of Equation IV.12 to these data. From "Invariant Properties of Masking Phenomena in Psychoacoustics and their Theoretical Consequences" by G. J. Iverson and M. Pavel, 1981, *SIAM-AMS Proceedings, 13,* p. 19. Copyright 1981 by American Mathematical Society. Reprinted by permission.

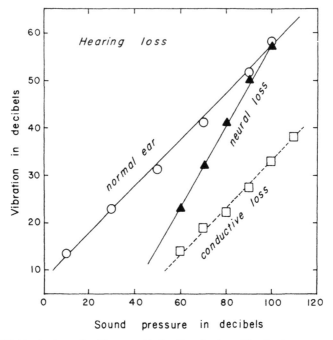

FIG. IV.16 A schematic of how two kinds of hearing loss affect loudness as measured by magnitude estimates. Neural loss refers primarily to hair cell, auditory nerve, and central damage, and conduction loss to failures of the mechanical parts of the system, especially in the middle ear. The difference in the two curves makes clear that hearing aids designed to compensate for hearing loss should amplify quite differently in the two cases. From *Psychophysics* (p. 133) by S. S. Stevens, 1975, New York: Wiley. Copyright 1975 by John Wiley & Sons. Reprinted by permission.

Research and development of hearing aids with highly nonlinear, frequency dependent amplification is under way and some are on the market. A generalized version of Stevens' law that describes such data is:

$$L(I, N) = AI^{\beta + \alpha}/(I^{\alpha} + BN^{\gamma}), \tag{12}$$

where N is an intensity measure of the noise (see Section V.5.2) and A, B, α, β, and γ are constants independent of both I and N. Note that for no noise, Equation 12 reduces to Stevens' law, Equation 10. The curves shown in Fig. IV.15 are calculated from Equation 12.

3.3.4 Magnitude Data from Individual Observers. As was noted, the results presented so far are all based on studies in which a number (10–30) of subjects each responded once or twice to each of 5 to 10 signals. Some researchers have approached the problem of collecting global data in much the same way as local studies are done, by studying very experienced individual observers using hundreds of presentations of each of 20 to 30 signals.

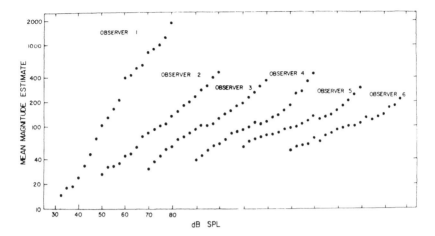

FIG. IV.17 Magnitude estimates of loudness for six different observers. Each data point is based on the geometric mean of 100 observations. The data are displaced horizontally 20 dB so as not to overlap. Note that Stevens' law is only partially supported and, to the extent that it makes sense to speak of slopes, they differ by as much as a factor of about three. From "Variability of Magnitude Estimates: A Timing Theory Analysis" by D. M. Green and R. D. Luce, 1974, *Perception & Psychophysics, 15*, p. 292. Copyright 1974 by The Psychonomic Society of America. Reprinted by permission.

Typical results from such a procedure are shown in Fig. IV.17. On the face of it, the fit of Stevens' law is clearly less satisfactory and the exponent β differs considerably over observers. Questions can be raised about whether these differences should be accepted at face value, and some research has attempted to decide whether or not the differences are real. The matter remains controversial (see Section IV.3.3.6).

3.3.5 Time-Intensity Trade-Off for Loudness.   Just as we were able to use equal-loudness methods to extend the curve of absolute thresholds to the entire domain of audible intensities and frequencies, we can use magnitude methods in a comparable way. The reason is, of course, that equal-loudness is really a special case of the magnitude methods. As an example of this, recall that in Fig. IV.9 we saw how intensity and duration trade off to yield just detectable signals. The natural generalization is to ask how intensity and duration jointly affect magnitude estimates of loudness. The results are shown in Fig. IV.18. As at threshold, durations beyond 150 ms have no effect on loudness, but below 150 ms the loudness drops off systematically as duration is shortened and intensity is held fixed.[9] From this plot, one can develop a plot of intensity versus duration for a fixed level

---

[9]The data for visual intensity are significantly different. Instead of there being a fixed time so that a time-intensity trade-off exists for durations below that cutoff, the time at which the break occur changes with intensity.

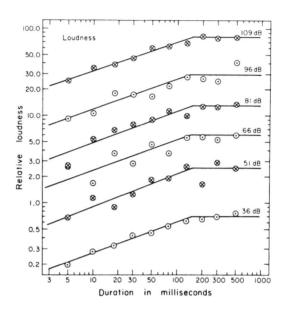

FIG. IV.18 Magnitude estimates of loudness as a function of both signal duration and signal intensity. As in Fig. IV.9, for durations less than about 200 ms there is an intensity-duration trade-off, but for longer durations magnitude estimates depend only on intensity and not on duration. From "Brightness and Loudness as Functions of Stimulus Duration." by J. C. Stevens and J. W. Hall, 1966, *Perception & Psychophysics, 1*, p. 324. Copyright 1966 by The Psychonomic Society of America. Reprinted by permission.

of loudness. As an exercise, do it for relative loudnesses of 2 and 10, interpolating intensity curves as needed, and plot these inferred data points together with the data from Fig. IV.9.

3.3.6 Stevens' Exponent.   One major question about Stevens' law is what interpretation to give to the exponent β. It is clear from Stevens' writings that he felt it to be a significant parameter of the sensory system. Some data seem to support this view. Consider the following argument.

Magnitude methods can, of course, be used with any sensory continuum, in particular with those that involve variation in intensity. This has been done, and Stevens' law describes the data quite satisfactorily, but with very different exponents for different modalities. Table IV.1 summarizes typical estimated values of the exponents. Several scientists have remarked on the very systematic relation between the exponents for different modalities and the dynamic range of the corresponding physical stimuli. By dynamic range, one means the ratio of the largest intensity tolerated by an observer to the threshold intensity for that modality. For example, the range of electric shock is quite small, considerably less than a factor of 10, whereas for sound and light it is very large. Conversely, the exponent is large for shock

TABLE IV.1
Estimated Stevens' Law Exponents for a Number of Different Modalities

Continuum	Measured exponent	Stimulus condition
Loudness	0.67	Sound pressure of 3000-hertz tone
Vibration	0.95	Amplitude of 60 hertz on finger
Vibration	0.6	Amplitude of 250 hertz on finger
Brightness	0.33	5° Target in dark
Brightness	0.5	Point source
Brightness	0.5	Brief flash
Brightness	1.0	Point source briefly flashed
Lightness	1.2	Reflectance of gray papers
Visual length	1.0	Projected line
Visual area	0.7	Projected square
Redness (saturation)	1.7	Red-gray mixture
Taste	1.3	Sucrose
Taste	1.4	Salt
Taste	0.8	Saccharine
Smell	0.6	Heptane
Cold	1.0	Metal contact on arm
Warmth	1.6	Metal contact on arm
Warmth	1.3	Irradiation of skin, small area
Warmth	0.7	Irradiation of skin, large area
Discomfort, cold	1.7	Whole body irradiation
Discomfort, warm	0.7	Whole body irradiation
Thermal pain	1.0	Radiant heat on skin
Tactual roughness	1.5	Rubbing emery cloths
Tactual hardness	0.8	Squeezing rubber
Finger span	1.3	Thickness of blocks
Pressure on palm	1.1	Static force on skin
Muscle force	1.7	Static contractions
Heaviness	1.45	Lifted weights
Viscosity	0.42	Stirring silicone fluids
Electric shock	3.5	Current through fingers
Vocal effort	1.1	Vocal sound pressure
Angular acceleration	1.4	5-Second rotation
Duration	1.1	White noise stimuli

Note: From *Psychophysics* (p. 15) by S. S. Stevens, 1975, New York: Wiley. Copyright 1975 by John Wiley & Sons, Inc. Reprinted by permission.

(over 3) and is small for sound and light (about .67 and .33). Shown in Fig. IV.19 is the plot, called a scatter diagram, of the estimated exponents versus the estimated range.

The theoretical curve was obtained as follows. Suppose the exponents are such that for all modalities the observer maintains the same dynamic range of numbers in making magnitude estimates, that is, if I_M denotes the maximum intensity for a modality and I_T its threshold intensity, then for each modality

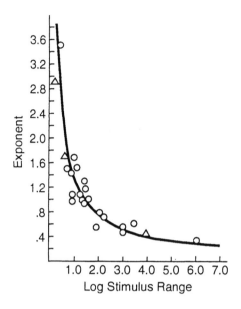

FIG. IV.19 Average exponents from magnitude estimates of a number of different intensive attributes as a function of the behavioral dynamic range, measured in dB, of each attribute. The behavioral dynamic range is defined to be the intensity ratio between the most intense acceptable level to the threshold level. Thus, for example, loudness and brightness have large dynamic ranges and electric shock a very small one. The smooth curve is the hyperbolic function of Equation IV.13. From "On the Exponents in Stevens' Law and the Constant in Ekman's Law" by R. Teghtsoonian, 1971, *Psychology Review, 78*, p. 73. Copyright 1971 by American Psychological Association. Reprinted by permission.

$$(I_M/I_T)^\beta = K, \qquad (13)$$

where K is a constant independent of modality. The function of Equation 13 is called a *hyperbolic* curve; it is shown in Fig. IV.19 with K chosen to fit the data as well as possible.

Such a result becomes plausible if one assumes that all sensory magnitudes are coded somewhere in the nervous system as firing rates of neural pulses, and that the several modalities have neurons that carry this intensity information to a common place in the brain where the comparisons can be made. Such a common neural intensity interface appears to exist in the forebrain. This explanation receives some support from cross-modal matching experiments described in the Section IV.3.3.7.

In Section IV.3.4, "additivity of loudness," we see another line of argument that seems to suggest that the exponent obtained by magnitude methods may be more than an artifact.

In contrast, however, are other data that say the exponent is quite malleable. For example, one study showed that if the experimenter selects a preassigned value for the exponent that is a factor of two larger or smaller than the value usually obtained, then using standard reinforcement methods the observer can be trained to respond according to that somewhat arbitrary function. Some have interpreted this to mean that the exponent has no clear meaning except as some sort of summary of the subject's previous experience. In particular, according to these scientists, it does not represent anything significant about the sensory system. Others say it simply arises because of the response flexibility of subjects under reinforcement.

Also, as we saw in Fig. IV.17, the exponents for individual observers appear to vary considerably, more than one might reasonably expect if the exponent were simply a reflection of sensory processing.

At this point, the evidence is conflicting about the interpretation to be given these exponents, and certainly no one has come up with a clear physiological explanation for these values.

3.3.7 Cross-Modal Matching.   As was mentioned earlier, one can think of both magnitude estimation and production as establishing matches between a sensory attribute and the number continuum in such a way that ratios are preserved. Because any two attributes of intensity, such as brightness and loudness, can each be matched to the number continuum, it is at least plausible that they can be matched to each other. Moreover, if a common intensity locus exists in the brain, such matching seems quite plausible. And indeed, when people are asked to do such matching, they do so with considerable consistency and regularity. Such a procedure goes under the name of **cross-modal matching.**

Assume for the moment that Stevens' law, Equation 10, does hold for each of two sensory attributes, which we identify by the subscripts 1 and 2. Then, matching attribute 2 to attribute 1 means finding for each value of I_1 that value of I_2 that causes the numerical scales to agree, that is,

$$A_2 I_2^{\beta_2} = L_2(I_2) = L_1(I_1) = A_1 I_1^{\beta_1},$$

or solving for I_2 in terms of I_1,

$$I_2 = A I_1^{\beta_1/\beta_2}, \tag{14}$$

where $A = (A_1/A_2)^{1/\beta_2}$. Thus, we conclude that if Stevens' law holds for magnitude estimation, then it should hold for cross-modal matching as well, with the exponent in the latter case being the ratio of the exponents from the estimation experiments.

Figure IV.20 presents cross-modal matching data between loudness and a number of attributes identified on the figure. Once again, the general form of Stevens' law is sustained by the data. The predictions of the cross-modal exponent from the magnitude ones are shown in Table IV.2, and for these group data the correspondence appears to be satisfactory. For individual subjects, the results are not as satisfactory, although no very comprehensive studies have been reported. One potential difficulty is that the estimation and production exponents are not the same (see Fig. IV.14), and both may be involved in cross-modal matching in the following way. Suppose that when I_1 is presented the subject magnitude estimates it and then uses that estimate to magnitude produce the corresponding I_2. Then the correct matching prediction would entail both the magnitude estimate exponent for the first attribute and the magnitude production exponent for the second attribute.

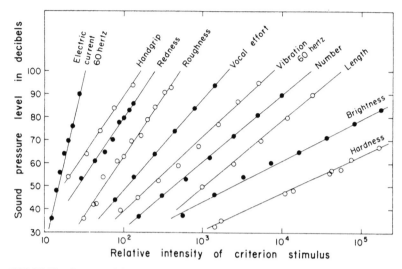

FIG. IV.20   Cross-modal matching of sound pressure in dB with 10 intensive attributes also measured in dB. From *Psychophysics* (p. 118) by S. S. Stevens, 1975, New York: Wiley. Copyright 1975 by John Wiley & Sons, Inc. Reprinted by permission.

TABLE IV.2
Exponents of Cross-modal Matches and the Predictions According to Equation IV.14

	Exponent obtained by handgrip	Predicted value	Difference in decilogs
Electric shock	2.13	2.06	0.14
Warmth on arm	0.96	0.94	0.09
Heaviness of lifted weights	0.79	0.85	0.32
Pressure on palm	0.67	0.65	0.13
Cold on arm	0.60	0.59	0.07
Vibration, 60 hertz	0.56	0.56	0.00
Loudness of white noise	0.41	0.39	0.22
Loudness of 1000-hertz tone	0.35	0.39	0.47
Brightness of white light	0.21	0.20	0.21
Average			$0.18 = 4.4\%$

Note: From *Psychophysics* (p. 113) by S. S. Stevens, 1975, New York: Wiley. Copyright 1975 by John Wiley & Sons, Inc. Reprinted by permission.

3.4 Additivity of Loudness

If two *independent* sources of sound are combined, it is plausible that the loudness of the combination should be the sum of their separate loudness. The operative word here is "independent," and it has taken some time to arrive at a suitable definition. Now we take independence to mean that the two sounds do not stimulate the same peripheral neurons. In terms of the peripheral tuning curves, we see that the two cases of panel a of Fig. IV.21 are not independent, whereas those of panel b are.

So we do not expect to obtain independence when the two signals are near to one another in the (I, f) space. In particular, independence will fail if the signals are of the same frequency and similar intensities. We do expect independence whenever two frequencies are widely separated and the intensities are not too great or whenever the two ears are separately stimulated.

The simplest experiment to perform is as follows: Alternate between presenting a tone to one ear (the monaural condition) and tones to the two ears (the binaural condition) of identical intensity and of the same frequency as was used in the monaural condition. The observer adjusts the intensity level of the pair until the loudness of the binaural presentation matches the loudness of the monaural one. In terms of dB, one finds the matching relation shown in Fig. IV.22. Note that at low intensity the

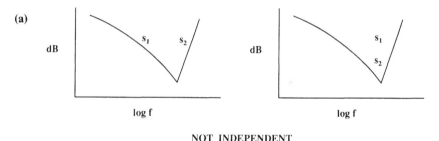

NOT INDEPENDENT

whereas the following are two are independent:

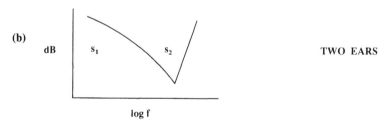

INDEPENDENT

FIG. IV.21 A schematic of typical auditory neural tuning curves showing two configurations of stimuli that are activating the same neuron, and so are deemed not independent, and two configurations—one monaural (single ear) and the other binaural (both ears)—in which signals do not activate the same neurons, and so are deemed independent. One expects additivity of loudness in the independent case.

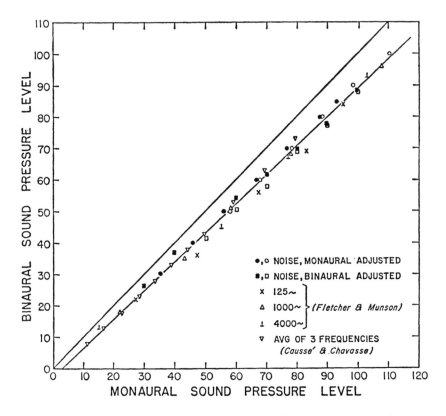

FIG. IV.22 A plot of the intensity, in dB, in a binaural presentation that matches in loudness the intensity, in dB, in a monaural presentation. The line with slope 1 represents identical intensities. It takes more intensity in one ear to seem as loud as an intensity in two ears. From "Binaural Summation of Loudness" by G. S. Reynolds and S. S. Stevens, 1960, *Journal of the Acoustical Society of America, 32,* p. 1341. Copyright 1960 by American Institute of Physics. Reprinted by permission.

difference is about 3 dB, but it increases to as much as 10 to 12 dB at high intensities. These data, however, tell us little about whether or not loudness is additive. To study that, a more complex procedure is needed.

The experimental procedure that can be followed is to let (s_1, s_2) denote the combined presentation of separate signals s_1 and s_2. The observer is then asked to judge whether presentation (s_1, s_2) is louder or softer than presentation (s_1', s_2'). Observe that this is a natural generalization of equal loudness judgments.

The mathematical analysis of such data is based on a method, called *additive conjoint measurement,* that shows how to construct an additive subjective scale, if one exists. Although it is too technical to describe fully here, we can report the results of two applications, one in 1972 to two-ear data and one in 1986 to widely separated frequencies. Additive scales were successfully constructed in each case so that (s_1, s_2) is judged louder than (s_1', s_2') when and only when

$$L(s_1) + L(s_2) > L(s_1') + L(s_2').$$

Furthermore, the loudness scale constructed in this way satisfies Stevens' law—it is a power function of I with an exponent near 0.3, as in the magnitude methods. Because nothing about the additive method forces power functions, some scientists interpret this as converging evidence in support of Stevens' method and his empirical generalization.

4. BRIDGING LOCAL
AND GLOBAL PSYCHOPHYSICS

The methods and results of the two types of psychophysics—local and global—are really quite distinct. The nearest thing to a bridge between them that we have seen so far is the Weber function, which describes how the local results vary over the entire space. But, as was remarked earlier, that is really only a local result, because the experiments used to determine any Weber fraction are entirely local in character, involving stimuli that differ by only 1 or 2 dB (see Figs. IV.4–7). So we need some additional methods. Two have been suggested.

One is to collect magnitude estimation data from individual observers using many signals and many magnitude estimates for each signal, as was true for the data shown in Fig. IV.17. Then one can examine the variability of the responses when the stimuli span a large range and ask how that variability relates to the variability discovered in local experiments. Research of this type has been done, but the results are moderately complex to describe, especially because there are very significant sequential effects, that is, the response to a stimulus is affected not only by that stimulus but also by previous stimuli and responses. So we confine our attention to the other method, which is to generalize the two-alternative absolute identification procedure.

4.1 Absolute Identification[10]

Recall that local absolute identification experiments involve trials on which one of two nearby signals is presented at random and the observer is required to try to identify which one has been presented. This is repeated

---

[10]These experiments are sometimes called *absolute judgment,* although "judgment" seems a misnomer for what is involved.

many times to get estimates of the probability of correctly identifying each signal. When there are only two signals and they differ only in intensity, this amounts to saying whether the signal presented is the more or less intense one.

This method can be generalized to a design in which there are N signals, each of which has an equal chance of being presented on a trial, and the observer is to identify which of the N it is. If the signals differ in just one attribute, such as either intensity or frequency but not both, then they are ordered from the least to the most intense or from the lowest to the highest frequency. That ordering can be used as one way of identifying each signal. Each time a signal is presented, the observer is asked to state which ranked position it holds in the series. One way is to provide an ordered set of N response keys and instruct the observer to press the key corresponding to the signal presented. Usually the signals are spaced in equal dB steps, which is true of the data shown here.

The data from such an experiment can be thought of as forming a table of percentages in which the rows correspond to the possible signal presentations and the columns to the possible responses. Thus, there are N rows and N columns. The cell entry of row i and column j is the percentage of times that response j is made when stimulus i is presented. The entry in cell (i, i) is the percentage of correct responses made when signal i is presented; all of the other cells in row i constitute errors of varying degrees of incorrectness.

4.1.1 Intensity Identification.   Figure IV.23 shows the percentages of correct responses in a study using $N = 10$ signals, where successive ones were spaced 5 dB apart. It is characteristic of absolute identification data that the most extreme signals are correctly identified much more often than are those in the middle of the range. This is not a question of which physical signals happen to be the end ones, because when the region spanned by the signals is changed, whatever signals happen to be the ends of the range in use are identified better than the others. The last statement is true provided the observer knows the range; however, if after some hundreds or thousands of trials, the experimenter changes the range without letting the observer know that a change has been effected, then the new endpoints continue to be just as poorly identified as they were when the range was larger. Results of this sort strongly suggest that at least some of what goes on is determined in the central nervous system, not in the periphery.

It is obvious that if we reduce the number of signals over a fixed range, then the percentage of correct responses will increase. In the extreme, with only two signals, any range beyond, being generous, 5 dB produces perfect identification. So, it is interesting to see how performance varies with both range and number of signals. The data in the literature report performance in terms of various measures that are suggested by certain theories. To

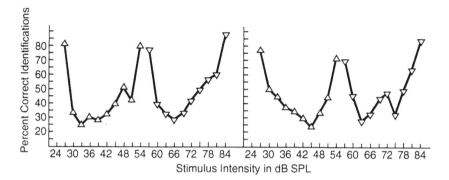

Stimulus Intensity in dB SPL

FIG. IV.23 Percent correct identifications in a 10-stimulus absolute-identification experiment in which signal intensity was varied. Each panel represents the data of an individual subject run in two conditions. In the one the 10 signals were spaced 3 dB apart in the range 27 to 54 dB SPL and in the other from 57 to 84 SPL. Each data point is based on 1,200 presentations of that intensity. Note the pronounced end effects: The ends of the range are correctly identified 80% of the time whereas those in the middle are correct as little as 25% of the time. Adapted from "Effects of Practice and Distribution of Auditory Signals on Absolute Indentification" by D. L. Weber, D. M. Green, R. D. Luce, 1977, *Perception & Psychophysics, 22,* p. 228. Copyright 1977 by The Psychonomic Society, Inc. Adapted by permission.

explain them fully would require an extended discussion; suffice it to say that they are closely related to percent correct.

Figure IV.24 shows performance as a function of the number of signals (in logarithmic coordinate) for a fixed range of 95 dB. (To get the number of signals, raise 2 to the power of the number shown; thus 3 in the figure corresponds to $2^3 = 8$ signals.) The diagonal line corresponds to perfect

FIG. IV.24 A measure of absolute identification performance as the number of signals equally spaced in dB over a 95 dB is varied. The number can be obtained from the "input information" by raising 2 to that power (i.e., input information $= \log_2 N$, where N is the number of stimuli). Note the lack of improvement in performance once the number exceeds about 7. From "The magical number seven plus or minus two: Some limits on our capacity for processing information" by G. A. Miller, 1956, *Psychological Review, 63,* p. 84. Copyright 1956 by the American Psychological Association. Reprinted by permission.

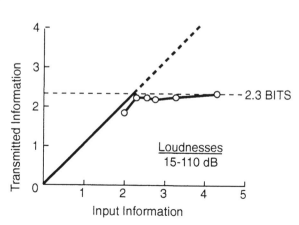

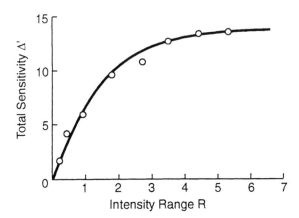

FIG. IV.25 A measure of absolute identification performance as the range of 10 signals equally spaced in dB is varied. The range is measured in dB/10. Note that the rate of improvement in performance diminishes rapidly with increasing range. From "Intensity Perception II: Resolution in One-interval Paradigms" by L. D. Braida and N. I. Durlach, 1972, *Journal of the Acoustical Society of America, 51*, p. 491. Copyright 1972 by American Institute of Physics. Reprinted by permission.

identification. We see that up to about 7 signals, which means that adjacent ones are spaced slightly more than 15 dB apart, identification is perfect. But adding more signals creates a pattern of confusion so that performance measured in this way remains constant and percentage correct for each signal decreases.

Figure IV.25 shows another measure of performance against signal range (measured in Bels, where one Bel = 10 dB) where the number of equally spaced signals was always 10. Despite the fact that the signals become more separated as the range increases, they do not become much more identifiable. The rate of improvement in performance is far greater when the range is 20 dB or less than it is when it is 50 dB, despite the fact that the stimuli are very closely packed when the range is small.

4.1.2 Frequency Identification and Absolute Pitch.   Results similar to those just described are found on all sensory dimensions, and they seem to reflect something basic about the way the central nervous system processes signal information.

The only partial exception to this generalization is that a small fraction of the population exhibit something called *absolute pitch*—a remarkable ability to listen to an isolated tone and to identify its frequency, as a note on the standard scale, with great accuracy. One study reported data on seven people who claimed to have absolute pitch and seven control subjects who made no such claim. All were run in an absolute identification experiment. The data, which are shown in Fig. IV.26, are plotted in a

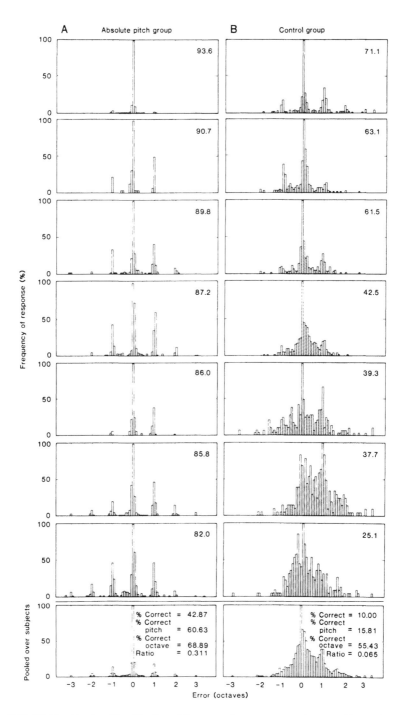

FIG. IV.26 Absolute identification of frequency for two groups of seven subjects. One group was composed of people claiming absolute pitch and the other was a control group of people making no such claim. The most frequent response is plotted as 100% and the others are relative to it. Note that those claiming absolute pitch do indeed have it to a large degree and that a substantial fraction of their errors are octave (factor of 2) mistakes. From "People with Absolute Pitch Process Tones Without Producing a P300" by M. Klein, M. G. H. Coles, and E. Donchin, 1984, *Science, 223,* p. 1307. Copyright 1984 by American Association for Advancement of Sciences. Reprinted by permission.

slightly unusual fashion. The performance is described by setting the most probable response at 100% and all others as a percentage of that. These percentages are plotted against the magnitude of the error shown on the abscissa, with its unit shown as octaves,[11] that is, factors of two in frequency. We see not only that the subjects who say they have absolute pitch are far more accurate than are ordinary subjects, but also that a large fraction of their errors are octave errors — they know the note, but not always the octave.

4.2 The Conundrum

The effect for auditory intensity may be summarized as follows:

Any two signals 5 dB apart can be correctly identified 100% of the time in a 2-stimulus identification experiment. Yet those same two signals are badly confused when they are adjacent in a 10-stimulus identification experiment.

This is a bit of a conundrum for several reasons.

First, it is certainly not true that any 10 stimuli are necessarily confused: Anyone can absolutely identify more than 10 people (hundreds or thousands is more likely) or more than 10 words (something well over 50,000 in reality) or more than 10 phonemes (more like 40), the basic auditory units of speech (see Section VI.7.2.1). The result reported has something to do with the fact that the signals lie on just one dimension. With multidimensional stimuli, absolute identification improves markedly.

Second, the phenomenon described is by no mean unique to auditory intensity or even intensity in general; it appears to apply to any one dimension of sensory stimuli, with the partial exception of frequency.

Third, it is difficult to understand why the brain has no trouble in identifying the signals when only two are involved and great trouble when others are also involved. After all, as far as is presently known, the information available in the peripheral auditory nervous system, on the auditory nerve, is totally unaffected by what other signals *might* have been presented. Rather it depends only on the signal actually presented. Thus, we know from the two-stimulus case that the peripheral information is quite adequate to distinguish the signals perfectly. This argument applies to every pair of signals in the *N*-signal experiment. And yet they are, in fact, confused.

The question simply is: What generates the observed confusion when there are many signals?

---

[11]Section V.2 makes clear why it is reasonable to use octave measures.

4.3 Possible Explanations

Two major ideas have been proposed to explain the apparent inconsistency. Both, which are outlined briefly and qualitatively, assume that the relevant, but unobservable, sensory variable on which identification decisions are based can be thought of as a number that varies from presentation to presentation of the same signal.[12] For example, it might be an estimate of the neural firing rate on those neurons that are firing above the resting rate and below the maximum rate, or it might be the total number of neurons that are firing at maximum rate. Whatever the source of the number, it differs somewhat from presentation to presentation of the same signal. That is, some naturally occurring variability exists in the information available at the periphery. Moreover, as the signal intensity increases, these numbers tend, on average, also to increase.

So in the case of two signals, the brain need only set a **criterion** on the firing rate such that when the sensory variable exceeds the criterion the brain concludes it was the more intense signal and when that variable falls below the criterion the brain concludes it is the less intense signal.

Models of this type, which are associated with the name of L. L. Thurstone and in psychophysics are often called *signal detection models,* have been shown to be very accurate in accounting for absolute identification results in great detail.

However, when the same model is applied to the data from different ranges, one has to conclude that as the range increases either the representation of the signal becomes more variable or the criteria used to distinguish between adjacent signals becomes more variable or both. Several studies, which are too technical to describe here, suggest that both changes occur. Either interpretation, however, raises questions.

4.3.1 Variable Criteria. It is by no means clear why the brain cannot maintain the levels of, let us say, 9 criteria in a 10-stimulus experiment; this does not seem an excessive memory load. One line of argument about this failure assumes that the criteria tend to be shifted away from the most recently presented signal in an amount proportional to the available space to the boundaries of the signal range. Thus, the space around the most recently presented signal is opened, and all other intervals are proportionately narrowed. When many stimuli intervene between two presentations of the same signal, then the criterion can be shifted about quite a bit, which is a source of variability in the data. In other words, the criteria are not fixed numbers, but rather highly variable ones that depend on the exact past

---

[12]Technically, such a representation of the percept of a signal is called a *random variable.*

history of the experiment. Certain analyses of sequential effects in the data give considerable support to this idea.

4.3.2 Neural Attention.   The other idea is that the stimulus representation is, in fact, poorer on average when the range is large than when it is small. Indeed both processes may underlie the observer's performance.

As was noted earlier, one objection to assuming that the signal representation is increasingly more variable with increasing stimulus range is the fact that, as far as anyone knows, the peripheral neural activity resulting from an auditory signal is unaffected by what other signals might have been presented. If that is true, and it appears to be, then the reason for the reduced quality of information must lie not in the periphery, but more centrally.

One suggestion is that the central nervous system is unable to monitor simultaneously all of the information available in the peripheral system. Rather it must focus on only a part of the frequency-intensity "scene," sampling information about the rest of it much less fully. Such incomplete monitoring of most input information but with full monitoring of a limited portion is characteristic of hierarchial systems with executive control. In this case, one may think of this as monitoring all of a group of similar neurons versus monitoring only a fraction of them. Such focused or selective "attention" creates no difficulty when all of the signals are sufficiently close together so that they all activate the same set of neurons whose activity is then monitored fully. But when the signals are so separated that they activate different groups of neurons, then only one group can be monitored fully and the rest only partially. In analogy with vision, the region being monitored is perceived, like images on the fovea, in sharp detail, and the rest of the scene, like peripheral vision, is far fuzzier.

This idea of limited attention in the ability to monitor peripheral neurons provides a conceptual meaning to the distinction between local and global psychophysics. When the signals are sufficiently separated, then, no matter where the central system attends, some of the signals must fall outside that region and so they will be very imperfectly represented, not in the periphery but centrally. This situation is global relative to the case where all of the signals fall within the scope of a single neuron. Clearly, as the signals become more widely separated, the chance is greater that any one presentation falls outside the region of attention.

The latter idea suggested running a two-stimulus experiment on the absolute identification of frequency that has two unusual features. First, the signals were presented randomly at intensities spanning a large, 50 dB, range instead of being at one fixed intensity, as is usually the case in studying frequency discrimination. Second, that range was not spanned in the usual uniform way. Rather, all but two of the intensities were clustered into a subrange of 10 dB, an intensity interval that is well within the estimated width of the attention mechanism. The remaining two intensities were located at either 20 or 40 dB from the nearest edge of the 10 dB interval.

Three conditions were run, as is illustrated in Fig. IV.27. One had the 10 dB interval at the bottom, one in the middle, and the third at the top of the 50 dB range. According to the hypothesis, the attention mechanism will tend to focus itself on the 10 dB interval, because that is where most of the action is. If so, then the representation of those signals will be much better than for the outliers, and so frequency identification should be better for intensities in the interval than for those outside it. Note that each intensity that is an outlier in one condition is also within the 10 dB interval in another condition. Thus, the frequency identification performance for such an intensity level can be directly compared when it is an outlier and when it is a member of the 10 dB cluster. The data are shown in Fig. IV.28, where the outliers are shown in black and a line shows its deviation from the performance when it is in a cluster. In many cases the predicted deterioration in frequency performance for the outliers is observed.

Experimental attempts have been made to manipulate the attention mechanism experimentally through feedback and payoffs, but these have failed. Apparently such a mechanism, if it exists at all, is relatively involuntary and is affected primarily by stimulus patterns.

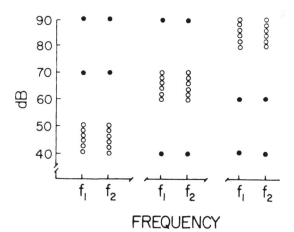

FIG. IV.27   The design of a two-frequency absolute identification experiment in which the signal intensities were selected at random from among eight levels. These levels were grouped in the three patterns shown. Each outlier is shown as a solid circle and appears in the cluster of one of the other patterns. From "Two Tests of a Neural Attention Hypothesis for Auditory Psychophysics" by R. D. Luce and D. M. Green, 1978, *Perception & Psychophysics, 23*, p. 369. Copyright 1978 by The Psychonomic Society of America. Reprinted by permission.

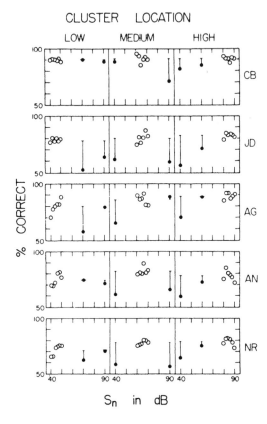

CLUSTER   LOCATION

FIG. IV.28 Percent correct responding for the design shown in Fig. IV.27. Again, the outliers are shown as solid circles with a line showing the drop from their behavior when that pair of signals is in the cluster. In some, but not all, cases, the loss predicted (see text) is observed. From "Two Tests of a Neural Attention Hypothesis for Auditory Psychophysics" by R. D. Luce and D. M. Green, 1978, *Perception & Psychophysics, 23*, p. 369. Copyright 1978 by The Psychonomic Society of America. Reprinted by permission.

Additional evidence is given in Section VI.3.2 on so-called critical bands that can be interpreted as being consistent with the idea of selective attention.

In order to discuss these and other experiments of interest, it is necessary to gain some understanding of signals more complex than pure tones. We turn in Section V to the physics of more complex sounds.

5. SUMMARY

Both behavioral observations and the patterns of neural activity seen in the peripheral auditory system suggest that one must make a local-global distinction. Local experiments are those for which the stimuli involved mostly activate the same neurons, whereas global ones involve the activation of quite distinct groups of neurons. Within the local context, one attempts to study the quality of the performance using detection, discrimination, and identification designs resulting in such things as Weber fractions and functions and estimates of percent correct responding. The behavior is highly consistent among subjects for intensity (a prothetic dimension) and considerably less so for frequency (a metathetic dimension). All of the local designs admit the possibility of feedback and rewards because there are correct and incorrect responses.

The global methods, with one exception, are different in that they ask observers to make judgments that are neither correct or incorrect; the judgments are what the observers say they perceive. Among these methods are equal attribute contours, magnitude estimation and production, and cross-modal matching. Some of these results have focused on the subjective scaling of loudness, and two "laws" – the logarithmic one of Fechner and the power one of Stevens – have played a controversial role.

The only method common to the two domains, absolute identification, leads to a quandary. Two stimuli that can be correctly identified 100% of the time when they are tested alone become highly confused when embedded in an experiment with numerous other stimuli varying in the same attribute that must also be identified when they are presented. This is a quandary because, so far as anyone knows, the peripheral representation of the signals is totally unaffected by what other signals might have been presented. Thus, in principle, there is no more or less information when a particular signal is presented in a 2-stimulus or in a 10-stimulus experiment. But, functionally, there is a vast difference. Explanations in terms of variable criteria and limited monitoring capability were outlined.

6. FURTHER READING

Boring (1950) is the classic history of experimental psychology up to midcentury, but the theoretical debates of local psychophysics are better summarized in the first eight chapters of Link's (1992) comprehensive treatment. The theory underlying ROC curves and procedures for data analysis are given in considerable technical detail in at least three places: Egan (1975), Green and Swets (1974), and Macmillan and Creelman (1991). Green and Swets is the classic in the field, but for beginners Macmillan and Creelman is probably more accessible. Laming (1986) developed a sweeping, novel view of local psychophysics. Although his book is not excessively mathematical, it is subtle and sophisticated.

Global methods are not as comprehensively surveyed as the local methods. Stevens (1975) presented his views in a highly readable form, but some of his views are considered quite controversial by others. A very different view, not much represented in the present text, is Anderson (1981, 1982). Bolanowski and Gescheider (1991) is a collection of papers from a conference focused on Stevens' approach to the scaling of magnitude.

Critiques, with commentary, of the scaling issue are by Kreuger (1989) and Lockhead (1992).

The issues of bridging the local and global results are mostly discussed in the journal literature, and I am not aware of a good secondary source. The classic paper that first brought the issue of bridging the two domains to wide attention is Miller (1956). Luce and Nosofsky (1984) described both the variable criterion and attention models and some of the data that bear on them. Further references on the variable criterion approach are Marley and Cook (1984, 1986), Treisman (1985), and Treisman and Williams (1984).

PART V

Descriptive Physics of Complex Sounds

This part concerns how several pure tone waves combine physically to form more complex sounds, such as notes with overtones and chords in music and, potentially, even speech. Various aspects of their interaction play an important role in our hearing. But, there is much about the hearing of complex sounds that cannot be accounted for by the physics of the situation or by that knowledge coupled with what we know about the peripheral nervous system.

1. SUPERPOSITION

1.1 Basic Principle of Superposition

If we have two or more simultaneous waveforms, then at each point in space and time a very simple superposition principle holds, namely **amplitudes add.** For sound waves, this means that the pressures add. This result is a consequence of the simple principle that if two forces are applied in the same direction, the resultant force is their sum.

1.1.1 Pulses. A simple example of such superposition of waves can be demonstrated with a rope or wire. Suppose it is held taut at opposite ends by two people and they simultaneously snap it in the same direction, each thereby initiating an identical one-sided pulse. So the two pulses are moving in opposite directions on the wire. Figure V.1 illustrates several "snapshots" of the situation. One sees that as the pulses come together, the one can be

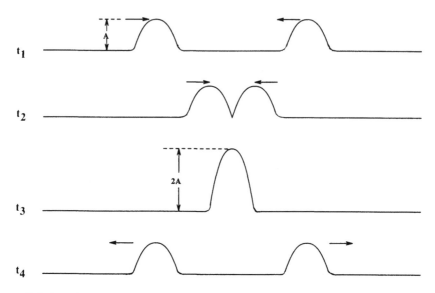

FIG. V.1 Two positive pulses of identical size and shape propagate along a wire toward each other at time t_1, reaching each other at time t_2, then superimposing so that at time t_3 the two amplitudes simply add, and at time t_4 they are moving away from each other.

thought of as climbing over the other, with the amplitudes adding, and then they come apart and continue on their separate ways.

Consider what happens if the two people snap the string to the same degree, but in opposite directions. One creates a pulse with a positive amplitude and the other one with an equal, but negative, amplitude, as in Fig. V.2. Here, again, the one pulse climbs over the other. However, because they have opposite amplitudes, instead of doubling the amplitude, they simply cancel each other and then move on.

1.1.2 Waves of Same Frequency. We next consider the simple case of two waves, each of the same frequency. They are the lighter curves; their sum is the darker curve. Three different snapshots taken at different phases are shown in Figs. V.3–5. With the same phase, Fig. V.3, there is simple summing of the two identical waves, thus producing a wave of the same frequency but double the amplitude. Turning next to two waves that are 90° out of phase, Fig. V.4, amplitude addition creates a more complex, but still periodic pattern. Continuing to change phase, when we get to 180°, Fig. V.5, the two waves are exactly opposed to one another, and their addition simply results in 0 amplitude throughout time.

Obviously, the difference of being in phase and completely out of phase is enormous – from doubling the amplitude to wiping it out.

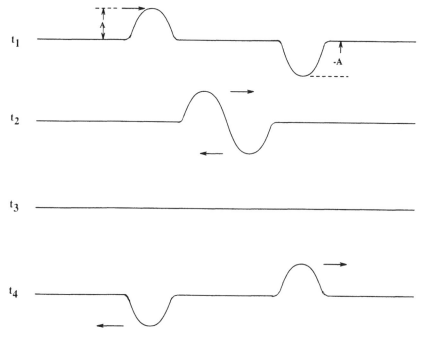

FIG. V.2 As in Fig. V.1, two pulses of identical size and shape, except that one is positive and the other is negative, propagate along a wire toward each other at time t_1, reaching each other at time t_2, then superimposing so that at time t_3 the two amplitudes simply cancel, and at time t_4 they are moving away from each other.

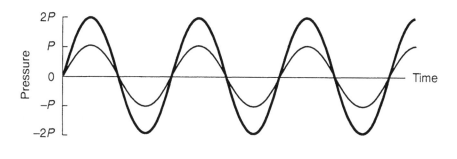

Phase Angle 0

FIG. V.3 Two identical sine waves of the same phase (shown as a single light curve) superimpose to produce a sine wave of double the amplitude (shown as the darker curve).

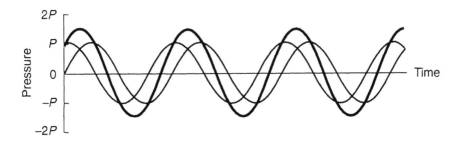

Phase Angle π/2

FIG. V.4   As in Fig. V.3, two identical sine waves are superimposed, but now they are 90° out of phase (the two lighter curves). The sum (the darker curve) is no longer a sine wave.

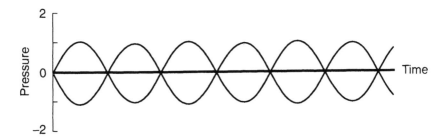

FIG. V.5   The phase separation of Fig. V.3 is now increased to 180° (the ligher curves), and the sine waves completely cancel each other everywhere (the darker line).

1.1.3 Application: Loudspeakers in an Open Field.   Let us assume that we have two loudspeakers, each playing the same pure tone. In order to avoid problems of reflected sound, which as is explained in Part VI makes a substantial contribution, consider them in an open field, shown from above in Fig. V.6. The curves show a snapshot of a horizontal slice of two patterns of spherical waves, centered on the two speakers. Similar transverse waves on the surface of water can, indeed, be photographed. The circles indicate the location of the maximum amplitude. The dots show the intersections of these maxima, which therefore are points of **constructive interference**—the maximum amplitudes add together. The crosses locate some of the points where the two waves are out of phase (phase angle $= \pi$), that is, where a peak of one and a trough of the other intersection, in which case we speak of **destructive interference**—the amplitudes cancel each other.

To get some idea of how these events are spaced, suppose f is the frequency of the pure tone. Because $c = 344$ m/s, we have the following pairings of frequency and wavelength:

FIG. V.6 Looking from above at a cross-section of the spherical wave patterns produced from two loudspeakers each emitting the same sine wave. The points of maximum pressure in a "snap shot" of each wave front are shown as (segments of) circles. The points of minimum pressure are circles located exactly half way between successive curves. Points of total maximum air pressure are where the solid curves intersect, a few of which are marked by dots. The points at which the pressure change is 0 are where a maximum and a minimum intersect, several of which are shown as crosses. (The plot ignores the decay of pressure with distance from the speakers.)

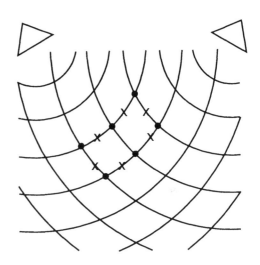

f(Hz)	λ
34.4	10m
344	1m
3440	10cm

At first, this appears to mean that there are serious interaction effects on the loudness of frequencies well within the normal range of voices and music. However, the situation is not as bad as it first seems because loudspeakers are usually found in rooms where the summation pattern is vastly more complex because of reflections off the walls, ceiling, and floor. And so although the interference is always present, it does not have a clear-cut, bad effect as in the special situation of out-of-doors loudspeakers.

1.2 Mathematics of Adding Waves

1.2.1 Same Frequency but Different Phase. If two sine waves of the same frequency and amplitude but different phase, say,

$$p_1 = P \sin 2\pi ft$$

and

$$p_2 = P \sin (2\pi ft + \phi),$$

are simultaneously present, then, because superposition simply means that the pressures add together, we obtain

$$p_1 + p_2 = P[\sin 2\pi ft + \sin(2\pi ft + \phi)].$$

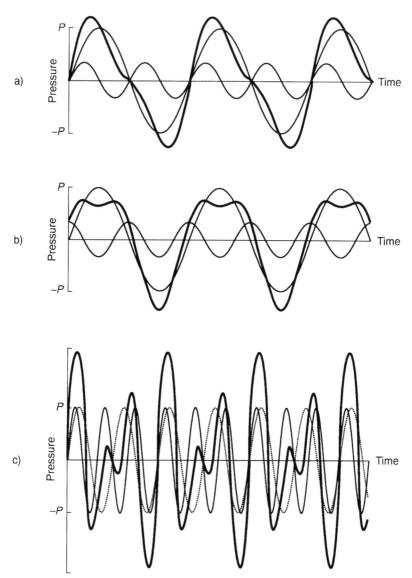

FIG. V.7 Superposition (darker curve) of waves *(f, P)* and (2*f, P*/3) (shown as lighter curves). Panel a shows the case where they are in phase. Panel b shows the case where the second wave is displaced by π/2 relative to the first. Note how different the resultant waveform appears with the change of phase. Panel c shows two waves *(f, P)* and (3*f*/2, *P*), which yields a more complex, but periodic waveform.

For the phase angles $0 = 0, 2\pi, 4\pi, \ldots$, the waves are said to be *in phase* and their sum is maximally constructive:

$$p_1 + p_2 = 2P \sin 2\pi ft.$$

For the angles $0 = \pi, 3\pi, 5\pi, \ldots$, the waves are said to be *out of phase* and their sum is maximally destructive:

$$p_1 + p_2 = 0.$$

1.2.2 Different Frequencies and Phases.   The previous mathematics changes very little if waves 1 and 2 have different frequencies, say f_1 and f_2. The picture, however, can get considerably more complex, as shown in Fig. V.7. Thus, we see that how two waves combine differs hugely depending on their phase. Surprisingly, the ear is remarkably insensitive to this, although not totally.

1.2.3 Beats.   One special case of considerable importance is when the two waves have nearly the same frequency. In that case, the overall envelope of the wave exhibits a periodicity at the difference frequency $f_1 - f_2$. This is shown in Fig. V.8. If the difference in frequencies is sufficiently

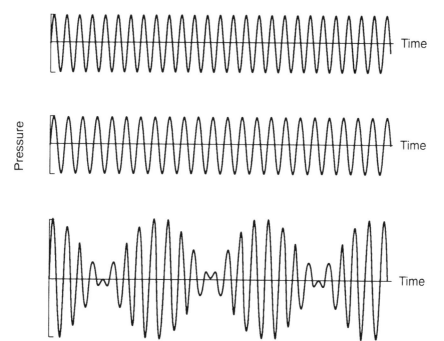

FIG. V.8   The superposition of two waves of the same amplitude, P, but a small difference in frequency of about $\Delta f = 1.57$ Hz. The resultant wave has an amplitude envelope that varies from 0 to $2P$ with the frequency Δf. This slow waxing and waning of the amplitude can be heard and is called beating.

small, only a few Hertz, then one is quite aware of the periodic waxing and waning of the sound. This pronounced fluctuation in the sound intensity is called **beating,** and can be heard in Demonstration 4. Subsequently, we find signs of beating in studies of the psychology of hearing complex sounds. Before turning to that, however, there are other issues about the physics of complex sounds.

1.3 Diffraction

Consider a sound source in a room with an open door or window, as illustrated in Fig. V.9. As the sound passes through each point of the door, it acts like a local source and generates a spherical wave front. Several are shown spanning the doorway. In addition, there are an infinity of others from each point in the doorway. The net result is for destructive interference to be worse the farther one is off the perpendicular from the middle of the door, as sketched in the sound distribution. The exact mathematical analysis of the infinity of interferences involved is complex, but the answer is simple. If d_{AC} denotes the distance interval of significant sound along a line parallel to the side of the room at the distance D from the doorway of width W, then it can be shown that:

$$d_{AC} = 2Dc/Wf,$$

where c denotes the speed of sound, f is the frequency of a pure tone sound source, and where all distances, including that involved in c, are in the same units.

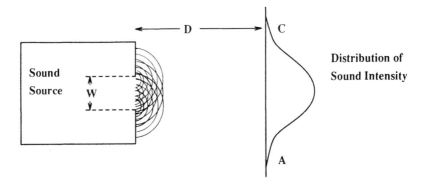

FIG. V.9 A top view of sound generated in a room exiting a relatively small opening, such as a door. In effect, there are a series of sources of spherical waves all across the door, and these superimpose to produce some maximum pressure at every point outside. The distribution of such pressures along a line is shown, and the text provides a formula for the distance AC as a function of the other distances and frequency of the source.

Observe that, because f appears in the denominator, low frequencies disperse more widely than do high ones. A numerical example is useful. For this we suppose $D = 10W$ and $c = 344$ m/s:

f	d_{AC} (in m)
100	68.8
1,000	6.88
10,000	0.688

As one can see, the effect is substantial. The low frequencies really do disperse far more than do the high ones, which are virtually focused. This has an obvious differential effect on complex sounds, such as speech. Only the low frequencies of speech spread through a door. Section VI.7.1 establishes that the loss of high frequencies does not greatly affect the intelligibility of speech.

2. STANDING WAVES

We turn next to the physics that underlies all musical instruments, namely wave motions that remain fixed over time in some physical object such as a wire under tension or a vibrating air column.

2.1 Transverse Reflections

2.1.1 Pulse on a Wire.   Suppose we have a wire rigidly fixed at one end, as illustrated in part a of Fig. V.10. If a symmetrical pulse is initiated and runs down the wire toward the wall, we get the sequence of temporal snapshots shown in parts b through e. Note that the pulse is reflected at the wall, and then returns as a pulse in the opposite phase, in the sense that the reduced amplitude precedes the increased one.

2.1.2 Wave on a Wire.   Next suppose that instead of a pulse, one produces a sine wave, which is really a train of pulses. Then as each pulse is reflected, it encounters not the unmoving wire of the previous example but rather the continuing input wave. Thus, the situation is exactly the same as the superposition of two waves of the same frequency and amplitude, but varying phase. The result will vary in time from the flat string, to the superposition of the two in phase, thereby doubling the amplitude, then again to an absence of any response, and so on.

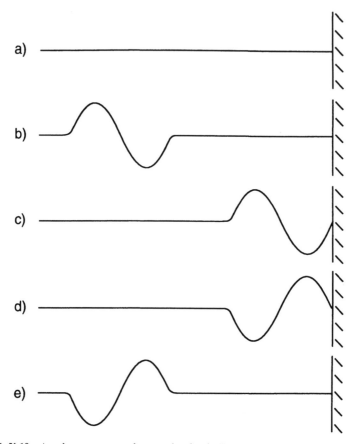

FIG. V.10   A pulse propagates along a wire that is firmly attached to the wall. When the pulse reaches the wall, it is reflected and propagates back along the wire. This is readily demonstrated.

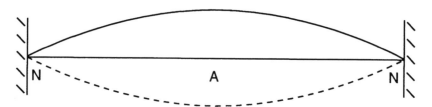

FIG. V.11   Plucking a wire that is attached firmly at both ends generates pulses in both directions and they reflect at the walls, resulting in a complex series of superpositions. The net effect is a pattern of vibrations known as a standing wave, and the overall amplitude pattern is a portion of a sine wave that has zero amplitude at each fixed point of the wire. These points of zero amplitude are called nodes, N, and those of maximum amplitude antinodes, A. The simplest pattern can be described as NAN and is called the fundamental frequency, or first harmonic, of the wire.

2.2 Transverse Standing Waves

2.2.1 Fundamental Frequency.   The next more complicated case is a wire held rigidly at both ends, and the pulse is initiated by deflecting the wire exactly in the middle. In that case pulses go forth from the middle to both ends, reflect, and return, continually interacting with each other. The net result of the interaction of the initiated wave and its reflection from the walls is to produce the envelop of wire positions, with two stationary points, one at each wall, shown in Fig. V.11. These stationary points are known as **nodes,** and are denoted by N. The point in the middle of maximum amplitude is known as an **antinode,** and it is denoted by A. This is an example of a transverse standing wave, known as the **first harmonic** of the wire or, equivalently, as its **fundamental frequency.** You can readily produce an example of such a standing wave using a rubber band around your thumb and forefinger.

2.2.2 Harmonics (or Overtones).   Other standing wave patterns are possible. For example, the **second harmonic,** also called the **first overtone,** exhibits the envelope shown in panel a of Fig. V.12. So the second harmonic has the node/antinode pattern of NANAN. In like manner, the third harmonic or second overtone has the pattern NANANAN shown in panel b. The general case of the ***n*th-harmonic** consists of *n* NAN loops, as in panel c.

2.2.3 Harmonic Frequencies and Length of a Wire.   Observe that the distance between successive nodes, a NAN distance, is one half the wavelength of the standing wave. Thus, if there are *n* such loops on a wire of length *L,* and if λ_n denotes the wavelength, then necessarily:

$$L = n(\lambda_n/2) \leftrightarrow \lambda_n = 2L/n. \tag{1}$$

As we know, a transverse pulse on a wire has a characteristic speed *c,* and we recall (Section II.3.2.2) that wavelength and wave frequency are related by

$$\lambda_n = c/f_n. \tag{2}$$

Eliminating the wavelength from Equations 1 and 2 and solving for the frequency, we find the frequency of the *n*th-harmonic is:

$$f_n = n(c/2L). \tag{3}$$

Observe further that

$$f_n = nf_1, \tag{4}$$

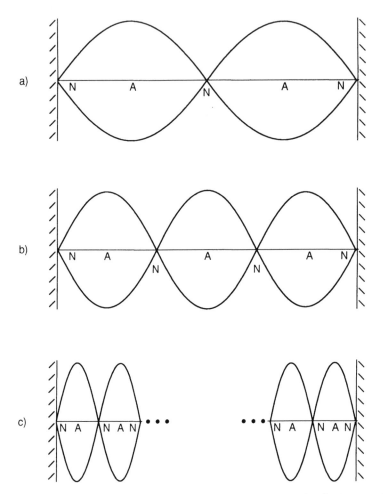

FIG. V.12 Higher harmonics of a wire with fixed ends. Panel a is the second harmonic, with the next possible pattern NANAN. Panel b shows the third harmonic. And Panel c the general patterns of a standing wave.

that is, the frequency of the nth-harmonic is exactly n times that of the fundamental frequency.

There are, therefore, two possible ways to control the value of the fundamental frequency, f_1, of a string of an instrument: vary either L or c or both. In the case of the piano and the harp, the value of L is determined structurally; whereas in the so-called stringed instruments, such as the violin and the cello, L is varied by the bridge location and by fingering. The value of c is determined by two primary factors, namely, the tension, τ, on the wire and the density, ρ, of the material composing it. Specifically, it can be shown that:

$$c = k(\tau/\rho)^{1/2}, \qquad (5)$$

where k is a constant. Clearly, c is not subject to change during the performance, but its value can differ among the several strings on an instrument.

Which harmonics are produced is determined by the exact way the performer activates the string during the performance. Learning to control this at will is a large part of the technical skill required to play an instrument such as a violin.

2.3 Compression (or Longitudinal) Waves

2.3.1 In a Room with Reflecting Walls.   Consider a room with reflecting walls and sound source at one wall and consider a pressure wave originating at a source at one end of the room. If the standing wave shown in Fig. V.13 is set up, then clearly there is a null in the middle of the room, which amounts to destructive interference. As an example, consider a room that is 10 m long, then by Equation 3 such a null will occur when:

$$\begin{aligned} f_2 &= 2(c/2L) \\ &= c/L \\ &= (344 \text{ m/s})/(10 \text{ m}) \\ &= 34.4 \text{ Hz.} \end{aligned}$$

Thus, it occurs in an ordinary size classroom only for very low frequencies. Note that as the size of the room is reduced, higher frequencies can exhibit such destructive standing waves.

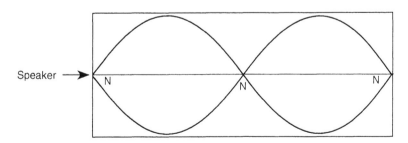

FIG. V.13   A standing wave in a room showing the case where there is a null in the middle of the room.

2.3.2 In a Half-Open Tube.   An example of a half-open tube is an organ pipe. The situation is diagrammed, with the compressive feature of air symbolized as a spring in panel a of Fig. V.14. Note that activation takes place at the open end of the tube, and it is here that one gets maximum amplitude. So it is an antinode. If we plot the amplitude of the compression, shown in panel b, we see the node/antinode pattern NA and that the wavelength of the first harmonic is four times the length of the tube. The next possible node/antinode pattern, bounded by N at the one end and by A at the other, is NANA, which is illustrated as panel c. Note that this wave is the third, not the second, harmonic of the fundamental. The second is impossible because it would place a node at the open end of the tube.

Of course, the general pattern is NAN . . . A, and so any odd harmonic can arise. If λ_n denotes the wavelength, then the following relations hold:

$$L = n(\lambda_n/4) = n(c/4f_n), \ n = 1, 3, 5, \ldots \tag{6}$$

$$f_n = n(c/4L) = nf_1, \ n = 1, 3, 5, \ldots \tag{7}$$

Note that no even harmonic can arise using a half-open tube.

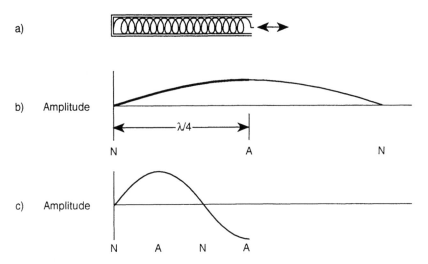

FIG. V.14   The generation of standing waves in a half-open tube. Panel a shows a model of the compression wave as a spring with one fixed end and the other being moved. Panel b shows the simplest standing wave, the fundamental, which has the pattern NA, with the antinode necessarily at the open end. The next possible pattern, shown in Panel c, is NANA, which corresponds to the third, not the second, harmonic of the fundamental. It is impossible to generate even harmonics with a half-open tube.

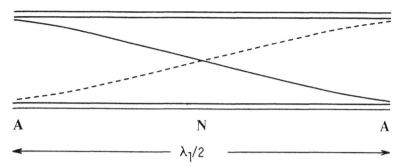

A   N   A

$\lambda_1/2$

FIG. V.15   The generation of standing wave in an open tube. There the pattern of the fundamental is ANA, which involves the same wavelength as the NAN pattern a string fixed at both ends. This formal identity, with N replacing A and A replacing N, holds for all harmonics.

2.3.3 In an Open Tube.   An example of an open tube is a horn. Here the pattern involves antinodes at both open ends, so the simplest one is ANA, as illustrated in Fig. V.15. The next possible pattern with A at both ends is ANANA. Clearly, the situation is formally identical to a string, and so all harmonics can arise and the same equations hold, in particular Equation 3, relating length, velocity, and frequency.

Of course, with wind instruments the value of c, in this case the speed of sound in air, cannot be manipulated, so the primary control of frequency is by means of the length of the tube and which harmonic is generated. The length can be controlled by either making it adjustable, as in a trombone, or by having the opening at one end controlled in some way by the performer. The control over the harmonics is in the mouth action in the case of wind instruments and horns.

3. SYNTHESIS OF A COMPLEX WAVE IN TERMS OF HARMONICS

It is clear that by adding to a wave a number of its harmonics in varying amplitudes, one can generate quite complex wave patterns. The problem addressed and solved in what is called **Fourier analysis** — named after an important French physicist from the early 19th century — is to find a recipe for combining the harmonics to produce any given periodic wave. A **periodic wave** is an amplitude pattern that repeats itself with some period T: If $p(t)$ denotes the pressure wave as a function of time t, then the condition is that for each t, $p(t + T) = p(t)$. Obviously a sine wave of period T meets this definition, as does the superposition of any finite number of its harmonics. We illustrate the Fourier decomposition in several special cases.

3.1 Spectrum of a Wave

3.1.1 Square Wave.   Our target candidate is a wave of the type shown in Fig. V.16. It is reasonably clear that a sine wave of period T, and so frequency $f = 1/T$, and amplitude P is a fair first approximation to the square wave. Of course, the square corners are going to have to be built up from higher frequency waves.

Consider, first, the second harmonic with frequency $f_2 = 2f_1$. Figure V.17 shows one period of it, somewhat enlarged to make the details clearer,

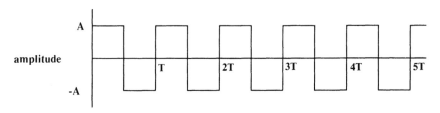

FIG. V.16   The waveform of an ideal square wave. The amplitude has the value A for a duration $T/2$ followed by $-A$ also for duration $T/2$, and so the period is T.

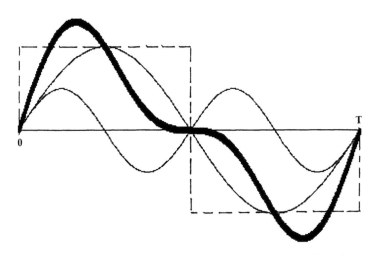

FIG. V.17   An attempt to approximate the square wave by superimposing a sine wave with period T and its second harmonic, using half the amplitude. The superposition fails to approximate the square wave because it introduces inappropriate asymmetries. This will happen if any of the even harmonics are added.

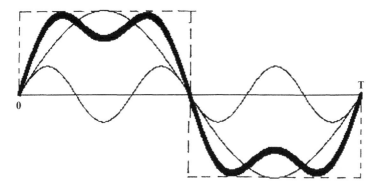

FIG. V.18 An attempt to approximate the square wave by superimposing a sine wave with period T and its third harmonic, using one third the amplitude. This approximation, while still far to go, exhibits the appropriate symmetries and is beginning to fill out the corners.

together with the fundamental and their sum. It is evident that the resulting asymmetry within each square is going in the wrong direction. Whatever is added should be symmetric around the loops of the fundamental. Thus, we omit f_2 from the recipe. And by an extension of this argument, we omit all of the even harmonics.

Figure V.18 shows what adding the third harmonic can do. Note that it is definitely a move in the correct direction; it is beginning to fill in the corners.

Without giving a proof, it turns out that by superimposing all of the odd harmonics with the nth-harmonic having peak pressure P/n yields the square wave. So, formally, the recipe is:

$$\text{Harmonic } f_n \text{ appears with amplitude } \begin{cases} 0 \text{ if } n \text{ is even} \\ P/n \text{ if } n \text{ is odd.} \end{cases}$$

If a wave is generated from the superposition of harmonics in varying amplitudes, then the graphical plot of these amplitudes is called the **spectrum** of the resulting wave.

Thus, from what we already stated, the spectrum of a square wave is as shown in Fig. V.19.

3.1.2 Sawtooth Wave.   Consider a wave of the sawtooth form shown in Fig. V.20. The spectrum in this case turns out to be every harmonic n in the amount P/n, which is plotted in Fig. V.21.

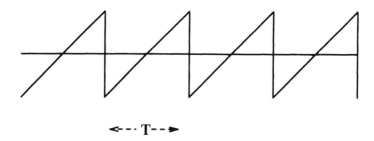

FIG. V.19 The plot of the amplitudes of the harmonics that when superimposed in these amounts reproduce exactly the square wave. This plot is called the spectrum of the square wave. All even harmonics have zero amplitude. Note that no phase information is provided by the plot, but to produce the square wave it is necessary that all harmonics be in phase.

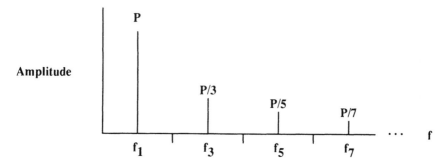

FIG. V.20 The pressure waveform called a sawtooth wave.

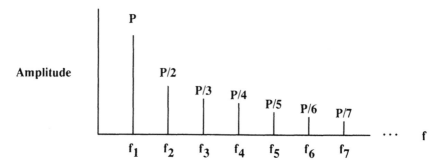

FIG. V.21 The spectrum for the sawtooth waveform.

3.1.3 Pulse Train.   A pulse train modifies the square wave in the sense that the durations of its maximum and minimum values are not the same. As shown in Fig. V.22, the period is T but the maximum pressure holds not for $T/2$, but some value $W < T$. Of course, it becomes a square wave when $W = T/2$.

The spectrum of such a pulse train is shown in Fig. V.23. Observe that the harmonics are at the values of n/T, but on top of that the spectrum has a damped oscillatory pattern in which the amplitude drops to zero at integer multiples of $1/W$.

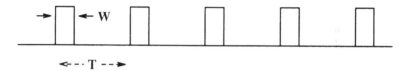

FIG. V.22   The pressure waveform of a pulse train. During each period T, the amplitude is A for a time interval of length W and 0 for the remaining time, $T - W$. (This wave becomes a square wave when $W = T/2$.)

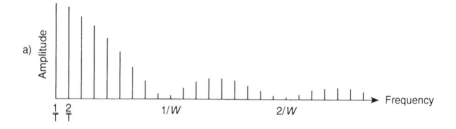

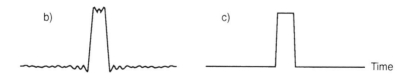

FIG. V.23   (a) The first 50 terms of the spectrum of a pulse train in which $W = T/10$. The amplitudes are all at harmonics, that is, frequencies of the form n/T, but the envelope has an overall pattern with minima at integral multiples of $1/W$. (b) One period of the pulse train reconstructed using the first 50 terms of the spectrum. (c) The same as panel b using the first 100 terms.

3.2 Spectral (or Fourier) Analysis

3.2.1 Fourier's Theorem.   Assuming the kinds of waves that can arise physically—those that do not change too abruptly—it is possible to prove mathematically that the kinds of recipes just given always exist for any periodic wave. That is, if wave has frequency f, then it can be reconstructed as a superposition, in appropriate amounts, of all of the harmonics of a sine wave with frequency f. This is quite a remarkable result. In essence it says that one can replace any periodic (sound) wave by a superposition of the harmonics of a pure tone having the same frequency as the given wave. This greatly simplifies many analyses, and it is widely used throughout physics and in its areas of applications. There are explicit formulas, beyond the scope of this text, for computing the amplitudes of the harmonics needed to reconstruct the given wave. There is also an empirical way to determine these amplitudes, which is described in Section V.3.2.3.

3.2.2 Loss of Phase Information.   Notice that from a spectrum one knows the frequencies and amplitudes of the components but nothing whatsoever about their phases relative to the fundamental. It is clear that from a single spectrum, one can produce, quite literally, an infinity of waveforms through the choices of the phases for the various harmonics. Put another way, for each spectrum, there is a family of "equivalent" wave-forms that look very different, but all have the same spectrum. The issue of phase will come up from time to time, and in some problems it is important to specify it.

3.2.3 Spectrum Analyzer.   Suppose a complex wave has the spectrum shown in panel a of Fig. V.24, and suppose a filter (see Section II.10.3) has the characteristic response pattern shown in panel b, then passing the input wave through the filter yields the wave that has only the part of the original spectrum that can pass the filter, namely that shown in panel c.

Thus, if a band pass filter has a sufficient high value of Q so that it spans less than the frequency of the fundamental of the wave, as shown in panel d, then passing the original wave through this filter will pass just the fifth harmonic of the Fourier decomposition of the input wave.

A **spectrum analyzer** is a machine that is composed of a collection of high Q band pass filters centered at a variety of frequencies in such a way that they do not overlap each other. The input wave is split into as many copies as there are filters, amplified, and then simultaneously each amplified copy is run through one of the filters. The outputs of the filters give an approximation to the spectrum of the periodic input wave—the degree of approximation depending on the number, spacing, and quality of the filters. The more filters, the more narrowly they are spaced, and the better

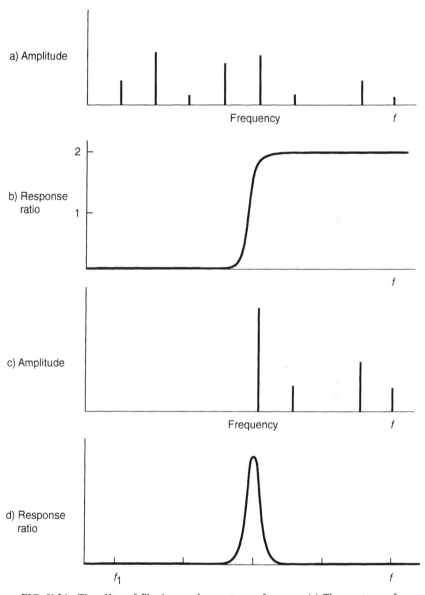

FIG. V.24 The effect of filtering on the spectrum of a wave. (a) The spectrum of a wave. (b) The response characteristic of a high pass filter. (c) The filter of panel b is applied to the wave of panel a to produce a waveform with the spectrum shown. Note that all frequencies of the original wave less than the filter cutoff are eliminated, and those above it are doubled in amplitude. (d) A high quality, narrow-band filter that, depending on where it is centered, passes at most one frequency of the spectrum in panel a. This is the basis of constructing a spectrum analyzer.

their quality, then the more accurate the spectral analysis – and the more costly the analyzer.

3.2.4 The Ear as a Spectrum Analyzer.   Because it is clear from our experience with music that the human ear is a facile processor of tones and harmonics, one natural question to raise is whether it is reasonable to think of the auditory system as primarily a spectrum analyzer. Some evidence suggesting that the ear may exhibit some aspects of a spectrum analyzer is provided in Demonstration 5. In this demonstration, a 200 Hz tone along with its first 20 overtones is used. To show the degree to which one can listen selectively to the harmonics, the following pattern is used. The complex sound is alternated with itself less one of its harmonics. This is done in the demonstration for each of the first 10 harmonics. Under this manipulation one can clearly hear the harmonic that is being switched on and off. However, the effect become less apparent for the higher harmonics.

So, such demonstrations provide some limited evidence that we carry out a Fourier analysis of sounds, although something is clearly amiss with the higher harmonics. In Part VI we gain some understanding of why that is so, as well as encountering some phenomena that remain mysterious from the perspective of Fourier analysis (Sections VI.4–6).

4. NONLINEAR DISTORTION

Even if the physical stimulus is a pure tone, it is quite possible, for the auditory processing to generate overtones via some form of nonlinear distortion. The possibility of transducers introducing distortion is an all-too-familiar problem encountered in audio equipment. One of the reasons for the expense of high fidelity equipment is to avoid just such distortion. Measured levels of the magnitude of harmonic distortion are regularly reported for amplifiers.

Our interest in this phenomenon stems from the possibility that the ear itself engenders such distortion. The purpose of this section is to gain some understanding of the types of distortion products, as these unwanted frequencies are known, that can arise from nonlinear distortion.

Any transformation of one variable X into another Y that is of the form of a straight line relationship between the two variables, that is,

$$Y = aX + b,$$

where a and b are constants, is said to be **linear.** The graph of a typical linear function is, of course, a straight line of slope a and Y-intercept b.

Any transformation that is not linear is said to be **nonlinear.** Thus, almost any relationship between variables is nonlinear; the linear case is exceptional. We have previously encountered at least two classes of nonlinear relations, the power functions of Stevens' law and the logarithmic function of Fechner's law.

Nonlinear transformations of sound waves are a serious problem in that they introduce new frequencies that were not there to begin with. To illustrate that fact, we consider two special cases of nonlinear transformations:

4.1 A Symmetric Nonlinear Transformation: The Square Root

The square root function is defined by:

$$Y = \begin{cases} X^{1/2}, \text{ for } X \geq 0 \\ -(-X)^{\frac{1}{2}}, \text{ for } X < 0. \end{cases}$$

The plot of this function is shown in Fig. V.25.

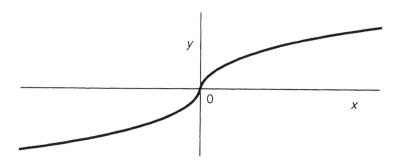

FIG. V.25 The plot of the square root transformation
$$Y = \begin{cases} X^{1/2}, \text{ if } X \geq 0, \\ -(-X)^{1/2}, \text{ if } X < 0. \end{cases}$$

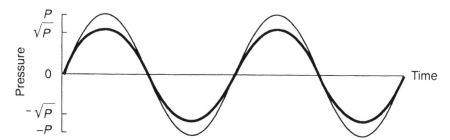

FIG. V.26 A sine wave (lighter curve) subjected to a square root transformation (darker curve). Note that the wave after the transformation is no longer a sine wave, although it still has the same period. This means that its spectrum must include higher harmonics of the original sine wave.

Suppose now that we have a pure tone (sine wave) and subject it to this square root transformation. As we can see in Fig. V.26, the transformed wave retains the same period, but it is itself no longer a sine wave. Because it is periodic and not a sine wave, its reconstruction will necessarily involve harmonics not present in the original wave. Indeed, by the same argument used in reconstructing the square wave, this distorted wave has a spectrum involving only odd harmonics.

An example of such nonlinear distortion is provided in Demonstration 33 (Track 64) in which:

1. A 440 Hz tone is subjected to a square root transformation.
2. The resulting distorted tone is alternated with the third harmonic of 440 Hz, namely, 1,320 Hz.

The question is whether you can hear that harmonic in the transformed tone. Most listeners can.

4.2 An Asymmetric Transformation: Half-Wave Rectification

Half-wave rectification is a linear transformation with slope 1 for positive values, so it does not change those values, and it is also linear, but with slope 0, for negative values. Thus, all it does is to replace every negative value by 0 while leaving the positive ones unchanged. The transformation is shown in Fig. V.27.

If a sine wave, the lighter curve in Fig. V.28, is subjected to the

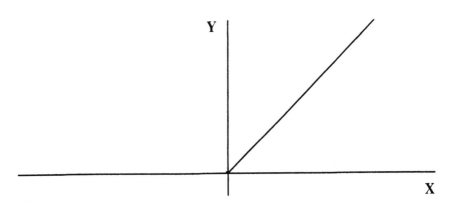

FIG. V.27 The plot of a half-wave rectifier. Positive values are unchanged and negative ones are changed to the corresponding positive value.

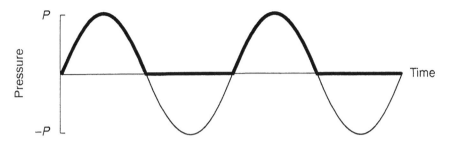

FIG. V.28 A sine wave subjected to half-wave rectification. It is periodic with the same frequency as the original sine wave. Because of its asymmetry, its spectrum has only the frequencies $2nf$, that is, just the even harmonics of the original wave.

half-wave rectification of Fig. V.27, then we obtain the solid curve of Fig. V.28. Observe that although the original sine wave and the half rectified wave have the same period, because of the asymmetry of the rectified wave its spectrum is dominated by the even harmonics of the original wave. This transformation is also illustrated in Demonstration 6 where:

1. The 440 Hz tone is subjected to half-wave rectification.
2. The resulting distorted tone is alternated with the second harmonic of 440 Hz, that is, = 880 Hz.

The question is whether in Case 2 one can select out the second harmonic of the distorted tone, as in Fourier analysis. Again, most people can.

4.3 Distortion of Sums of Waves

Consider a sound wave formed by adding two sine waves of frequencies f_1 and f_2. If the resulting wave is nonlinearly distorted, the result is more complex than carrying out the same distortion on each wave separately and then adding the distortion products. The reason is simply illustrated by a little algebra. Suppose the pressures at time t are:

$$y(t) = p_1(t) + p_2(t).$$

If these values are subject to a squaring (symmetric) nonlinear distortion, then we see:

$$y(t)^2 = [p_1(t) + p_2(t)]^2$$
$$= p_1(t)^2 + p_2(t)^2 + 2p_1(t)p_2(t).$$

Thus, all of the distortion products expected from the two component sine waves will be present, but in addition the term $2p_1(t)p_2(t)$ introduces frequencies other than the harmonics of f_1 and f_2. In particular, it can be shown that the frequency $2f_1 - f_2$ will be part of the decomposition. (The proof involves trigonometric manipulations.) These frequencies that involve the difference of harmonics of the two input tones are known as **combination tones.**

So, for example, if $f_1 = 700$ Hz, $f_2 = 1,000$ Hz, then $2f_1 - f_2 = 2 \times 700 - 1,000 = 400$ Hz. Demonstration 33 (Track 66) uses these signals:

1. The wave formed from the superposition of pure tones of frequencies 700 and 1,000 is subjected to a symmetric distortion.
2. This distorted wave is then alternated with 400 Hz.

Again the question is whether or not one hears the 400 Hz component in the distorted sum. Most people do.

So far, the evidence is not inconsistent with the idea that our hearing systems are carrying out a spectral analysis of the distorted waves, although clearly some trouble exists in isolating the higher harmonics.

In Part VI we examine evidence suggesting that the hearing process has to be more complex than just being a spectrum analyzer.

5. NOISE

5.1 Noise Spectrum

5.1.1 Construction of Noise from Pure Tones. Recall that we have asserted that any periodic wave can be represented as a sum of harmonics of the pure tone having its period equal to the period of the given wave. The plot of the amplitudes of those harmonics is called the spectrum of the wave. A typical spectrum and its corresponding waveform are shown in Fig. V.29.

There is, of course, no reason why one cannot combine a collection of pure tones of frequencies that are not harmonics of any common fundamental. Moreover, the pattern of their amplitudes can also be shown as a similar spectral plot, except that the amplitudes are not integral multiples of a frequency, an example of which is shown in Fig. V.30. Because the tones being superimposed are not harmonics, the resulting sound wave *cannot* be periodic. For if it were periodic, then by the Fourier theorem its spectrum would necessarily consist just of harmonics of the frequency of the wave.

A simple example of such sounds are aharmonic chords, such as three pure tones that do not share a harmonic relation.

Going to the other extreme, the spectrum might involve every frequency

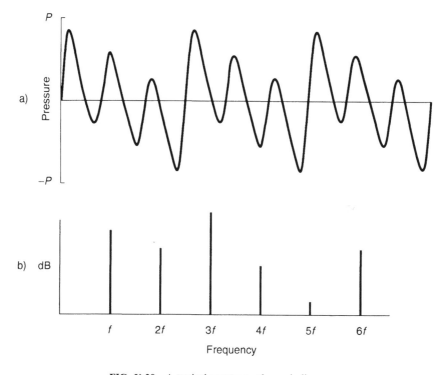

FIG. V.29   A typical spectrum of a periodic wave.

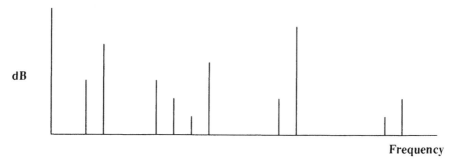

Frequency

FIG. V.30   A spectrum that results in a waveform that is not periodic, because these frequencies are not harmonics of a common frequency.

in which case the spectrum can be represented as a continuous curve such as that shown in Fig. V.31.

If in addition, the curve represents a statistical average in the sense that at each instant in time the intensity at each f varies at random but with some fixed average value over time, then the resulting sound is called **noise.** Noise

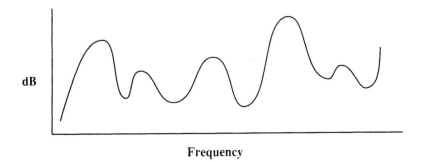

Frequency

FIG. V.31   A continuous spectrum of some noise.

typically sounds like steam escaping from a leaky pipe or the "shushing" sound one makes to quiet children or talkative neighbors at the theater.

5.1.2 White Noise.   If the average spectrum of the noise is flat over the audible frequencies, as shown in Fig. V.32, then the noise is called **white noise.** (This terminology arises in analogy to light, where monochromatic lights correspond to pure tones and a flat spectrum corresponds—more or less—to ordinary daylight, white light).

5.1.3 Filtered White Noise.   If one has a low-pass filter, such as shown in panel a of Fig. V.33, then passing white noise through that filter produces low-pass noise whose spectrum is shown in panel b.

Similarly, a high-pass filter, panel a of Fig. V.34, results in high-pass noise, with the spectrum of panel b.

Finally, a band-pass filter, panel a of Fig. V.35, yields the band pass noise of panel b.

Examples of filtered white noise are provided in Demonstration 7.

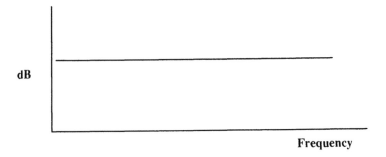

Frequency

FIG. V.32   The continuous spectrum of what is called white noise.

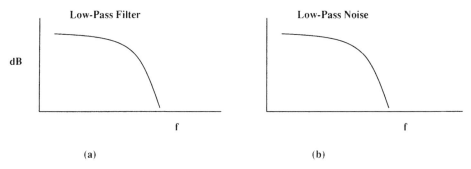

FIG. V.33   Low-pass noise constructed by subjecting white noise to low-pass filtering.

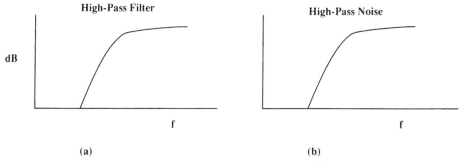

FIG. V.34   High-pass noise constructed by subjecting white noise to high-pass filtering.

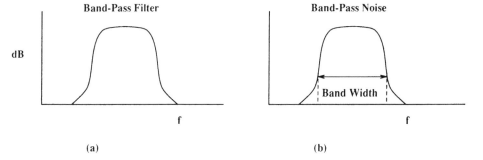

FIG. V.35   Band-pass noise constructed by subjecting white noise to band-pass filtering.

5.2 Intensity of Noise

If N is the total power of band-passed white noise and W is the bandwidth in Hz, then the **noise power density** in dB is defined to be

$$N_0 = 10 \log N/W.$$

If a pure tone signal has power P and duration D, then the **signal energy** measured in dB is

$$E = 10 \log PD.$$

The quantity $E - N_0$ is the key variable for the detection of a pure tone in wide band noise. For the region

$$250 \leq f \leq 4{,}000 \text{ Hz}, \ 10 \leq D \leq 200 \text{ ms},$$

an empirical generalization is that the detection threshold is given by

$$E - N_0 = 2(f/1{,}000) + 8.$$

For example, if $f = 1{,}000$ Hz, $D = 100$ ms, then $E - N_0 = 10$ dB (which is true up to ± 1 dB).

The general empirical curves of detectability in noise are shown in Fig. V.36.

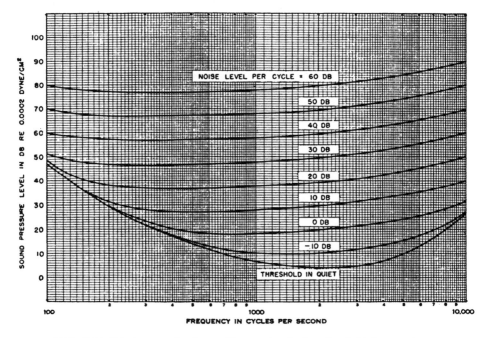

FIG. V.36 The impact of noise masking on the absolute threshold for pure tones. From "The Masking of Pure Tones and of Speech by White Noise" by J. E. Hawkins and S. S. Stevens, 1950, *Journal of the Acoustical Society of America, 22,* p. 9. Copyright 1950 by American Institute of Physics. Reprinted by permission.

5.3 Methods of Noise Reduction

Noise is mostly a problem to be eliminated or at least suppressed. It plagues us in at least three ways: in the reproduction of sound from tapes and records; in the transmission of information over telephone lines and in computers; and in the intrusion of unwanted sounds from trucks, airplanes, ventilating systems, and so on in our daily lives. Various schemes have evolved to deal with the problem in each context, and we describe them briefly.

5.3.1 Dolby Suppression.   Analogue systems of recording — tapes and records — inherently involve some background hiss as the result of the mechanical nature of the processing. When the sound — for example, music — being recorded is moderately loud, the signal-to-noise ratio is large and the hiss creates no problem. One simply does not notice it. But for soft passages in the music, the hiss can be quite noticeable and unpleasant. These two facts underlie the solution devised by the Dolby Laboratories, Inc.

At the time the music is recorded on the tape, the Dolby system subjects it to an intensity transformation in which the loud sounds remain unchanged and the softer ones are boosted considerably — to the point where the signal-to-noise ratio on the tape is sufficient so that one ignores the hiss. Of course, if this transformed sound were played back through a normal linear amplifier, the music would be most distorted. So one must build into the amplifier the exact inverse of the boosting transformation, namely one that reduces the soft sounds (plus noise) by the very amount the signal was boosted at the time of recording. That reduces the loudness of the music and the noise by the same amount, thereby maintaining the desirably high signal-to-noise ratio.

This scheme is implemented in many tapes and film sound tracks, and it is quite effective.

5.3.2 Digitizing the Signal.   A digitized version of a signal is constructed as follows. One first selects an intensity versus time grid. In the example shown in Fig. V.37, intensity is partitioned into five distinct levels, which is very coarse but still retains a great deal of information about the signal, and time into successive intervals of duration Δt, a parameter whose value greatly affects the quality of the process. The value $1/\Delta t$ is called the *sampling rate*. Table V.1 gives some idea of the range of sampling rates commonly encountered.

Figure V.38 represents the sort of digital code that partially encodes the information in the original signal. Thus, the result of such digitizing is to approximate the signal by a *step function*.

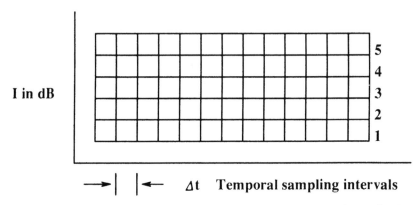

I in dB

$\longrightarrow$| |$\longleftarrow$ Δt **Temporal sampling intervals**

FIG. V.37 An intensity-time grid used in digitizing a continuous waveform. Time is divided into equal intervals of duration Δt and intensity is divided into, usually equal, dB intervals up to some maximum.

TABLE V.1
Common Sampling Rates

	Sampling Rate	
Δt in μs	Hz	kHz
1,000 (= 1 ms)	1,000	1
100 (= .1 ms)	10,000	10
1	10^6	1,000

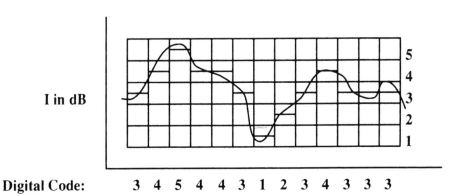

I in dB

Digital Code: 3   4   5   4   4   3   1   2   3   4   3   3   3

FIG. V.38 A typical waveform subjected to the digitalization grid of Fig. V.37. The digital code simply shows for each time interval which intensity interval includes most of the signal intensity over that time period.

The digitizing of signals is very important today in signal transmission for four major reasons:

- People are relatively insensitive to digitization when the sampling rate is sufficiently high. This is examined in greater detail in Section VI.7.1.4.
- It is far more economical to transmit a sequence of numbers than it is a continuous function.
- Digitized signals are, of course, highly compatible with digital computers, which makes it convenient both to generate and to process such signals.
- Finally, such a representation of the signal is resistant to the addition of a certain amount of noise to the signal.

Observe in Fig. V.39 just how much one can jiggle the pressure waveform without altering the digital code. Both of the pressure waves shown would be digitized as the same number. Thus digitization serves to reduce the vulnerability of the signal to erosion by noise. In some systems, a series of repeater stations are used to keep restoring the digital quality of the signal.

5.3.3 Noise as Antinoise.   Explosive combustion and the rapid movement of air through narrow ducts is a general source of noise in our society, and great efforts are made to reduce it and to ameliorate its effects. Reduction efforts are, however, limited to a considerable degree by the very nature of the processes that underlie propulsion systems used in automobiles, trucks, and aircraft and in air movement systems. The noise is inherent to the processes.

Until recently, most of the effort has gone into ameliorating the effects of noise by using impedance mismatches (Section II.9) one or more times, both

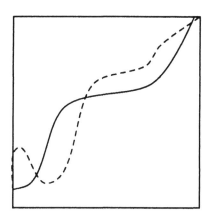

FIG. V.39 A blow up of one cell of the digitizing grid showing two different waveforms that would receive the same code. One may think of these as a signal and that signal after it has been modified by noise.

in the form of walls to separate the listener from the source and of mufflers to limit the output of sound from the source. Neither is perfectly effective, as we are all aware.

There is, in principle, a perfect solution to this type of noise problem. If the sound that is produced has the pressure pattern $p(t, x, y, z)$ as a function of time t at the location x, y, and z in three-dimensional space, and if we could generate the sound pressure wave $-p(t, x, y, z)$, then the simple superposition of the two yields

$$p(t, x, y, z) + [-p(t, x, y, z)] = 0,$$

that is, total suppression. We may speak of $-p(t, x, y, z)$ as *antinoise* to the noise $p(t, x, y, z)$. This possibility for suppressing noise has been known for years, but no effective use of it was possible because of the great and unpredictable complexity of the sounds resulting from turbulent flows. It was, of course, apparent that if the following three conditions could be met, the idea could be implemented:

1. One must have detailed measurements of the sound as it is being produced.
2. One can solve the equations of sound propagation in the moving exhaust gasses in the exhaust pipe and predict the pressure wave, $p(t, x, y, z)$, for some region in the pipe not very far from the source. Moreover, the solution has to be worked out before the sound actually gets there, which means exceedingly rapidly.
3. One can design a sound source to be located at (or really around) this region in the exhaust pipe that is capable of producing the predicted $-p(t, x, y, z)$ over the region.

Because of the amazing development of very powerful computers along with equally remarkable advances in instrumentation technology, these three conditions are increasingly being satisfied. As of 1992, research on and development of such antinoise devices for fixed-location noise sources, as occur in a variety of industries, is underway. Research on those suited to moving sources, such as automobiles and jet aircraft engines, is also underway. Some luxury cars are expected to be equipped with it in 1993. It is an extremely promising avenue of research and may, ultimately, significantly reduce if not eliminate one of the offensive aspects of living in a technological society.

6. SUMMARY

Pressure superposition of pure tones was the major theme in developing some understanding of the physics of complex sounds. It is the source of the standing waves — natural resonances — of wires and tubes that are the basis of musical instruments. It is central in Fourier analysis where it is shown that any physically realizable periodic wave can be constructed by super-positioning a pure tone of the same frequency plus its higher harmonics. The recipe for the amplitudes of these harmonics is known as the spectrum of the wave. The amplitudes and frequencies of the reconstruction are provided, but not the phases. Sometimes this has to be given separately. Superposition coupled with nonlinear distortion gives rise to not only the harmonics of the input frequencies, but also to combination tones such as $2f_1 - f_2$. And finally, it provides a compact way to describe such non-periodic waveforms as noise, again using a recipe for construction in the form of a spectrum of frequencies. Understanding superposition leads to methods for combatting noise in the context of tape recordings, the transmission of information, and an environment of engines and fans.

7. FURTHER READING

The references for this chapter are the same as for Part II. In particular, at the level of the present text, consult Johnson, Walker, and Cutnell (1981). For more advanced treatments, go to Rossing (1982) or Halliday and Resnick (1978). Additional material connected with noise and dealing with it, as of some years ago, are discussed in Burns (1968) and Kryter (1970). Alper (1991) gives a clear nontechnical discussion of antinoise.

PART VI

Psychophysics of Complex Sounds

This last part of the text explores some phenomena of hearing that arise only with sounds more complex than pure tones. A fundamental issue is the degree to which facts that we know about the physical stimuli or about the neural coding of signals account for behavioral findings. One aspect of this is the degree to which the hearing system acts like a spectrum analyzer and thereby reduces the phenomena in question to the study of pure tones. The answer is "to some degree," but we encounter a number of important auditory phenomena having no explanation in terms of the physics of the stimuli or of the peripheral physiology. Presumably they involve higher centers of the brain engaged in functions not yet understood.

1. EXAMPLES WHERE THE PHENOMENON IS PHYSICAL

We begin with two simple examples in which the physical stimulus seems to determine the percept and a third, related to the second, where it is unclear what is happening.

1.1 Combination Tones

We have seen (and heard in the demonstrations) some evidence that the hearing system is able to isolate the pure tones (at least the lower ones) that make up a complex periodic wave. For example, one demonstration showed that when two frequencies f_1 and f_2 are both presented, nonlinear distortion allows the combination frequency $2f_1 - f_2$ to be heard (Demonstration 6.

This is explicable in terms of the Fourier components that are present as a result of the distortion.

1.2 Beats

When two pure tones are within a few Hz of each other, they produce a waveform that has a highly prominent low frequency pattern in overall amplitude. One can easily see the waxing and waning of the resultant waveform (Fig. V.8 of Section V.1.2.3) as well as hear it (Demonstration 4. Section VI.2.1.2 discusses how beating interacts with the masking effect of one pure tone on another, making it easier to detect the signal than would otherwise be expected.

1.3 Binaural Beats

The next question asks what happens when two tones of similar frequencies are presented to the different ears. The most prominent effect occurs only for low frequencies, below 1,500 Hz. As the signal separation is increased to an optimal value – about 30 Hz at 400 Hz – the fused sound appears to oscillate in the head from one side to the other at about the frequency of the separation. This is called *binaural beating,* but it should not be confused with (physical) beating that involves oscillations in intensity. In the binaural case, the oscillation is in the lateralization of the sound. It is heard as if the relative sound intensity in the two ears is varying, but that is not actually happening. This phenomenon can be heard, using earphones, in Demonstration 8. As the tones are further separated, at first the sound becomes increasingly diffuse until ultimately one hears the two tones separately, each in the ear to which it is presented. There is no accepted theory for the phenomenon.

2. PURE TONE MASKING AND FACILITATION

We turn next to a phenomenon that is not explicable on the basis of physical properties of the stimulus but that makes some sense in terms of the peripheral transduction into electrical activity.

2.1 Upward Spread of Masking

2.1.1 Demonstration. The phenomenon of one pure tone masking another can be heard in Demonstration 9. Two tones, at 1,200 Hz and 2,000 Hz, are used. In the first demonstration the 1,200 Hz tone serves as the masker. It is held at a constant, moderately high intensity, and is pulsed eight times (200 ms on, 100 ms off). The 2,000 Hz test tone is added to every other pulse. In each sequence of eight pulses the signal remains at the same intensity, but in successive sequences it decreases by 5 dB except that the first drop is 15 dB. As long as the eight pulses seem to alternate one is continuing to hear the 2,000 Hz test tone; but once all eight sound alike, then the test tone has been successfully masked. The data are the number of steps required until the 2,000 Hz tone disappears, that is, is successfully masked by the 1,200 Hz tone.

Next the roles of the tones are reversed—the 2,000 Hz tone serves as the masker at a constant intensity. The procedure is identical to that just described, except for interchanging the tones. Once again, the data are the number of steps until the 1,200 Hz tone disappears.

Typically, one finds that the lower (1,200 Hz) tone masks the higher (2,000 Hz) far better than the other way round.

2.1.2 Systematic Data.   Suppose, as in the demonstration, the masker (I_M, f_M) is fixed, and for each test signal frequency f_T we determine the intensity I_T just needed to detect the test in the presence of the masker. The data are shown in Fig. VI.1 for a masker of 80 dB at 1,200 Hz. Exactly as

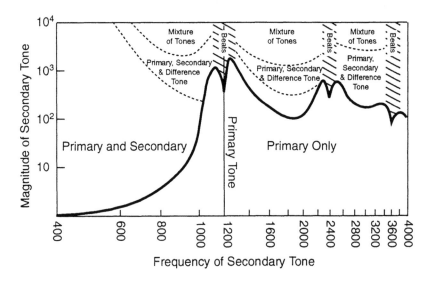

FIG. VI.1   With an 80 dB, 1,200 Hz tone as masker, the curve of the intensity needed to detect a tone of frequency f in the presence of the masker. The intensity is measured in dB above the absolute threshold (dB SL) for each f. The local improvement at 1,200, 2,400, and 3,600 Hz is attributed to beating between the signal and the masker and its first few harmonics. The improvement elsewhere is attributed to difference tones arising from distortions (see Section V.4.3). From "The Auditory Masking of One Pure Tone by Another and Its Probable Relation to the Dynamics of the Inner Ear" by R. L. Wegel and C. E. Lane, 1924, *Physical Review, 23,* p. 272. Copyright 1924 by American Physical Society. Reprinted by permission.

was found in the demonstration, a very pronounced asymmetry exists. When the test tone is well below the masker, it is readily detected. As it gets quite near the masker it becomes more difficult to detect and in the region above the masker it remains difficult to detect to well above 4,000 Hz.

Notice that there are decided dips, that is, improvements, in the detectability of the tone when the test tone is near either the masker frequency or its first or second harmonic. This arises from the occurrence of both combination tones and beats. Beating can occur, although it is somewhat less pronounced, between a tone whose frequency is near one of the higher harmonics of f_2, namely, the frequencies nf_2, where $n = 2$, 3, ... The beats, being amplitude oscillations at very low frequencies, are unaffected by the masker, thereby making the signal more detectable than it could otherwise be. Thus, we see the effects of the beats at the masker frequency, 1,200 Hz, at its second harmonic, 2,400 Hz, and at its third harmonic, 3,600 Hz.

2.2 Psychophysical Tuning Curves

Another way to study how effectively one tone masks another is to fix the test tone (I_T, f_T) and for each masker frequency f_M to determine what masker intensity I_M is just sufficient to mask (I_T, f_T). A plot of I_M, converted to dB, versus $\log f_M$ is known as a **psychophysical tuning curve.** Note that this procedure is just the opposite of the demonstration—there (I_M, f_M) was fixed and I_T was varied.

Empirically, this is a totally different measurement procedure from the physiological measurements of neural spike rates that led to the tuning curves of Section III.4.2.4. The reason they have been given the same name (with adjectives "neural" and "psychophysical") is the fact that the two curves are very similar. Figure VI.2 shows a comparison between a neural tuning curve obtained from a cat and a human psychophysical tuning curve.

Presumably there is a good reason for the obvious similarity. If two tones activate the same group of neurons, then the resulting firing pattern is some mixture of the effects from each of the signals and, as we have seen earlier, it cannot be a simple summation of the two effects. Rather, some complex interaction occurs within the neuron, and this is believed to be the source of the behavioral masking. If the two tones activate different families of neurons, then the brain receives information about each signal uncontaminated by the other, and so no masking of this sort is to be expected.

The asymmetry of masking—lower frequencies mask higher frequencies better than the other way round—follows directly from the great asymmetry of the neural tuning curves. Recall that these tuning curves extend far below the CF, but not much above it. Thus, the neurons with the CF of the higher frequency tone will respond also to a masker of much lower frequency,

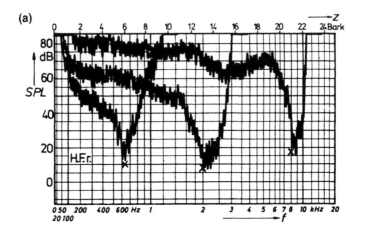

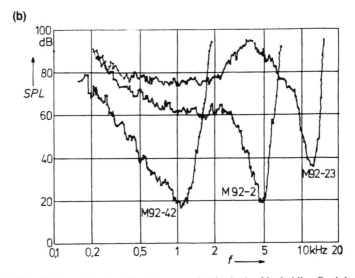

FIG. VI.2 (a) A psychophysical tuning curve that is obtained by holding fixed the test tone and for each frequency finding the intensity just sufficient to mask the test tone. (b) Several neural tuning curves for cats for comparison with the human psychophysical tuning curves of panel a. Note the striking similarity in the shapes of these curves from from different species using different methods. From "On a Psychoacoustical Equivalent of Tuning Curves" in *Facts and Models in Hearing* (p. 134) by E. Zwicker, 1974, Berlin: Springer-Verlag. Copyright 1974 by Springer-Verlag. Reprinted by permission. Panel b was originally presented by Kiang and Moxon at a 1973 von Békésy symposium.

thereby producing some interaction, whereas the neurons with the CF of the lower frequency tones do not react to tones of significantly higher frequency.

If a complex signal includes harmonics that do not interact in the sense that each lower harmonic fails to mask the next higher one, then each

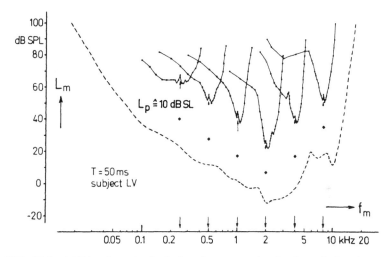

FIG. VI.3 Additional psychophysical tuning curves showing how similar they are throughout the entire frequency band when they are plotted in terms of log *f*. From "Pure Tone Masking; a New Result From a New Method" in *Facts and Models in Hearing* (p. 147) by L. L. M. Vogten, 1974, Berlin: Springer-Verlag. Copyright 1974 by Springer-Verlag. Reprinted by permission.

harmonic activates a separate neuron group. Thus the brain can isolate and react to each harmonic separately. Because the psychophysical tuning curves are all similar when plotted against log *f* (not *f*), as is evident in Figs. VI.2 and VI.3, a separation Δf that does not result in masking at low frequencies may well do so at higher frequencies. This fact was in evidence in Demonstration 5 where one tries to isolate particular harmonics in a chord composed of a 200 Hz tone and its first 20 harmonics. This is done by alternating the full chord with that sound minus the harmonic one is trying to isolate. If the change can be detected, one is successfully isolating the harmonic that is intermittently absent. For the lower harmonics neither the fundamental nor any lesser harmonic masks them and so they can be isolated, whereas the higher harmonics are masked by those below them and they are much more difficult to isolate.

We conclude, therefore, that the hearing system is only partially a Fourier analyzer.

2.3 An Effect of Amplitude Modulation

A somewhat different way to study the impact of one tone on a person's ability to evaluate a change in another, perfectly detectable, test tone is to use a procedure known as **amplitude modulation** (abbreviated

AM).[1] Introduce a slow, sine wave variation in the amplitude (or intensity) of the test tone, and ask what is the least modulation that is detectable. When the modulated carrier tone is all alone, the classical result is that the Weber fraction — the proportion that the amplitude of the tone must be changed to be detected by a person — is about 0.05.

Suppose such a test tone is of frequency 1,000 Hz and that another tone, say at 4,000 Hz, again called the "masking tone," is present. By what we have just seen from the detection studies, we might anticipate that detection of the modulation of the test tone would not be affected by the higher frequency masking tone. Certainly there is no effect of the higher tone on a person's ability to detect the lower tone in a simple detection experiment. And, indeed, that is also the outcome when detecting the modulation provided that the masking tone is steady. The surprise is not that, but that when the masking tone is also modulated in the same way as the test tone, the test tone is masked: The just detectable modulation of the test tone must be increased by from 10 to 20 dB above the case where the masker is steady.

A second surprise is that exactly the same results are found when the roles of masker and test tone are reversed. That is, when the 4,000 Hz tone is the test tone and the 1,000 Hz is the masker, then, in contrast to the detection result, the low frequency masker does not affect the detection of the modulation in the 4,000 Hz tone unless the 1,000 Hz tone is itself modulated in the same way as the test tone.

These results differ appreciably from the effect of a masker on the detectability of a signal. Masking or not in the detection of modulation is symmetric whereas in the detection of the existence of the test tone it is highly asymmetric. This difference strongly suggests that the interference of one tone with another differs depending on just what aspect of the test tone is in question. Apparently, some substantial difference exists between absolute detectability and modulation detectability.

These matters are subtle and far from fully understood. One source of the difference in masking is the fact that an amplitude modulated pure tone has a complex spectrum, with frequencies other than the carrier frequency on both sides of that frequency. Thus, if the masker fails to mask any of these side frequencies, there is an opportunity to detect the modulation. When the masker itself is also modulated to the same degree, it too has additional frequencies and these can then mask the corresponding side frequencies of the modulated test tone.

---

[1]Rapid amplitude modulation is the way that information is carried by radio stations located on the so-called AM band of frequencies. They are called this not because of any very special feature of these frequencies but because they have been agreed on as the ones that will carry information in this way. The much higher frequency band called FM for frequency modulation involves using a single frequency as a carrier and modulating the frequency rather than the amplitude of the wave. In both cases, a band of frequencies centered on the carrier must be assigned to each station.

2.4 Facilitation Using Profile Analysis

2.4.1 The Experiment. A variant on amplitude modulation that does not introduce a complex spectrum is to have a carrier frequency present whose amplitude may or may not be increased for a brief time, such as for 100 ms. This is equivalent to saying that a 100 ms pure-tone signal is added in phase to an existing ongoing carrier tone of the same frequency. Note that in this case the spectrum is a single frequency with or without an increase in amplitude, which, as was just noted, is not what happens with amplitude modulation. Using, for example, a two-alternative forced-choice design, the problem for the subject is to detect in which interval the signal has been added to the carrier.

Now, introduce on either side of the carrier tone other frequencies of, let us suppose, the same intensity as the carrier.[2] For example, suppose that the signal and carrier are at 1,000 Hz and 10 frequencies are added on each side, spaced equally in log f from 300 to 3,000 Hz. Given the masking results described earlier, one might anticipate that those frequencies below the carrier frequency will reduce the detectability of the signal. The data are otherwise: Adding these flanking signals facilitates detectability considerably.

This is a very different result from either the masking of one pure tone by another or the modulation results. Depending on the exact condition, in these earlier studies either the masker had no impact on performance or it deteriorated it. In contrast, when the amplitude of a single frequency is changed, the existence of the flanking tones improves detectability considerably.

One may ask, does the spectrum or the waveform really matter? This is easily tested because the spectrum tells us nothing about the phase relations among the several frequencies, and so the phases relative to the carrier frequency can be varied from presentation to presentation while holding the spectrum constant. Doing so has a large effect on the waveform, as we saw in Figs. V.2–4. Empirically, the detectability of the signal is unaffected by these phase changes. Thus, it is the spectrum, not the waveform, that matters.

In the case described, the carrier and signal were the middle frequency of the profile of 21 frequencies. Given the earlier questions about the symmetry or asymmetry of one tone masking another, it is natural to explore what happens when the carrier and signal is one of the other tones. The result is simple: The improvement in detectability is least when the carrier is at the extremes and best when it is in the center of the profile. The difference is substantial, about 10 dB.

---

[2]Studies have been carried out in which these intensities vary and similar effects occur, although there are subtle differences that we do not go into here.

Studies of this character are called **profile analysis,** where the term refers to the fact that the entire frequency profile — the spectrum — is involved in evaluating what really is a change of only a single component of that profile.

2.4.2 Spectral Weights.   A natural question to raise is how the observer uses the flanking tones to help in detecting whether or not the signal has been added to the carrier. One important additional fact is that the results really do not depend on the absolute level of intensity; the overall intensity of the profile can be varied from trial to trial without greatly affecting the enhancing effect of the flanking frequencies. In some sense, the listener must use the flanking tones to estimate what the carrier tone would be without the addition of the signal and then compare that estimate with what is observed on each trial. When the discrepancy between what is observed and what is predicted from the flanking tones is sufficiently large, the listener concludes that the signal was added.

To be more specific, let us denote the m frequencies of the profile by f_i, where in the case mentioned $m = 21$ and $i = 1, \ldots, 21$. Denote by L_i their perceived intensities. If the index of the signal and carrier frequency is s, then the test observation is of the form:

$$z = L_s + a_1 L_1 + \ldots + a_{s-1} L_{s-1} + a_{s+1} L_{s+1} + \ldots + a_n L_n.$$

The first question is to select weights so that in the absence of a signal, the expected value of z is zero. Once done, the observer then determines a value of z on each trial and when it is sufficiently larger than zero reports that the signal was added to the carrier. Of course, chance fluctuations in the percepts L_i may cause z to be large when no signal is added or to be small when a signal is added, thereby generating errors. For equal intensities, it has been established that the weights estimated from the behavioral data are very close to the theoretically optimal values, which can be shown in this case to be $a_i = -1/(m - 1)$.

3. NOISE MASKING AND FACILITATION

3.1 Varying Bandwidth

As we are all well aware, signals are more difficult to detect when noise is present than when it is not. A familiar example is trying to listen to music in a moving car with the windows open. Noise masks other sounds, like tones, speech, and music.

Given that pure tones mask other pure tones, it is no surprise that noise masking occurs. One question to be asked about such masking is how it varies with the bandwidth of the noise. H. Fletcher first posed this question in the 1920s. At that time the answer came as a surprise, although it no longer seems much of a mystery given what we know about neural tuning curves. He, and subsequently others, demonstrated that only a somewhat narrow band of noise matters. Increasing the bandwidth beyond some critical value does not increase the masking effect of noise. It is important not to confuse this fact, namely, that after a certain bandwidth is reached noise has no additional ability to mask a pure tone, with a second fact, namely, that the overall loudness of the noise increases steadily as the bandwidth increases. Beyond a certain point, the increased loudness of the noise simply has no further effect on detectability.

Demonstration 10 uses a staircase, or count-down, procedure for detecting a 2,000 Hz signal in noise of various bandwidths: broad band, 1,000, 250, and 10 Hz. The procedure is as follows: The 2,000 Hz tone is run through 10 steps of decreasing intensity, 5 dB per step. During each sequence, one counts the number of steps for which one can hear the 2,000 Hz tone. The first sequence is run without any masking. Following that, the tone is imbedded in noise of various bandwidths, all of which are centered on the 2,000 Hz tone. For each bandwidth, the sequence of 10 intensities is run through twice. One uses the average count to construct a plot of that value versus bandwidth.

Systematic data on noise masking are shown in Fig. VI.4. This plot is simpler than it first seems. Focus initially on just one pure tone frequency, say 2,000 Hz, and find the points (downward pointing triangles) corre-

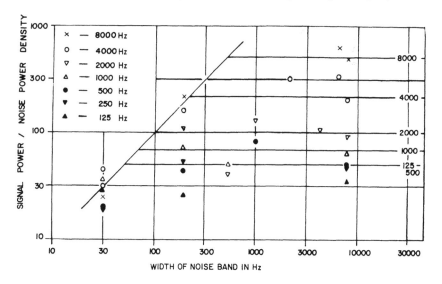

FIG. VI.4 Evidence that supports the critical band hypothesis is provided by plotting for each of several frequencies the signal-to-noise ratio (in dB) required to detect the signal in the presence of noise. The abscissa is the bandwidth of the noise that is centered on the frequency in question. The key observation is that once the critical band is reached, which depends on frequency, a further increase in bandwidth does not affect the detectability of the signal. From "Auditory Masking" in *Handbook of Perception: Vol IV. Hearing* (p. 343) by R. D. Patterson and D. M. Green, 1978, New York: Academic Press. Copyright 1978 by Academic Press. Reprinted by permission.

sponding to it. The independent variable in the plot is the bandwidth of the masker, which, in this case, is centered at 2,000 Hz. We see that as the bandwidth changes from about 100 Hz to 8,000 Hz the masking effect does not change, but the detectability improves markedly as the band narrows below 100 Hz.

3.2 Critical Bands

The width of a noise band after which no further effect is noticed is called a **critical band.** On discovery, these were viewed as something of a mystery. Now we believe that a critical band corresponds to the width of neural tuning curves having their CFs at the frequency of the to-be-detected tone. We know that frequencies outside the tuning curve cannot interact at the periphery with the test tone and so do not mask it directly. Noise affecting neurons unresponsive to the signal simply does not add to the masking effect. Thus, the physiological data lead us to expect behavioral critical bands, and we observe them. But as is pointed out in Section VI.3.4, matters really are not quite this simple.

Figure VI.5 shows the value of the estimated width of the critical band as a function of its center frequency.

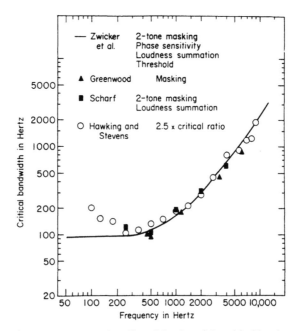

FIG. VI.5   Estimates from several studies of the size of the critical band as a function of signal frequency. From "Critical Bands" in *Foundations of Modern Auditory Theory* (Vol. 1, p. 161) by B. Scharf, 1970, New York: Academic Press. Copyright 1970 by Academic Press. Reprinted by permission.

Observe that these masking results — both the fact that lower frequencies mask higher ones better than the other way round and the existence of critical noise bands — have no physical explanation, although they are quite comprehensible in terms of what we know about the peripheral neural encoding of signals.

3.3 Binaural Masking

The first observation about binaural masking is that the degree of masking is unaffected by whether the presentation is monaural or binaural, provided only that the binaural input to both ears is exactly the same as the monaural input to a single ear. Second, three variants of the binaural procedure yield very marked — up to 15 dB — reductions in the masking effect: (a) present the signal just to one ear and the same noise to both ears; (b) present the signal and the noise to both ears, but have the signals 180° out of phase; and (c) present the signal and the noise to both ears but with the two signals in phase and the identical noise waveform shifted somewhat in time, as they would be if the signal and noise sources are at different locations and the listener faces the signal source. Using earphones, the first two cases can be heard in Demonstration 11. As with binaural beats, the phenomenon is more pronounced at lower frequencies and it all but disappears at 4,000 Hz and higher.

Observe that if in case (a) we were to calculate the physical difference in the waveforms at the two ears, the noise is completely cancelled and the signal remains. In case (b), the noise once again cancels but the signals add, doubling their pressure. In case (c), adding the inputs on average reduces (although does not completely cancel) the noise, and again the signals sum. Just how the brain carries out the (near) equivalent of these operations using the outputs of the two auditory nerves is unclear. But functionally, adding or subtracting the inputs seems to happen.

Such reduced binaural masking may well be related to our ability to overcome the masking effect of background noises when listening to a specific person talking.

3.4 Comodulation Effects

There are a series of studies, mostly carried out in the 1980s, showing that the noise outside a critical band does indeed still have a very significant effect under appropriate conditions. The basic idea is to see what happens when the noise is slowly amplitude modulated (see Section VI.2.3). We consider two kinds of studies.

3.4.1 Comodulation Masking Release. As we know from Section VI.3.1, the detection of a pure tone of, say, 1,000 Hz in a noise band centered on the signal is unaffected once the bandwidth of the noise exceeds about 130 Hz. However, if the noise amplitude is slowly modulated, but fast enough so that several cycles of change occur during the signal duration, then for a noise bandwidth of 1,000 Hz the detectability of the signal becomes markedly easier, by as much as 20 dB, which is a huge effect.

To gain some additional information about this phenomenon, studies have been run in which the signal is centered in a band of masking noise that is 100 Hz wide, and well separated from that band is another noise band of similar width, called a flanking band, which lies in a distinct critical band either below or above the masking band. When the amplitudes of both bands are modulated in exactly the same way—they are said to be **comodulated**—the signal becomes easier to detect by some 5 to 12 dB. Moreover, the effect is largest when both bands are at the same intensity level and largely disappears when they are more than 20 dB apart. If multiple flanking bands are used, the detectability increases even more, but the evidence supports the idea that the band nearest the stimulus has the greatest effect. Phenomena of this type are grouped together under the label **comodulation masking release.**

The effect, to some degree, involves central rather than peripheral processing. This can be demonstrated by having the signal and the masking band of noise presented to one ear and the flanking band of noise to the other ear. Again, the detectability of the signal increases with comodulation, although not as much as when they are all presented to the same ear. This result can only arise through a central comparison of what is happening at each ear.

One can modulate the frequencies of the spectrum rather than their amplitude, as in FM radio, and no such increase in detectability is found.

3.4.2 Comodulation Detection Difference. Consider the problem where the signal is not a pure tone, but is a narrow band of noise whose presence or absence is to be detected. Moreover, suppose a flanker noise band is also present that is outside the critical band of the signal. If the noise to be detected and the flanker are comodulated, then it becomes considerably more difficult to detect the signal than when the modulation does not exist or it is uncorrelated between the two noise bands. This is called the **comodulation detection difference.** Again, it provides evidence that noise outside the critical band of the signal can indeed have a significant effect, in this case a negative one.

These two results—comodulation release of masking and comodulation detection difference—may at first seem contradictory, but they are not.

Indeed, the fact that the comodulation of the two noise bands makes the salient one less detectable suggests that it should, therefore, become less effective as a masker for a pure tone. So, in that sense, the results are actually consistent.

Although several theories have been proposed for how people use the modulation to improve the detectability of the pure tone, none has yet been widely accepted and so we do not try to explain them. Suffice it to say that the data make clear that the information outside the critical band of the signal being detected is not simply ignored. The same conclusion was reached from the profile analysis work described in Section VI.2.4.

4. ILLUSORY PITCH
(OR THE MISSING FUNDAMENTAL)

We turn next to a practically important phenomenon that is not understood in terms of either the physics or properties of the peripheral neurons.

4.1 Early Results Using Sirens

In 1841 A. Seebeck performed an experiment, using a simple siren, whose outcome was very difficult to understand in terms of Helmholtz's place theory. The unhappy fact is that we still do not understand it.

A siren can be created by constructing a disk with one or more holes at a constant distance from the center, rotating the disk at a constant speed, and applying air pressure through a tube located so it goes through the holes as they pass by (see Fig. VI.6). This generates a square wave of the form shown, along with its spectrum (see Section V.3), in Fig. VI.7. The experimental result is that when people are asked to select a pure tone having the same pitch as the square wave produced by the siren, they choose one of frequency $1/T$. This is as it should be from the perspective of spectral analysis.

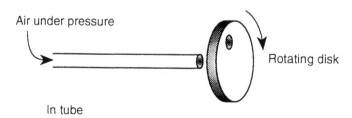

FIG. VI.6   A schematic of a disk with a hole in it rotating at constant angular velocity in front of a pipe with air under pressure. When the hole passes in front of the tube, the air rushes through the hole, thereby producing a pulse train that is heard as a siren.

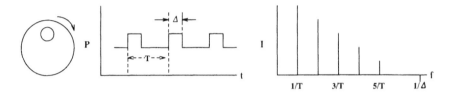

FIG. VI.7 The pressure pulse train produced by a rotating disk with one hole and the corresponding spectrum.

Next consider a siren in which there are two holes in the disk and they are exactly opposite each other on a diameter of the disk. Thus the wave and its spectrum are as in Fig. VI.8. The pitch of this siren is matched by a pure tone of frequency $2/T$, that is, its pitch is an octave above that in the first siren. Again, this is as it should be.

Finally, consider a third siren that is like the previous one in that it has two holes, but let them deviate ever so slightly from being at opposite ends of a diameter. So there are two periods between successive sounding, say T_1 and T_2, where $T = T_1 + T_2$ and $T_1 \neq T_2$. Thus, the resulting sound has the waveform and spectrum shown in Fig. VI.9.

Even if T_1 and T_2 differ by only a few *micro*seconds, the perceived pitch in the third case is the same as that of the first, namely $1/T$, not that of the second, $2/T$. This is surprising in two respects. First, from the perspective of the waveform, the third case is far more similar to the second than to the first. Second, there is hardly any energy at $1/T$ to be heard.

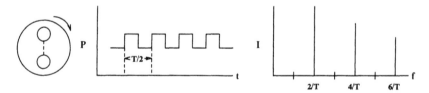

FIG. VI.8 The pressure pulse train produced by a rotating disk with two holes at opposite ends of a diagonal of the disk and the corresponding spectrum.

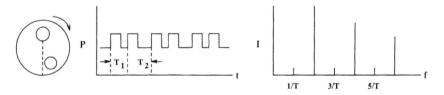

FIG. VI.9 The pressure pulse train produced by a rotating disk with two holes almost at opposite ends of a diagonal, but slightly displaced from the diagonal, and the corresponding spectrum. Note the this spectrum is very similar to Fig. VI.8; however, the perception of pitch is that of Fig. VI.7, not VI.8, which is an octave higher.

The problem in understanding this finding is that if the hearing system were only to carry out a Fourier analysis, then because there is hardly any energy at $1/T$, it should not conclude that the fundamental pitch is $1/T$. Although, this discovery caused some scientific consternation at the time, it was gradually forgotten until well into this century.[3]

4.2 Modern Results

4.2.1 The Telephone as a Band-Pass Filter.   The phenomenon was accidentally rediscovered in this century largely because of the telephone. To hold down transmission costs, which are proportional to bandwidth, telephone companies wanted to transmit only that much of speech as is absolutely necessary to maintain intelligibility and, possibly, identifiability of the speaker. Empirically, it was found that the band from 300 to 3,000 Hz, which is the bandwidth of existing telephones, is quite adequate.

That this bandwidth is in fact satisfactory seems surprising. Measurements on human voices show that for most people, especially men, the fundamental vocal frequency is well below 300 Hz—something like 125 to 175 Hz. Thus, the phone is a band pass filter that does *not* pass the fundamental frequency of the voice. Nonetheless, we do not hear each other on the phone as if we are speaking in falsetto. How is this possible?

4.2.2 Experimental Explorations.   These facts led a Dutch scientist, J. F. Schouten, at the Phillips laboratories, to study the phenomenon in the 1930s using the then new ability to generate in the laboratory pure tones of various precise frequencies and intensities. In essence, he presented sounds composed of only the higher harmonics of a fundamental that was not there. An example is shown in Fig. VI.10. When people are asked to match a pure tone in pitch to such a complex, they select the fundamentals, 200 Hz, as the match, despite the fact that the signal has no energy whatsoever at this frequency. Demonstration 12 illustrates this phenomenon. What is the reason for it?

4.2.3 Nonlinear Distortion Is Ruled Out.   One initial idea was that the effect is due to nonlinear distortion. This says that because of distortions in the hearing system, probably in the ear itself, there really is energy at 200 Hz even though there is none in the input signal itself. The induced energy arises because of the distortion products or combination tones such as $2f_1 - f_2$. Thus, for example, the frequencies $f_1 = 1,000$ Hz and $f_2 = 1,800$ Hz in the signal produce the combination frequency $2f_1 - f_2 = 200$ Hz.

---

[3]It is not uncommon in the history of science to see data ignored, at least for a while, when they do not fit into an accepted theoretical scheme.

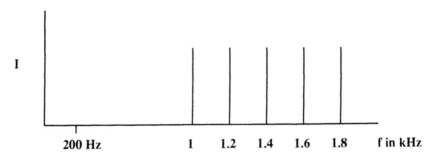

FIG. VI.10   The spectrum of a sound generated by the superposition of the fifth through the ninth harmonic of 200 Hz.

If so, then this apparent illusion really is no illusion at all, but has a physical origin. That account was vividly shown to be incorrect in 1954 by the late American psychophysicist and computer expert J. C. R. Licklider. His demonstration that there really is no significant energy at the missing fundamental can be heard in Demonstration 13.

His idea, like so many decisive ones, was very simple. If we hear the pitch of 200 Hz because of energy at 200 Hz, then low pass noise with an upper cutoff at 500 Hz should mask the pitch just as it does a pure tone at 200 Hz. Equally, high pass noise (with a lower cutoff at 500 Hz) that is sufficient to mask the higher harmonics being presented in the experiment, should leave unaffected any energy that exists at 200 Hz. So the prediction of the nonlinear distortion hypothesis is that low frequency noise should mask the missing fundamental and high frequency noise should leave it unaffected. If, however, there is no energy at 200 Hz and the pitch is somehow induced from the harmonics, then exactly the opposite is predicted. In summary, the predictions are:

		At 200 Hz	
		Energy	No Energy
Noise	Low	MASKS PITCH	PITCH REMAINS
Frequency	High	PITCH REMAINS	MASKS PITCH

The demonstration and the data are unambiguous. Low frequency noise does not affect the illusory pitch at 200 Hz, whereas high frequency noise eliminates it completely. The illusory 200 Hz pitch seems to sit on top of the noise, almost as if it exists in a domain completely separate from the noise.

The conclusion is that the inference of a low pitch from the harmonic complex is just that, an inference made by the brain. It is not based on there being energy at that frequency. It truly is an auditory illusion. To this day we do not know exactly how it arises.

Some evidence indicates that it is probably not something that is acquired with auditory experience but rather a fundamental feature of the hearing system. Studies on very young infants — which are based on the fact that they tend, when alert and happy, to turn to novel stimuli — indicate that infants perceive the missing fundamental at 200 Hz when only 1,000, 1,200, 1,400, 1,600 Hz are present.

4.2.4 An Engineering Example.   A practical example of illusory pitch occurred in the 1960s after Congress mandated a significant reduction in the annoyance levels of jet engines. The engineers were faced with the problem of attenuating the noise as much as possible with as little increase in weight, cost, and fuel usage as possible. Thus, it was crucial to determine as well as they could which frequency bands most annoy people. Their initial interview studies told them that the main objection was to the low pitch rumble of the taking off jet; however, their physical measurements told them that there was, in fact, comparatively little energy at the frequencies about which people complained. After a period of some perplexity, consultation with hearing experts led them to realize that the rotating fans were producing the harmonics of lower frequencies and missing fundamentals were what people described as the source of the annoyance, when in fact the energy activating their hearing was at much higher frequencies. Thus, only the higher frequencies needed to be attenuated physically.

5. ECHOS AND REVERBERATION

5.1 Echos

A plaster wall reflects some 80% to 90% of the sound energy impinging on it. As a result, often there is more reflected energy than direct energy at some points in a room. A vivid example of this occurs in many domed rooms — two famous ones are the Capitol building in Washington and St. Paul's cathedral in Rome, and other less famous examples include some Paris metro stations[4] — where a hushed conversation in one location is heard with perfect clarity at a distant point because the reflected waves converge (see Fig. VI.11).

In any echo situation, each indirect path is necessarily longer than the direct one, so the echo of any sound is necessarily delayed relative to the sound received directly. The delay is roughly 3 ms for each additional meter travelled. We can calculate that from the fact that sound travels at 344 m/s and so

---

[4]An anonymous reviewer of the manuscript cited this location, remarking ". . . where I've occasionally heard interesting conversations of couples standing on the opposite platform!"

Domed room

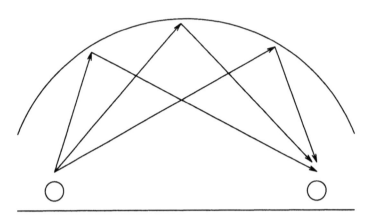

FIG. VI.11 Sound reflections in a suitably domed room focus sounds at a place symmetrically located relative to the sound source.

$$(1/344 \text{ s/m}) \times (1{,}000 \text{ ms/s}) = 2.91 \text{ ms/m}.$$

The simple sum of all these delayed waves is, of course, an enormously complex pressure wave. Whatever it is, one might expect a priori that all these echos would create a serious problem for the listener. And, to a degree, they sometimes do. In highly reverberant rooms — those with plaster walls, lots of glass, tile floors, no curtains or carpets — many people, particularly older ones, find the sound quite unpleasant and speech can be difficult to understand. However bad that may seem, the negative aspects do not seem nearly proportionate to the complexity of the physical stimulus itself at the ear.

This suppression of echos can be heard in Demonstration 1 using some rather ordinary sounds, such as a hammer hitting a hard surface, which were recorded in rooms with different reflective properties. These tapes are played both as recorded and then backward. The remarkable feature of the backward version is the long sound — the echo — that precedes the percussive sound itself. This echo is hardly noticed at all when played as recorded, when it follows rather than precedes the primary sound. The echo is largely suppressed.

5.2 Not Hearing Echos: The Precedence Effect

5.2.1 Facts About the Precedence Effect.   The following are some of the raw empirical facts:

- No echo is heard at all if the delay is in the range of 20 to 30 ms, which corresponds to a room length of about 7 to 10 m. Moreover, the sound under these circumstances appears to be coming entirely along the shortest path, even when more energy actually arrives via reflections. This fact is referred to as the **precedence effect,** which only names the phenomenon; it is not an explanation. It means that the direct wave takes precedence over the reflected ones in the sense that one appears to hear just the direct wave.

- One hears some aspects of the reflected wave. To verify this, sit off center before a pair of balanced stereo speakers so that the sound appears to be coming just from the nearest speaker. Then have a friend disconnect the more distant speaker. A noticeable change in the quality of the sound will be heard as well as a roughly 3 dB drop in loudness, corresponding to the halving of the intensity.

- Echos, as such, are heard when the delay is from 500 ms to 1,000 ms, which is the equivalent of a room length of from 172 m to 344 m.

- Precedence is not the result of poor auditory acuity on the part of the listener. For example, two clicks presented successively in earphones are heard as two separate clicks when the temporal separation is greater than 2 ms. That time difference corresponds to a hand clap more than one meter from a plaster wall—and you can easily verify that you do not hear two claps.

- Precedence is not a result of the fact that, in general, the intensity of the reflected wave is somewhat less than that of the direct wave. This is readily verified by earphone experiments.

- Precedence is not easily maintained when recording sounds, a major problem for audio engineers. For example, take a tape recorder to a party and record what is going on near you. When played back, conversations are nearly unintelligible and the snap of a flip-top can opened 5 m away sounds like a minor explosion. Yet at the time of the taping little difficulty is experienced in understanding a nearby speaker and one is unlikely to be aware of the snap of the can.

- With delays falling between the two ranges discussed previously—more than 30 ms, below which no echo is heard, and less than 500 ms, above which the echo is distinct—there is a noticeable effect called *reverberation*. It is something heard in any large hall or auditorium. Depending on exact configurations and the nature of wall and ceiling materials, auditoria vary considerably in their degree of reverberation. This is an important feature in the musical quality of such halls.

- The precedence effect has no accepted theory. We do not know how the brain manages to ignore the echos as well as it does. In particular, we do not know how to build computer-based auditory equipment that is equally able to ignore echos.

5.2.2 Two Practical Applications of the Precedence Effect.

Conference Microphone Configuration.   How should one configure a microphone located on a conference table to record speech as well as possible? Panel a of Fig. VI.12 shows the traditional way. The difficulty with this arrangement, as indicated in panel b, is the reflections from the hard, smooth table top. Unlike the ear, the microphone does not exhibit the precedence effect. As a result, the taped sound is frequently quite unintelligible.

One solution, shown in panel c, is quite simple: Design the microphone so that reflections have little or no opportunity to occur. Put the microphone as close as possible to the table top. Another solution is to cover the table with a sound absorbant fabric, thereby eliminating both the amount of energy in and the coherence of the reflections.

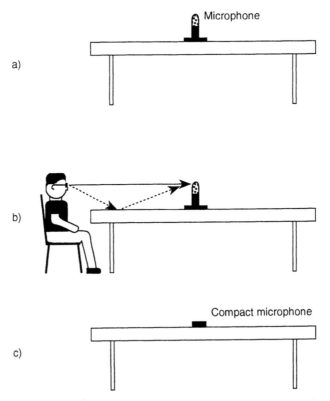

FIG. VI.12   (a) The usual configuration of a microphone at a conference table. (b) The reason that sounds reflected by the table are fairly prominent in this arrangement. (c) A modified configuration that largely eliminates the problem of table reflections.

Amplification in a Large Auditorium.   During the 1930s very large auditoria began to be constructed both for concerts and motion pictures (e.g., Radio City Music Hall). Their massive volume made sound amplification absolutely necessary. The obvious solution was to mass sufficient amplifiers and loudspeakers at the front of the hall to get the sound level up to the desired intensity. This solution, however, had three serious drawbacks:

- The most obvious difficulty is the inevitable substantial loudness gradient from front to back. Those in the front rows are overwhelmed with sound, whereas those in the back can barely hear it.
- Second, at the time it was difficult to build sufficiently large, distortion free amplifiers and loudspeakers to fill the room with quality sound when they were located only in the front.
- By far the most serious problem was that the dimensions of such halls were sufficiently great that echos, not reverberation, occurred.

The solution to all three problems is to take advantage of the precedence effect. This is done by placing speakers all along the side walls, which is now standard in movie theaters. It is reasonably clear that by having sufficient, only moderately powerful, loudspeakers, the space can be filled with relatively uniform sound levels. However, if one does this naively, then the sound seems to lack a clear source — it is diffuse and comes from all around the listener. That difficulty is readily solved by introducing sufficient delay — 10 to 30 ms — relative to the front speakers so that, according to the precedence effect, one hears the sound as coming from the stage, even though substantially more of the energy at the listener's ears is actually coming from the side walls.

This illustrates is a happy rarity in which a single engineering solution solved several problems simultaneously without undesirable trade-offs.

5.2.3 Interaction of Localization with Precedence.   Two clicks that are less than 2 ms apart are heard as a single sound. That does not mean, however, that the system is insensitive to their separateness. This can be demonstrated in an experiment in which we control the relative times of the first and the second pair of clicks to the two ears. Panel a of Fig. VI.13 illustrates one experimental situation.

If $\Delta t = 20$ μs (note, this is micro-, not milli-, seconds), the click is localized as being on the left. Now let us try to center the click by changing the order of the second click, as shown in panel b. For $\Delta t = 20$ μs, the value of $\Delta t'$ needed in order to center the click is -200 μs, that is, a factor of 10. Once again, that which gets there first is dominant.

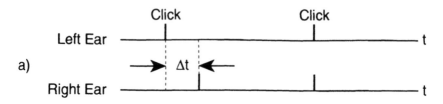

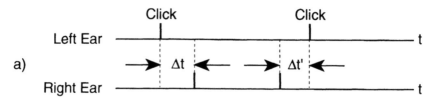

FIG. VI.13   (a) A pair of clicks are presented to each ear. The first arrives at the left ear Δt seconds prior to when the first one arrives at the right ear, and the second ones are simultaneous. With Δt sufficiently large, one perceives the click pairs as first to the left and then to the right ear. (b) The late arrival at the right ear is now compensated by having the second click arrive at the right ear $\Delta t'$ seconds prior to when the second click arrives at the left ear. The question is how large must $\Delta t'$ be in order that the two sounds are perceived as arriving at the same time.

5.2.4 Lack of Theory.   All of these precedence effects are obviously of great importance in hearing. Nevertheless, auditory scientists do not yet understand how the brain processes sounds to produce precedence and echo suppression. In particular, we do not know how to build machines to do the same thing. It would be a highly desirable feature if it could be achieved in hearing aids. That, however, may well not be possible if the phenomenon is truly central rather than peripheral.

6. PERCEPTUAL STRUCTURING OF SOUNDS

6.1 Signals Over Time

During the 1970s and 1980s, increasing empirical attention has focused on the ways in which we perceive complex, temporally patterned sound signals over relatively prolonged periods of time. The motivation for such studies is the obvious fact that a most important aspect of auditory perception is maintaining some degree of source continuity over time, even as the spectral distribution of frequencies changes considerably. This is an undeniable aspect of both speech and music. One can isolate single instruments in an orchestra and individual speakers in a noisy, crowded room.

The importance of temporal continuity has long been recognized, but the techniques for good experimental control of stimuli to study such phenomena only became available with the advent of relatively inexpensive, very powerful computers. Among other things, they permit the digital simulation of arbitrary waveforms, and therefore of very detailed experimental control.

We have already encountered some examples of systematic detection studies involving such complex sounds in Sections VI.2 and VI.3. Here we report a series of phenomena that are both striking and very poorly understood. We do not have anything approaching a theory for such perceptual structuring, but there are quite a number of empirical findings, some of which we can describe and demonstrate.

6.2 Perceptual Induction of Missing Sounds[5]

6.2.1 A Frequency Example: Tone Glides. A tone glide is a relatively rapid, continuous change in frequency with the sound being held at (approximately) a constant intensity. This is illustrated in panel a of Fig. VI.14. If one introduces temporal gaps into the glide, as illustrated in panel b, they are readily perceived. This can be heard in Demonstration 14. However, if the gaps are filled with broad band noise, as shown in panel c, then the ear does just what the eye does with the graph—it induces the missing segment as if the noise had blocked out the segment, and the glide does not seem to be interrupted by the noise (Tape Band 7b). Of course, one hears the noise bursts, but the tone glides right through them.

6.2.2 An Intensity Example. Suppose the signals are noise bands that are one octave wide (say, from f to $2f$) but of different intensities in different time intervals, as shown in part a of Fig. VI.15. Perceptually, this

---

[5]Most often the phenomenon to be described is called "restoration of missing sounds," but in fact "induction" is a far more accurate term.

(a)   f

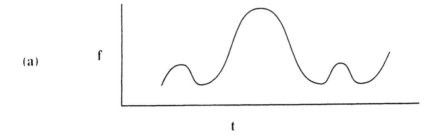

t

(b)   f

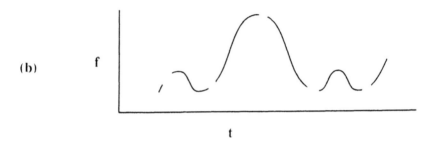

t

Noise bursts

(c)   f

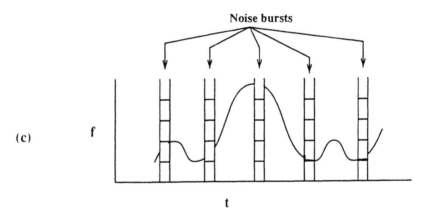

t

FIG. VI.14 (a) A typical frequency glide. (b) The same frequency glide with brief gaps. (c) The same as panel b except that the gaps are all filled with broad band noise. The gaps are noticeable in panel b but are not heard in panel c, that is, panel c sounds like the glide of panel a with noise bursts added.

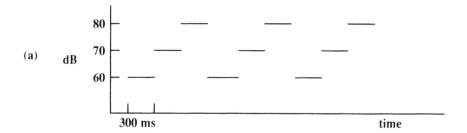

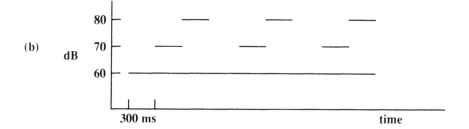

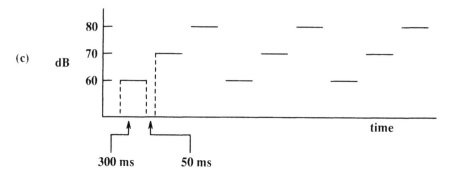

FIG. VI.15 (a) A repetition of three one-octave wide noise bands of increasing intensity and no gaps between their presentations. (b) The perception of panel a is that the lowest intensity is continuously present. (c) If, however, gaps as small as 50 ms are introduced, the percept is as shown, not as in panel b.

is heard as if the lower intensity is continuous, as is indicated in part b. Such induction fails to occur where there are gaps of at least 50 ms between noise bursts, as in panel c.

6.2.3 A Speech Example.   Suppose one takes a recording of natural speech and erases short segments that correspond to some of the basic speech sounds called *phonemes* (roughly, a consonant-vowel pair) about which more will be said later. Thus, this modified speech is full of silent gaps (similar to the glide example in Section VI.6.2.1). In one experiment sufficiently many gaps were introduced so that intelligibility (as measured by correct identification of words) was reduced to only 20% of its normal value. However, when the gaps were filled with broad band noise, intelligibility was restored to 70% of its normal value. Note that the noise does not in any physical sense restore the missing information; there was neither more nor less actual information than when the gaps were silent. Yet, perceptually it was as if the information had been partially restored by the noise.

6.2.4 The Induction Principle.   The following empirical generalization appears to be valid. Perceptual induction (restoration) occurs when the situation meets two conditions:

- The induction transforms something discontinuous or disrupted into something continuous or coherent; and
- Had the induced sound actually been there, the other sounds present would have effectively masked it.

One implication of this principle is that the induced sounds must lie in the same critical band (i.e., activate the same peripheral neuron group) as the apparent masker.

A second implication is that induction and masking data should agree. For example, let the masker be (80 dB, 1,000 Hz) and for each f find the largest value of I such that the masker just masks (I, f). This is usually done by presenting the masker in a series of pulses and adding the test tone (I, f) to alternate pulses. The intensity I is decreased until the sense of alternation vanishes. The data are shown in Fig. VI.16. These masking and induction data almost agree, except for discrepancies at 1,000 and 2,000 Hz, which are due to beats in the masking case that cannot occur in induction.

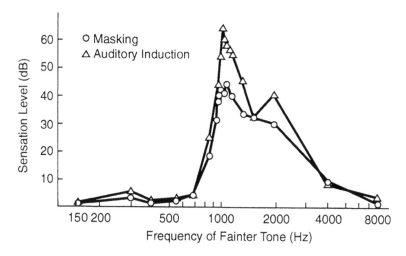

FIG. VI.16   A comparison of masking and auditory induction using an 80 dB, 1,000 Hz masker. The masking procedure and data are as in Fig. VI.1 and, as there, beating causes better performance near the masker than would otherwise be expected. In the auditory induction procedure one determines the intensity as a function of frequency that is just sufficient for induction to occur across a gap. From "Auditory Induction: Perceptual Synthesis of Absent Sounds" by R. M. Warren, C. J. Obusek, and J. M. Ackroff, 1972, *Science, 176,* p. 1149. Copyright 1972 by American Association for the Advancement of Sciences. Reprinted by permission.

6.3 Fusing and Streaming

6.3.1 Fusing.   When several tones are presented at once, they usually **fuse** into a single, rich sound that is not separated into its Fourier components. Certainly, this is true for a tone with its overtones (harmonics) and for musical chords.

6.3.2 Streaming.   Although fusing is the natural tendency, situations exist in which it can be disrupted and replaced by what is called (temporal) **streaming.** When this happens, one or more of the component frequencies is peeled off the complex and is heard as a pure tone. A simple example of two streams of slightly varying tones can be heard in Demonstration 15, part 1. Conceptually it is as shown in panel a of Fig. VI.17. If, however, the successive tones are connected by pitch glides, as in panel b then, as one can hear in Demonstration 15, parts 2 and 3, streaming is blocked. Whether or not streaming occurs also depends on the rate of alternation, which is also demonstrated.

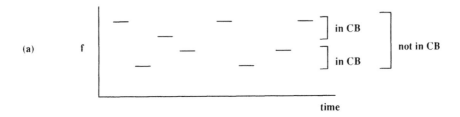

(a)   f

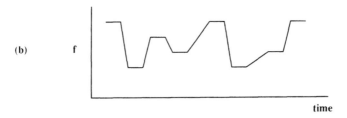

(b)   f

time

FIG. VI.17   (a) A sequence of tones at four levels of frequency, with the top two within one critical band, the bottom two within one critical band, but the top and bottom separated by more than a critical band. The perception is streaming. (b) The same tones connected together to form a tone glide. The perception is as a tone glide, not as in panel a.

6.3.3 Crucial Role of Critical Bands.   Suppose we have a pair of pure tones alternating with a single intermediate frequency such that no pair of frequencies lies in a critical band, as shown in panel a of Fig. VI.18. The perception, as is demonstrated in part 1, Demonstration 16, is of a pure tone of the middle frequency alternating with a distinct, fused sound composed of the top and bottom frequencies. If, however, the upper two frequencies are in the same critical band, as shown in panel b, then the perception is of two separated sounds, the higher one streaming continuously and the lower one a pure tone that is pulsed on and off (part 2). The role of critical bands in streaming is also illustrated in Demonstration 17 of the Phillips disc.

6.3.4 Temporal Coordination.   Suppose that a sequence of triples of tones is such that the triples stay in some fixed frequency ratio relative to one another, for example, 3:4:5, as they rise and fall together in frequency. Let a fourth tone rise and fall in a temporal pattern completely independent of the triple of tones. This is diagrammed in Fig. VI.19. As in Demonstration 18, the percept is of the triple (shown as lighter lines) fused together as a chord on top of which the fourth (shown as a heavier line) is heard as a sequence of discretely shifting tones that is isolated from the fused chord.

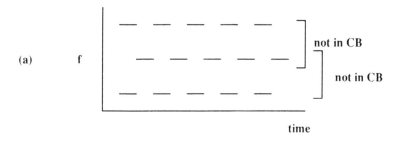

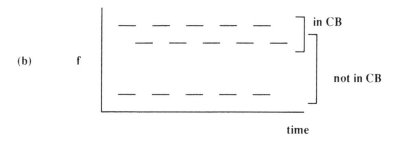

FIG. VI.18 (a) Three levels of frequency, no two in the same critical band. The top and bottom are presented together and alternate with the middle one. This is perceived as a chord alternating with a pure tone. (b) The same arrangement as panel a except that the top and middle tones are in a critical band and the middle and the bottom are not. The perception is of the top two tones streaming and the lower one pulsing.

6.3.5 Segregation Due to Induced Continuity.   Suppose three tones, no pair of which falls in a critical band, are repeated in a fixed order, as shown in panel a of Fig. VI.20. Perceptually it is difficult to decide whether the top pairs are presented in the same order or if they are reversed. The second of these pairs is not well segregated from the lower frequency "distractors." However, suppose that the low frequency distractor is made highly distinctive and more continuous, as in panel b. Then the perception is of a segregated lower frequency, and as a result the judgment of temporal order is much easier (Demonstration 19).

6.3.6 Binaural Fusing and Dominance.   Consider an alternating sequence of low and high frequency tones, for example, 400 and 800 Hz. The sequence is presented to both ears, but shifted by half the period, so that the ear pairs are (low, high) followed by (high, low), then by (low, high), and so on. Using earphones, one can listen to this in Demonstration 20. One perceives the high tone pulsing on and off in one ear and the low tone pulsing on and off in the other. Moreover, it does not matter which ear

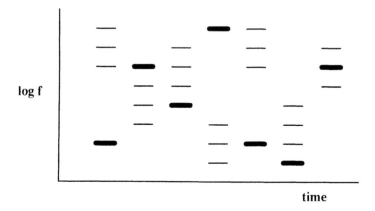

FIG. VI.19 Groups of four tones are presented together. They consist of a triple of tones that maintain the same frequency ratios (lighter lines) as the triple rises and falls, and the fourth moves independently of the triple. The perception is of the three being fused as a changing chord and the fourth tone moving independently of the chord.

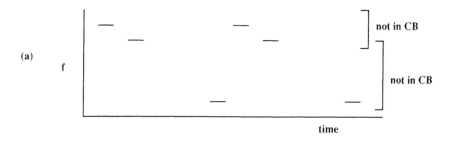

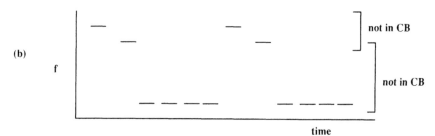

FIG. VI.20 (a) Three levels of frequencies no two of which are in a critical band are presented top, middle, a gap of three times the length of the tones, and bottom. This is repeated. Under these conditions it is difficult to tell the order in which the top two frequencies occur. (b) If the gap is filled with three of the bottom tone, then the bottom one becomes segregated and it is easier to tell the order of the top two.

first heard the high frequency, the segregation of the high frequency is always to the same ear.

But which ear hears the high frequency? Right-handed subjects generally hear the high tone in the right ear and left-handed individuals split about 50:50. This may have something to do with the dominance in right-handed people of the left hemisphere for speech.

Quite clearly, the phenomenon is an auditory illusion because each tone is in each ear half the time, but is heard in only one ear. We do not currently understand why this happens in terms of our knowledge of the brain.

7. SPEECH:
A SPECIAL PERCEPTUAL ABILITY

A certain amount of empirical evidence has led some scientists to the view that speech production and analysis is a special ability, quite distinct from the processing of other nonspeech sounds. Such a special system must, of course, draw on basic peripheral processes of hearing, but it goes far beyond that. One can reasonably ask whether music perception also involves a distinctive auditory subsystem, and certainly it is plausible that it does, but the evidence is not so strong. However, be aware that not all auditory experts agree even about the separate, modular nature of speech. It is a matter of ongoing controversy.

One indication of specialization is that when conflicting speech signals are presented to the two ears, the right ear typically dominates and one perceives only what is in that ear. Because the main neural fibers from the auditory nerve cross to the opposite hemisphere, this implicates a left hemisphere location for speech. (The phenomenon discussed in Section VI.6.3.6 is probably related to speech dominance.)

This is further confirmed by clinical evidence. Damage to appropriate regions of the left hemisphere has deleterious effects on speech, whereas similar damage in the right hemisphere has little or no effect on speech. Substituting musical inputs reverses the pattern.

Whether or not speech is modular, there certainly are a number of speech phenomena that are quite distinct from anything we have encountered so far.

7.1 What Aspects of Speech Signals Affect
Their Perception?

Attempts to answer this question have been the focus of a good deal of research throughout the past 50 years, and the area is still extremely active.

It is of great interest to computer specialists working with voice-activated inputs to computers.

7.1.1 The Pressure Waveform. Speech perception is surprisingly insensitive to some gross aspects of the pressure waveform. The most apparent, if not very revealing, evidence is that one understands quite different productions of the same word or sentence. Not only are there large variations from speaker to speaker, but also one speaker's productions vary considerably from occasion to occasion. Clearly, no very specific waveform is associated with a particular speech interpretation.

If it is not the waveform that controls intelligibility, then what does? Some insight is gained, first, by systematically distorting the speech in various ways, of which we describe three; and, second, by examining how speech is produced and what is controlled by the speaker (Section VI.7.2).

7.1.2 Filtered Speech. Speech can be run through a low pass filter with an 1,800 Hz cutoff or through a high pass filter with an 1,800 Hz cutoff resulting in an accuracy score of about 67% in each case. With a band pass filter of only one octave from 1,000 Hz to 2,000 Hz, accuracy is about 90%; with a band pass of 300 to 3,000 Hz (the filter characteristic of a telephone) it is 100%. The differences in the appearance of the pressure wave before and after such filtering is very great, but that seems to affect neither the intelligibility nor the ability to recognize the speaker.

For obvious reasons, a number of these studies were carried out at the AT&T Bell Laboratories.

7.1.3 Peak Clipping. A common failing of much inexpensive audio equipment is what is known as peak clipping. This is illustrated in Fig. VI.21. Such a distortion of the pressure waveform has little effect on the intelligibility of speech. This is demonstrated most vividly in the next section.

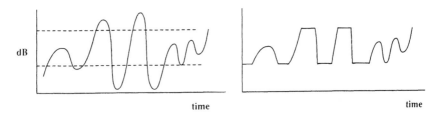

FIG. VI.21 Peak clipping of a waveform involves upper and lower thresholds, and any part of the wave above the upper threshold is replaced by the threshold value, and similarly for the lower one.

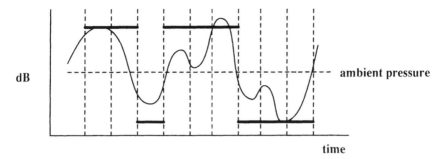

FIG. VI.22 Using a digitizing grid in which intensity is partitioned into just two levels—positive and negative—tends to preserve the information about the zero crossings of the original wave. Just how accurate this is depends on the fineness of the temporal grid.

7.1.4 Digitized Speech. It was remarked in Section V.5.3.2, which focused on the digitization of signals as a means of noise suppression, that people are insensitive to digitization provided the sampling rate is sufficiently high. This is illustrated in Demonstration 21 in which speech is presented using several levels of digitizing and sampling rates. With a sampling rate of 10 kHz, the number of binary levels of intensity are given in bits, where the actual number of levels is 2 raised to the power of the number of bits. [Thus, one bit equals $2^1 = 2$ levels, 2 bits is 4 levels, 4 bits is $2^4 = 16$ levels, and 12 bits is $2^{12} = (2^4)^3 = 16 \times 16 \times 16 = 4,096$ levels.] Also, at a sampling level of 12 bits, four sampling rates are used: 10, 5, 2.5, and 1.25 kHz.

The demonstration establishes that intelligibility suffers by reducing the sampling rate, but hardly at all by reducing the levels of digitizing. The rate is so important probably because at high sampling rates, binary digitizing provides fairly accurate information about where the pressure wave crosses the ambient air pressure, as is diagrammed in Fig. VI.22. Recall that these crossing values are called *zero crossings* because they are the times at which the wave, which is deviations from the ambient pressure, passes through the ambient pressure (see Section II.2.2.4). The data seem to suggest that the pattern of zero crossings carries much of the information in speech.

7.2 Speech Production

To a crude first approximation, the vocal tract is a long "tube-like" cavity open at the mouth and activated by air under pressure from the lungs being

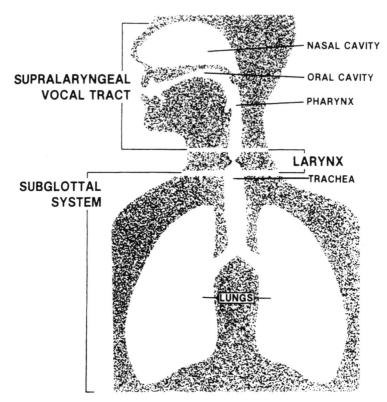

FIG. VI.23   A schematic of the human vocal system. From *Auditory Perception: A New Synthesis* (p. 157) by R. M. Warren, 1982, New York: Pergamon Press. Copyright 1982 by Pergamon Press, Inc. Reprinted by permission.

forced rapidly through a narrow slit, called the **glottis,** that is formed by the vocal folds (see Fig. VI.23). The glottis is controlled by muscles. When it is open, a buzz is produced, which is the source of the speech sounds that are called **voiceless.** An example is the nasalness of some consonants. Otherwise, it opens and closes rapidly, producing a sound with a fundamental frequency that varies from 75 to 100 Hz for men and from 150 to 200 Hz for women. The resulting sounds are called **voiced** and include the vowels. The sex difference lies in the length and thickening of folds.

The sounds emanating from the glottis are then modulated by manipulations of the opening to the nasal cavity, the tongue, and the lips. These manipulations primarily alter the resonance characteristics of the vocal track. One can think of the resulting resonances as a system of acoustic filters through which the emitted sound is passed and thereby modulated. The following principle holds:

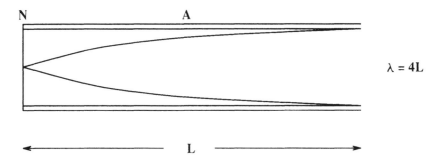

FIG. VI.24   The pressure envelope of the fundamental resonance frequency of a half open tube.

Those harmonics of the basic activating buzz approximately equal to a resonance frequency of the vocal tract are amplified by the resonance.

A highly simplified model of the vocal track is as a half open tube with natural resonances (see Fig. VI.24). Thus, we can calculate the fundamental resonance frequency of the track:

Males	Females
L = 17.5 cm	14 cm
F_0 = (344 m/s)/(4 × 17.5) (1/100)	344/(4 × 14) (1/100)
= 491 Hz	= 614 Hz

Note that F_0 for males is the fourth harmonic of 123 Hz and the fifth harmonic of 98 Hz. For females it is the third harmonic of 205 Hz or the fourth harmonic of 153 Hz. Recall, that a half-open tube has only odd harmonics — $3F_0$, $5F_0$, ... So the natural frequency of the vocal track is approximately some harmonic of the modulation of the fundamental buzz. Thus the resonance has the effect of amplifying some harmonics of the buzz and suppressing others.

7.2.1 Formants.   It follows that only a limited number of frequencies will be present in the vocal output at any one time. These resonances are called **formants**. In identifying formants neither the harmonic number of the modulated buzz nor the harmonic number of the resonance is used. Rather, the following unusual convention is employed: The lowest (narrow) frequency band for which there is substantial energy is called the **first formant**, and denoted F_1. The next one with any substantial energy is called the **second formant**, denoted F_2, and so forth. Thus, if one speech sound has formants at 500, 1,500, and 2,500 Hz (i.e., the first, third, fifth harmonics of resonance), they are referred to as formants F_1, F_2, and F_3, and if another speech sound has formants at 500, 1,500, and 3,500 (first, third, seventh) they are also referred to as F_1, F_2, and F_3.

7.2.2 Pictorial Representations of Formants.   The graphical problem is how best to represent spectral amplitude as a function of both time and frequency. Recall, spectral amplitude simply means how much pressure or intensity occurs at each frequency at each instant. An example is shown in Fig. VI.25. For a relatively sustained sound the plot is the simpler one of Fig. VI.26.

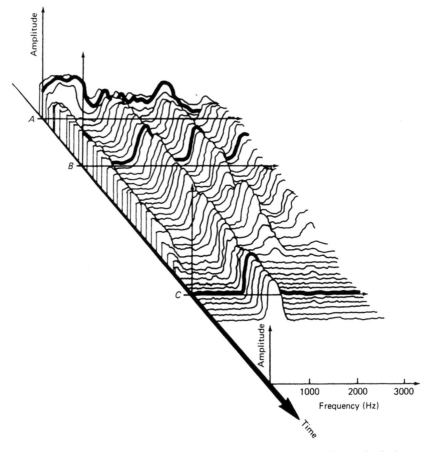

FIG. VI.25   A three-dimensional — amplitude and frequency versus time — of a ringing telephone. From *Fundamentals of Sensation and Perception* (p. 521) by M. W. Levine and J. M. Shefner, 1991, Pacific Grove, CA. Brooks/Cole. Copyright 1991 by Wadsworth, Inc. Reprinted by permission.

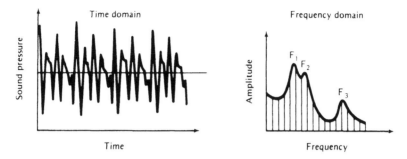

FIG. VI.26 A sample of a speech amplitude waveform and the corresponding spectrum. Note the three amplitude peaks in the spectrum that are identified as the formants F_1, F_2, and F_3. From *Fundamentals of Hearing* (p. 190) by W. A. Yost and D. W. Nielsen, 1985, Orlando: Holt, Rinehart & Winston. Copyright 1985 by Holt, Rinehart & Winston, Inc. Reprinted by permission.

We know from Section VI.7.1.4 that a very crude digitization of the intensity dimension does little to affect speech perception, so a plausible way to summarize the desired three-dimensional graph is to use a binary digitization of intensity and only show the *(f, t)* regions where that intensity is exceeded. An example of this is shown in the top of Fig. VI.27. These exact digitized plots are then idealized into what are called **painted spectrograms.** The manufacture of such idealizations that actually reproduce acceptable speech is rather more complex than just looking at actual spectrograms of the phoneme and estimating an equal amplitude contour for, say, the 50% level. Rather they are formed by making trial-and-error drawings that are then used to construct sounds electronically, and one accepts the painted spectrogram that best reproduces the desired speech sound, which in the case shown is the phrase "to catch pink salmon."

Much artificial speech you hear today is done in this manner. For example, with a few exceptions, the voice on the Phillips Demonstration Disk is that of a noted auditory expert, Ira Hirsh. In some cases his voice was taped; in others it was simulated artificially. It is not easy to tell which is which, even for someone who knows him.

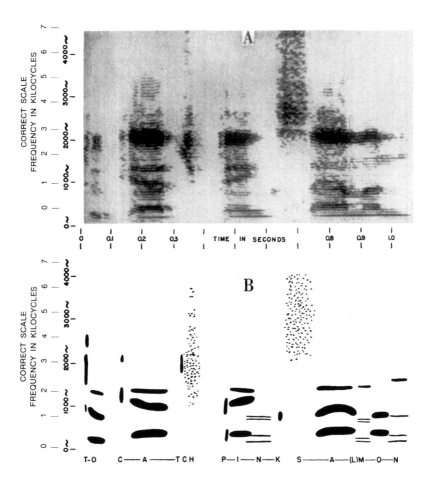

FIG. VI.27 The spectrogram and resulting formant structure of the phrase "to catch a pink salmon." Panel a is the measured spectrogram, and panel b is the resulting idealized or "painted" spectrogram that makes the formant structure more obvious. From "The Role of Stimulus-Variables in the Perception of the Unvoiced Stop Consonants" by A. M. Liberman, P. C. Delattre, and F. S. Cooper, 1952, *American Journal of Psychology, 65,* p. 498. Copyright 1952 by American Journal of Psychology. Reprinted by permission.

7.3 Isolation of Elementary Components of Speech: Phonemes

Once this technique for the analysis and synthesis of speech sounds was developed in the 1950s—primarily at the Haskins Laboratory associated with Yale University—it became possible to search for patterns characterizing particular speech sounds. As we know, no fixed pattern can describe a phoneme because physically it varies considerably from person to person and from occasion to occasion. Nevertheless, we expect to be able to find something invariant among all instances of what native speakers say are the same speech segment.

In many cases, the pattern concerns primarily the first two formants, F_1 and F_2. Figure VI.28 shows the pattern for three syllables. In all cases, the initial segment of both formants increases to a constant that is the same for all three syllables. They differ only in the rate of rise of the initial segment. A slightly different pattern is exhibited by Fig. VI.29—note that the initial approach to F_1 and F_2 differs.

Another way of saying the same thing is that syllables are composed of two parts—a constant one, corresponding to the vowel, and a changing one, corresponding to the accompanying consonant. But as becomes evident, it is not quite so simple.

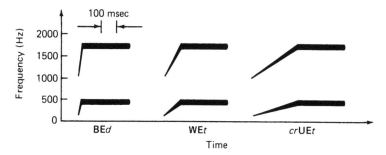

FIG. VI.28 Painted spectrograms in which the approach to the same vowel formant structure is varied from a steep rise to a slow one, yielding the three sounds BEd, WEt, and crUEt. From "Tempo of frequency change as a cue for distinguishing classes of speech sounds" (p. 130) by A. M. Liberman, P. C. Delattre, L. J. Gerstman, & F. S. Cooper, in (1952) *Journal of Experimental Psychology* 52. Copyright 1952 by America Psychological Assoc. Reprinted by permission.

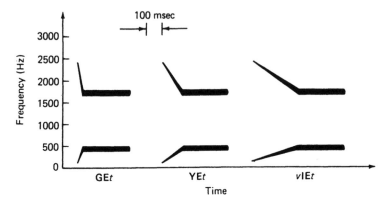

FIG. VI.29   Painted spectrograms in which the approach to the same vowel formant structure is varied from steep to shallow, but unlike Fig. VI.28, the upper one is a decrease and the lower one an increase, yielding the three sounds GEt, YEt, and vIEt. From *Fundamentals of Sensation and Perception* (p. 130) by M. W. Levine and J. M. Shefner, 1991, Pacific Grove, CA: Brooks/Cole. Copyright 1991 by Wadsworth, Inc. Reprinted by permission.

7.3.1 Effect of Context.   First, a particular stimulus pattern does not necessarily have a single interpretation. For example, the same consonant pattern of rising or falling formant leading into the vowel is heard as different sounds depending on the vowel. This is illustrated in Figs. VI.30 and VI.31. More of this later.

Second, phonemes do not exhibit a great deal of physical invariance. Fig. VI.32 shows the same vowels when spoken by men and by children. The pattern is similar, but the frequencies differ considerably. Yet, we hear them as the same phoneme.

Figure VI.33 shows spectrograms of the short sentence "I can see it" broken into individual words, and those same three words spoken in isolation. The lack of invariance is again clear.

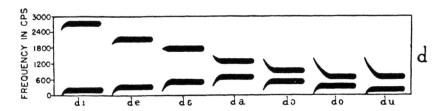

FIG. VI.30   A series of syllables obtained by systematically varying both the approach and the location of the vowel segment. The distinct sounds are shown. Note that the initial consonant is perceived as identical in all cases, despite its radically different shape in the spectrogram. From "Acoustic Loci and Transitional Cues for Consonants" by P. C. Delattre, A. M. Liberman, and F. S. Cooper, 1955, *Journal of the Acoustical Society of America, 27,* p. 770. Copyright 1955 by Acoustical Society of America. Reprinted by permission.

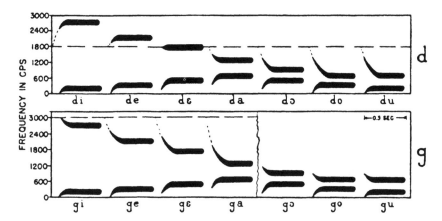

FIG. VI.31 Another example of systematic changes that leave the initial consonant invariant. From "Some Results of Research on Speech Perception" by A. M. Liberman, 1957, *Journal of the Acoustical Society of America, 29*, p. 121. Copyright 1957 by Acoustical Society of America. Reprinted by permission.

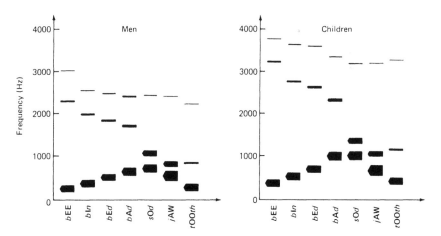

FIG. VI.32 Formant patterns for seven vowels. The left panel is the pattern of a typical adult male and the right one of children. Note the structural similarity, but the quite different frequencies that are involved for the second and, especially, the third formant. From Fundamentals of Sensation and Perception (p. 437) by M. W. Levine and J. M. Shefner, 1991, Pacific Grove, CA: Brooks/Cole. Copyright 1991 by Wadsworth, Inc. Reprinted by permission.

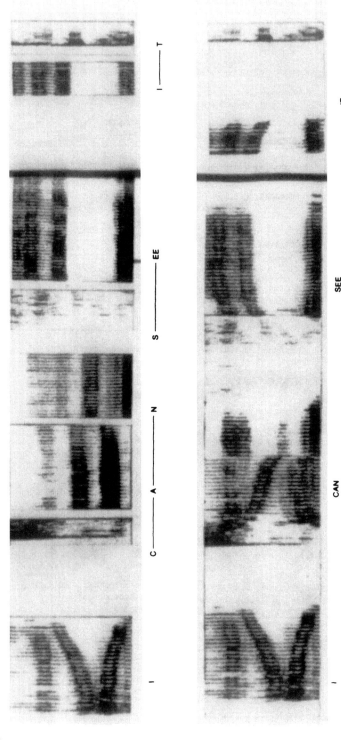

FIG. VI.33   The phrase "I can see it" as spoken one word at a time (lower half) and as a continuous sentence (upper half). From *Visible Speech* (p. 38) by R. K. Potter, G. A. Kupp, and H. G. Kupp, 1966, New York: Dover Publications. Copyright 1966 by Dover Publications. Reprinted by permission.

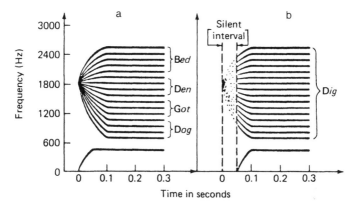

FIG. VI.34   The role of the onset to the second vowel formant in making phonemic distinctions. Panel a shows the onsets and how the initial consonants are categorized. Panel b shows the same sound except without the first 50 ms of each transition. Only a single initial consonant is heard. From *Fundamentals of Sensation and Perception* (p. 443) by M. W. Levine and J. M. Shefner, 1991, Pacific Grove, CA: Brooks/Cole. Copyright 1991 by Wadsworth, Inc. Reprinted by permission.

7.3.2 Categorical (or Quantal) Nature of Speech Perception.   The idea that speech is categorical simply means that continuous physical changes do not result in continuous perceptual changes, at least not when they are parts of speech sounds. Panel a of Fig. VI.34 illustrates the phenomenon. As the slope of onset to second formant is varied, the change from ba to da to ga is quite discontinuous. This is heard in Demonstration 22. If, however, the changing slope is presented in isolation, that is, without the vowel, then the change no longer seems discontinuous. It is necessary that it be connected to a vowel, and so become a phoneme, for the categorical nature of the sound to appear. This is also presented in the demonstration.

If the first half of the rise (50 ms) is erased, as in panel b of the figure, then only a single syllable is heard regardless of the physical changes.

Another example varies the silent interval between a voiceless fricative, s, and vowel, a. Two categories, SA and STA, are perceived. This is also heard in Demonstration 22.

The sharpness of transition from one speech sound to another is illustrated in Fig. VI.35. Here the variable is the time of onset of voicing — vibrating vocal folds — relative to release of the stop consonants b and p. The method used in this study is known as an ABX design, in which A and B represent two fixed stimuli and X represents a variable one that can be perceived as either A or B. On each trial the subject hears all three sounds and judges whether X best matches the first or second signal presented. The order of A and B is varied at random from trial to trial.

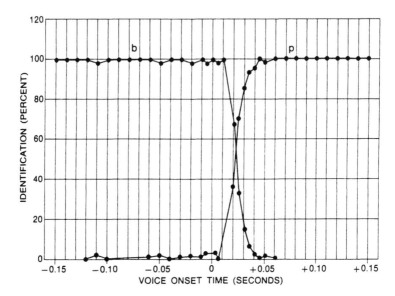

FIG. VI.35   The categorization into b and p sounds as a function of the time of onset of voicing, which is the vibration of the vocal chords, relative to the release of a stop consonant. Note that the shift from one to the other is almost discontinuous, requiring no more than a change of 30 ms. From *Language and Speech* (p. 69) by G. A. Miller, 1981, San Francisco: W. H. Freeman. Copyright 1981 by W. H. Freeman, Inc. Reprinted by permission.

7.3.3 Musical Analogues.   Several musical analogues exist to these speech phenomena. One is based on having the same, single note played on a number of different musical instruments. For an experienced musician, there is enough information in a single note to identify absolutely (without error) the type of instrument that produced it. However, if the first 50 ms, that is, the "attack" to the note, is deleted, then the note can still be identified, but the instrument cannot.

A second is a categorical classification of musical chords by musicians. Consider two chords, where the numbers are the component frequencies:

A minor (440, 523, 659)
A major (440, 554, 659).

These obviously differ only in the frequency of the middle frequency. So one uses the ABX design and varies middle frequency in small steps from 523 to 554 Hz. Musicians exhibit a sharp boundary line dividing a minor from a major chord. Untrained people do not. More surprising, a musician's ability to discriminate two such chords is better across the boundary than within a category. This appears to be either a partially learned skill or, perhaps, one for which there are substantial individual differences.

7.3.4 Are Phonemic Categories Learned or Built In?   Probably no one is fully confident of the answer to this question, but there are some data (albeit, controversial) on infants that argue for built in distinctions that are either reinforced or extinguished by the linguistic environment. (Any one language uses only a fraction of the phonemic distinctions made in at least one natural language.)

Such experiments are designed using the principle that infants tend to turn toward novel stimuli. To see if a simple physical difference is perceived as a distinction, the infant is exposed to one value until it does not respond (i.e., adapts to the stimulus). The question then is whether some small change that corresponds to a phonemic distinction made by adults and by children who are speaking also causes the infant to respond. Such experiments are very difficult to conduct because there is a lot of spontaneous head turning when the baby is awake and alert and none at all when the infant has fallen asleep or is crying. Some believe the data provide supporting evidence for in-built categorical perception, but that remains controversial.

7.3.5 Adaptation and Category Boundaries.   As was noted earlier, the switch from hearing ba to hearing da is effected somewhat discontinuously by varying the second formant attack. Suppose the experiment involves 10 levels of slope, and the switch normally occurs in going from level 5 to level 6. It has been shown that if a subject is adapted to either extreme, number 1 corresponding to ba or number 10, to da, for 40 trials, then the boundary shifts. In the former case it goes either to 3–4 or 2–3 and in the latter case to 6–7 or 7–8. Thus, the distinction is not firmly "wired" into the subject, despite the somewhat supportive evidence from the infant studies.

7.3.6 Selectivity of Adaptation.   In the typical pronunciation of ba and da there are four noticeable formants, and the ba/da distinction can be effected either by changing F_2 with F_3 fixed or by changing F_3 with F_2 fixed. So one can adapt to ba or da either by working on just F_2 or just F_3, and one can test for where the boundary is located by changing just F_2 or just F_3. The question to be considered is whether adaptation occurred in all cases. The summary of the data as to when the boundary is affected is:

		Test Formant	
		F_2	F_3
Adapting	F_2	YES	NO
Formant	F_3	NO	YES

From these data we may conclude that formant analysis is, in part, carried out on separate channels; and we may conjecture that this is because they lie in different critical bands.

8. SOME RELATIONS OF HEARING
TO OTHER SENSES, ESPECIALLY VISION

8.1 Separate "Channels"

There are at least two senses in which channels seem to occur in hearing. First, peripheral neurons do not respond to the entire audible region of *(I, f)* pairs. Rather, there is a characteristic region, characterized by the tuning curves, for which a neuron is responsive. One can group together those neurons that have roughly the same tuning curve and say that they form a single channel.

Second, parallel channels appear to exist higher up in the brain that are designed to carry out simultaneously quite different processing of auditory information. These separate analyses are then reassembled at some later stage of the process into coherent perceptions. Among those things that are widely believed to be carried out as distinct modules are:

> discrimination and detection
> identification
> localization
> echo suppression
> speech vs. other sounds
> formant analysis.

Somewhat analogous things obtain in vision and, possibly, in the other senses. We cite several that are well established.

• The visual cortex is now known to be highly structured and there are cells that respond only to selected orientations. This fact was discovered by D. H. Hubel and T. N. Wiesel in a group of studies for which they were awarded a Nobel Prize.

• There are cells elsewhere in the cortex that are so specific they respond only to one class of complex things such as faces, hands, or claws.

• There is a close visual analogy to neural tuning in what is called *spatial frequency* analysis. The stimuli are *spatial sinusoidal grids,* that is, parallel bars that vary from light to dark and back again in a sinusoid over space (see Fig. VI.36). Using masking procedures analogous to those in audition, there is comparable evidence for "critical bands" or "channels," as they are called in vision.

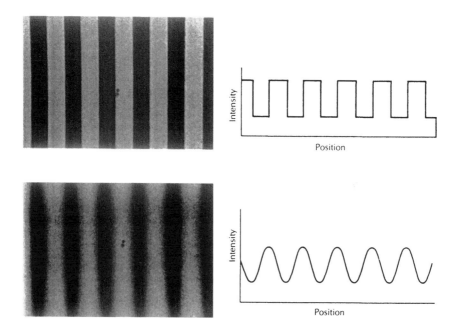

FIG. VI.36   Visual square and sine waves gratings shown both as seen and as intensity waveforms. From *Visual Perception* (p. 313) by T. M. Cornsweet, 1970, New York: Academic Press. Copyright 1970 by Academic Press, Inc. Reprinted by permission.

8.2 Notable Differences

We may cite two examples of substantial differences between the two systems.

First, vision is temporally sluggish. Consider that motion pictures are composed of a sequence of still photographs presented at a rate of 16 frames/s, that is 62.5 ms/frame. Nonetheless, we perceive such a presentation as completely continuous motion, encountering trouble only when something is rotating at a speed that is slightly different from some multiple of 16 Hz, in which case it appears to be rotating slowly, and sometimes in the wrong direction. The fact that this slow rate mostly works means that the temporal sensitivity of the visual system is measured in tens of milliseconds as compared with tens of microseconds for auditory phenomena.

Second, color is affected by changes in electromagnetic frequency. Single frequencies are called *monochromatic light* and as such they are in some ways analogous to pure tones. Adding together monochromatic lights of various intensities produces various colors, which is similar to the synthesis of complex sounds from pure tones, as in Fourier decompositions. But, unlike audition, many different combinations of monochromatic lights are perceived as the same, that is, as being *identical* in color. Indeed, any combination whatsoever of monochromatic lights can be matched by adjusting the intensities of three fixed monochromatic lights that are presented together.[6] Nothing remotely like this is true for sounds. Our visual system reduces the infinite-dimensional space of possible physical stimuli to a three-dimensional space of color perception; whereas, the auditory system apparently introduces no analogous reduction.

8.3 Interaction of Modalities

We give a number of more or less familiar examples of sensory interactions.

• One's speech production is modulated by our visual appreciation of the distance to our intended listener.
• Speech reception involves a good deal more lip reading than is commonly realized. If the environment is noisy, one finds that one is watching the speaker's lips to aid in understanding. A simple way to know if you are doing this is to note your frustration when the speaker's lips are obstructed. The following facts are interesting:

   o Lip reading in total absence of the speech sound tends to be rather poor — try it by turning off the sound on a TV set. However, some totally deaf people have been able to perfect lip reading to a high degree of effectiveness.
   o Lip reading supplemented by a sound that is unrelated to speech except for being at the fundamental frequency of the voice improves lip reading a good deal.
   o By dubbing sounds, the speech sound actually heard can be different from the (unheard) sound being produced by the lips. The perception is a compromise. For example, when one dubs ba-ba on a film of person saying ga-ga, then da-da is heard by 98% of adults and 80% of preschool children. However, if one simply close one's eyes, ba-ba is heard.

• The perceived location of a sound source is usually controlled by visual evidence, not by localization. For example, if you have ever listened to a simulcast of a TV program in which the TV sound is turned off in favor of your higher quality audio system, there is no problem in perceiving the sounds as coming from the TV even though the stereo speakers are to one side.

---

[6]One of the three may have to be added to the given light and then matched to the remaining two. This is interpreted as assigning it a negative weight.

8.4 Attempts to Substitute One Sense for Another

Again, we simply list some familiar examples:

* The blind learn, with varying degrees of mastery, to use auditory reflection to detect obstacles. They say that perceptually it does not seem like an auditory phenomenon, but rather like a tactile one. However, careful experiments prove otherwise; it is in fact entirely auditory.
* Attempts to encode ongoing speech as visual signals, other than as ordinary written text, have so far failed. For example, people simply cannot learn to "read" spectrograms, even "painted" ones, fluently.
* Some laboratory success has been achieved in converting visual and auditory information to touch on a large skin surface (the back), but this is currently impractical because of inconvenience and the size of the apparatus needed to carry out the translations.
* Perhaps the most promising, long-range approach for those with total hearing loss is direct electrical intervention on the auditory nerve and indirect intervention using ultrasonic bone conduction. Such work is highly experimental at present.

9. FURTHER READING

Because no single secondary source, save some of the general text books listed in the preface, treats most of the topics of this chapter, it seems best to list the topics individually. Many of the topics, at an advanced level but now somewhat dated, are treated in chapters of the edited volumes Carterette and Friedman (1978) and Tobias (1970, 1972). The handbook edited by Boff, Kaufman, and Thomas (1986) is more up-to-date.

Combination tones: These are discussed in the context of the illusory (or periodicity) pitch by A. M. Small in Chapter 1 of Tobias (1970).

Binaural beating and masking: Chapter 8 on binaural phenomena in Green (1976) is a good source, and more technical surveys are found in the Chapters 10 and 11, by N. I. Durlach and S. H. Colburn, of Carterette and Friedman (1978), Green and Yost (1976), and Chapters 9, 10, and 11, respectively by L. A. Jeffress, N. I. Durlach, and J. V. Tobias, of Tobias (1972).

Pure tone masking: The simplest results are covered in most texts. The work on amplitude modulation is due to Yost and Sheft (1989). Initial studies on profile analysis are summarized by its originator Green (1988), where one can also find detailed references to the literature. The theoretical idea of comparing the signal to a weighted average of the flanking tones was proposed by Durlach, Braida, and Ito (1986). Later Berg (1989) devised a method to estimate the weights, and Berg and Green (1990) established the closeness of the empirical weights to the optimal ones.

Critical bands: This topic is covered in all texts. Scharf (1970) summarized many of the basic results up to that date. Hall (1987) described the comodulation results.

Illusory pitch: As was mentioned, Seebeck (1841, 1843) first recognized the phenomenon and its importance. Schouten explored the topic in the late 1930s and that work is reviewed in Schouten, Ritsma, and Cardoza (1962). Licklider (1954) described his classic experiment, which can be heard on the demonstration disk. Summaries of the findings are in Chapter 7, by J. O. Nordmark, of Carterette and Friedman (1978) and Chapter 1 by Small in Tobias (1970).

Precedence effect: This is discussed briefly by B. Scharf and A. J. M. Houtsma in Chapter 15 of Boff, Kaufman, and Thomas (1986).

Perceptual structuring: This is a relatively new area of research, and there is not yet any very coherent understanding of all the phenomena involved. Some of the relevant research summaries in book form are Bregman (1990), Green (1988), and Kubovy and Pomerantz (1981). Warren (1982) is good on perceptual induction.

Speech production and perception: This is a sprawling area of research, full of interesting phenomena and much controversy. Two general books at about the level of the present text are Borden and Harris (1984) and Lieberman and Blumstein (1988). Both Green (1976) and Warren (1982) have broad introductory chapters without a lot of detail. Several expository chapters and articles are Liberman (1982), Liberman and Mattingly (1985), and Miller (1990). Basic books with somewhat different orientations are Fletcher (1953) and Massaro (1987). The general topic of categoricalness is explored in Harnad (1987). Perceptual induction was studied by Warren, Obusek, and Ackroft (1972).

Music perception: This topic, which is somewhat related to speech, was not taken up in any detail. Several leads into that literature are Chapter 12 of Carterette and Friedman (1978), Dowling and Harwood (1986), Krumhansl (1990), Pierce (1983), Roederer (1975).

Relation to other senses: Chapter 25, titled Intersensory Interactions, by R. B. Welch and D. H. Warren of Boff, Kaufman, and Thomas (1986) treats the entire complex of interactions, but without special attention to audition. I am not aware of a more focused source.

PART VII

Exercises

The exercises are organized by major subsections of the text; however, some questions involve issues encountered earlier in the text. A few questions are grouped at the end that cover the entire text.

Answers are provided for a few of the exercises (see pp. 278–280).

PART I. TRANSMISSION, TRANSDUCTION, AND BLACK BOXES

1. Consider communication from a source to a receiver. It can involve either the movement of an object, an impulse in a medium, or propagation as a field. In each of the following cases, explain which it is:
   (a) Electrical signals carrying information on a telephone line.
   (b) Communication between two people using sign language.
   (c) An odor (often a form of communication among animals).
2. (a) Give an example of a transducer other than those listed in Section I.3.
   (b) Explain why the example you have selected is properly called a transducer.
   (c) Does your example have an inverse transducer and, if so, what is it?
3. Cite three examples of "black boxes" that play a role in your life. In each case, is it also a transducer?

PART II. DESCRIPTIVE PHYSICS OF PURE TONES

Waves, Frequency, and Period

1. Convert the following periods into frequencies in Hz:
   (a) 2 ms, (b) 30 μs, (c) 5 hrs, (d) 1 min.
2. Suppose a sine wave has phase angle $-\pi/2$.
   (a) Express this same phase difference as a positive phase angle.
   (b) Sketch a clock diagram that shows how each arises and why they are equivalent.
   (c) Sketch the resulting waveform.
3. Suppose two pendulums 1 and 2 have lengths l_1 and l_2, masses m_1 and m_2, and frequencies f_1 and f_2, respectively.
   (a) Express f_1/f_2, in terms of l_1, l_2, m_1, and m_2.
   (b) If f_1 is twice f_2, m_1 is four times m_2, and $l_2 = 80$ cm, what is l_1?

Wave Propagation in Time and Space

4. If a wave in a medium has period 20 ms and wavelength 5 m, what is the speed of sound in that medium?
5. If a wave in air has wavelength 10 m, what is its frequency?
6. If a wave in a medium has a wavelength of 5 m and a period of 778.8 μs,
   (a) What is its frequency?
   (b) What is the speed of sound in the medium?
   (c) What is the medium?
7. A sound wave of frequency 1,500 Hz has a wavelength of 22.93 cm in air. Suppose it impinges on a thick wall of unknown material. In that wall, the wavelength is measured to be four times larger than it is in air, that is, 91.73 cm. What is the velocity of sound in the wall material?

The Doppler Effect

8. Suppose you are standing on a train platform, and a train that is approaching you at 27 m/s is emitting pulses at a rate of 200 per second. What is the frequency of the pulses that you perceive?
9. A sound source is emitting a pure tone of 1,000 Hz. Calculate the frequency heard by a stationary observer if the sound source is moving directly away from the observer at a velocity of 86 m/s.
10. Suppose that a sound source and an observer are both at rest relative to the ground, but a wind is blowing from the source toward the observer at velocity v m/s. If the source emits a pure tone of frequency f, what

is the frequency at the observer? Explain your answer. Keep in mind that the Doppler effect arises because of movement of either the source or the observer relative to air, not relative to the ground.

11. A police car has a siren that emits a 7,200 Hz tone when at rest. Suppose that, after passing another car at an intersection, the police car is moving east and the other car is moving west.

 (a) If the speeds of the two cars are the same, how fast must each be going so that an observer in the car going west hears the siren as 5,600 Hz?

 (b) If the observer continues to move at the same speed but the perceived frequency increases to 6,300 Hz, what is the new speed of the police car?

12. A police car is chasing a male suspect at 44 m/s, and its siren is emitting a 3,000 Hz tone.

 (a) What is the period of this sound when the police car is stationary?

 (b) If the suspect is standing still as the police car approaches him, what frequency does he hear?

 (c) At what speed must he flee in order to hear the actual frequency of the siren?

13. Certain sources of sound waves, such as dog whistles, cannot normally be heard by people because they produce frequencies above the upper threshold of human hearing. However, under certain conditions, they can become audible by making use of the Doppler effect. For a sound of 22 kHz and a person whose upper level of hearing is 11 kHz, determine precisely what the person must do to make the source just audible.

14. Suppose that you and your dog, both being young and having no noticeable hearing loss, are moving in air at 100 m/s in a silent vehicle that approaches and then passes a person who is sounding a "silent" dog whistle. It emits a tone of 22 kHz, which is quite audible to dogs but not to (most) people. Calculate the apparent frequency of the whistle before and after you pass it. Describe what you and your dog will hear in this situation.

Reflection and Refraction

15. Suppose that a sound wave passes from one medium of lower density ρ_1 and lower speed of sound c_1 through an interface into a second medium of higher density ρ_2 and higher speed of sound c_2. In each of the following sentences, indicate the phrase that makes the sentence true:

(a) The frequency in the second medium is (higher than, the same as, or less than) the frequency in the first medium.

(b) The wavelength in the second medium is (longer than, the same as, or shorter than) the wavelength in the first medium.

(c) The angle of refraction in the second medium is (larger than, the same as, or smaller than) the angle of reflection in the first.

16. Suppose a plane sound wave of frequency 2,000 Hz in air has an angle of incidence of 30° when it encounters a glass partition.

(a) What is its speed of propagation in air and in glass?

(b) What is the angle of refraction in the glass?

(c) What is its frequency in the glass?

17. Suppose a plane sound wave propagating in medium i (e.g., air) with speed of sound c_i encounters a partition (e.g., glass) at the angle of incidence θ_i. It passes through the partition at speed c_r and exits the partition into a third medium j (e.g., water) at angle of refraction θ_j and speed c_j.

(a) How is θ_j related to θ_i?

(b) What is this relation when the media are air, glass, and water?

(c) What is the relation when i and j are the same medium?

dB and Intensity

18. A jet aircraft at takeoff is emitting 30 dB more sound than an accelerating motorcycle. The intensity ratio of the motorcycle noise relative to 0.0002 dynes/cm^2 is 2×10^{10}. How loud is the jet measured in dB SPL?

19. Suppose that a sound X is eight times as intense as sound Y, that is, the intensity ratio is $I_X/I_Y = 8$. Suppose further that sound Y is 50 dB SPL. What is the intensity of X in dB SPL?

20. Indicate the correct answers in each case (none, one, or both may be correct):

(a) sin $(a + 180°) = $ sin (a) or $-$ sin (a)

(b) cos $(a + 90°) = $ sin (a) or $-$ sin (a)

(c) Suppose $a = b10^c$, where a, b, and c are positive numbers. Then, $c = $ log (a/b) or $(1/b)$log (a)

(d) log $5 = 1 - $ log 2 or ½

(e) log $1,500 = $ log 3 + log 5 + 2 or log 30 + log 50

(f) $10^{\log C} = C$ or log C

21. Suppose you are testing the balance of your stereo system by listening to a 2,000 Hz test tone (available on test records and tapes) played alternately through the two speakers. If the intensity level from the left speaker is 76 dB at your location and that from the right speaker

is 70 dB, then how much more or less intense is the right speaker compared to the left one as measured in
(a) dB;
(b) an intensity ratio I_R/I_L; and
(c) a pressure ratio P_R/P_L?
Compute the intensity I in dB sound pressure level (SPL) for the following sounds. Recall that SPL is defined to be $p_0 = 2 \times 10^{-4}$ dynes/cm², which is equivalent to $I_0 = 10^{-9}$ ergs/cm²–s $= 10^{-16}$ w/cm².
(a) Rustling leaves: $I = 1.585 \times 10^{-15}$ w/cm².
(b) Whispering at half a meter: $p = 1.125 \times 10^{-2}$ dynes/cm².
(c) Normal conversation at 2 m: $p = 2 \times 10^{-1}$ dynes/cm².
(d) Busy traffic intersection with surrounding buildings: $p = 1$ dyne/cm².
(e) Shouting at 1.5 m: $I = 10$ ergs/cm²–s.
(f) Jet taking off at 60 m: $I = 2.5 \times 10^{-4}$ w/cm².
(g) A pulse with amplitude equal to standard atmospheric pressure: $p = 10^6$ dynes/cm².

Sound Attenuation

23. Suppose a sinusoidal sound wave in air is propagating at an angle of incidence of 60° to a metal wall. Suppose that the ratio of the acoustical impedance in the metal to that in the air is $R = 99$.
(a) What is the angle of reflection of the sound wave?
(b) What fraction of the sound intensity is transmitted across the air–metal interface?

24. A pure tone of wavelength 68.8 cm is incident on a wooden wall from a direction perpendicular to that wall. The speed of sound in the wood making up the wall is 3.44×10^5 cm/s. The ratio R of the acoustic impedance in the wall to that in air is 4,000. For numerical answers, be sure to make clear how you arrived at the answer.
(a) What is the frequency of the incident wave?
(b) What is the frequency of the refracted (transmitted) wave?
(c) What is the wavelength of the refracted wave?
(d) What proportion of the sound energy is transmitted into the wall?
(e) What happens to the rest of the energy? (A three-word sentence is sufficient.)

25. Suppose a wall of homogeneous material separates two rooms. Thus, there are two air–wall interfaces. Consider a plane wave sound source far back in the one room with angle of incidence θ_i. Some of the sound intensity is transmitted through the wall into the second room, and it

will have some angle θ_r of refraction into the air. What is the relationship between θ_r and θ_i?

26. Consider the following partitions designed to attenuate transmission of airborn sounds from one side to the other:

   (i) A 2 cm thick steel plate.

   (ii) A 2 cm thick plasterboard wall.

   (iii) Two 1 cm thick steel plates separated by 4 cm of air.

   (iv) Two 1 cm thick steel plates separated by a 1 cm vacuum.

   (a) Rank partitions (i)–(iv) from best to worst as sound attenuators.

   (b) What is the acoustic intensity loss in dB due just to the impedance mismatch in case (iii)—two steel plates separated by air—on the assumption that the acoustic impedance ratio of steel to air, R, is 999.

27. Compute the proportion of incident sound energy that passes through an air–glass interface.

	glass	air
$\rho(\text{g/cm}^3)$	2.32	1.16×10^{-3}
c (cm/s)	5.64×10^5	3.44×10^4

What is the dB loss at an air–glass interface?

Localization

28. Two distinct mechanisms have been suggested as underlying the localization of the direction from which pure tone sound signals originate. Explain why the finding that sound localization is poorest for frequencies in the range 1,500 to 3,000 Hz is consistent with the hypothesis of these two mechanisms.

29. (a) The brain can localize sound in at least two distinct ways. What are they?

   (b) What are the strengths and weakness of each method of localization?

   (c) Why is it sometimes difficult to localize a loud, percussive sound such as a gun shot?

30. Suppose that a sound source is displaced 60 degrees to the right of an observer's straight-ahead direction and that, when a 1,000 Hz tone is emitted, it arrives at the left ear 0.5 ms later than the right ear.

   (a) What phase difference of the signals at the two ears corresponds to this time difference?

   (b) Suppose the same source begins to emit a 4,000 Hz tone, then what is its time difference at the two ears?

(c) According to the Duplex theory, what information would the listener use to localize the signal in case (b) (your answer should not exceed one sentence) and why is this information available (again, one sentence)?

Resonance and Filters

31. Although the human voice and hearing span at least the frequency range from 50 Hz to 15,000 Hz, a telephone system transmits virtually no energy below 300 Hz or above 3,000 Hz.
    (a) Discuss telephones as transducers.
    (b) What type of filter is a telephone?
32. Transducers often have inverse transducers (e.g., microphone and loudspeaker).
    (a) Is the same true of a filter? Discuss.
    (b) What can then be said about a device, such as a telephone, that is both a transducer and a filter?
33. The quality of a filter is defined as $Q = f/\Delta f$. See Fig. II.34. Another way to describe the quality is in terms of

$$Q' = f_2/f_1,$$

where $f_1 = f - \Delta f/2$ and $f_2 = f + \Delta f/2$. Show that Q and Q' are related as:

$$Q' = (2Q + 1)/(2Q - 1).$$

PART III. PROPERTIES OF THE EAR

Mechanical

1. (a) Define a transducer.
   (b) Name each of the distinct transducers found in the ear. State clearly what the input and output is for each.
2. In designing earplugs, whose purpose is to attenuate loud sounds reaching the tympanic membrane, what are the two most important considerations that you can think of and why are they important?
3. In designing an earplug aimed at sound attenuation, is it better to arrange for it to be in direct contact with the tympanic membrane or not? Explain your answer in a sentence or two.
4. Suppose that roughly cylindrical earplugs are made from a doughlike material with an acoustic impedance of 4,000 dynes-s/cm^3. Suppose they are inserted into the external auditory canal of the ear in such

a way that they do not make direct contact with the tympanic membrane. Assuming that all of the sound passing into the middle ear (and beyond) first passes through the earplug, what is the drop in sound intensity between the outer ear and the inner ear due to the earplug? Express your answer as
(a) an intensity ratio,
(b) a pressure ratio, and
(c) a dB loss.
(Recall, the acoustic impedance of air is 40 dynes-s/cm^3.)

5. Suppose that the attenuation effected by an earplug as a function of signal frequency is as shown in Fig. VII.1:

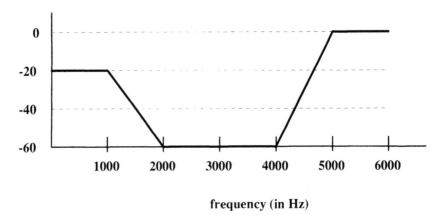

frequency (in Hz)

FIG. VII.1 The attenuation in terms of dB reduction effected by an earplug as a function of frequency.

What will the intensities at the tympanic membrane be for the following pure tone inputs:
(a) 1,500 Hz at 95 dB.
(b) 2,700 Hz at 55 dB.
(c) 4,000 Hz at 120 dB.
(d) 5,500 Hz at 85 dB.

6. For each of the following frequencies, compute the ratio of the length of the basilar membrane to its wavelength in the fluid of the cochlea. The speed of sound in the cochlea = 160,000 cm/s and the length of the basilar membrane = 3.5 cm.
(a) 20 Hz, (b) 250 Hz, (c) 1 kHz, (d) 2 kHz, (e) 5 kHz, (f) 10 kHz, (g) 20 kHz.

7. The resonance and reflection properties of the outer ear (pinna, external auditory canal, etc.) are such that the intensity of the sound is amplified (increased) or attenuated (decreased) as it travels from the pinna to the tympanic membrane, the exact amount of the amplification or attenuation depending on frequency. Figure VII.2 shows such a pattern of attenuation and amplification for a hypothetical ear. It is expressed as a dB difference between the intensity at the pinna and that at the tympanic membrane. Suppose at the pinna, sound A is a pure tone of 1,000 Hz at 30 dB SPL and sound B is a pure tone of 4,000 Hz at 20 dB SPL. What are the intensities (in dB SPL) of these sounds at the tympanic membrane?

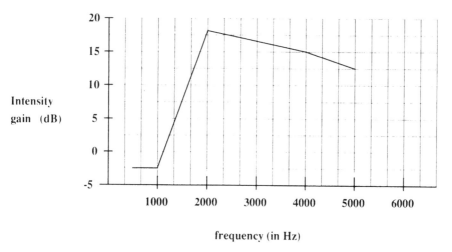

FIG. VII.2 The attenuation and amplification in a hypothetical ear between the pinna and the tympanic membrane.

8. A hearing aid amplifies (increases) the intensities of sounds as they enter the outer ear. Figure VII.3 shows the exact amount of amplification for a particular hearing aid as a function of frequency. In this graph, amplification is expressed as a pressure amplitude ratio, that is, the ratio of the sound pressure output by the hearing aid to the sound pressure incident on it (p_o/p_i).

(a) For a 300 Hz tone, what is the increase in intensity produced by the hearing aid? Give your answer both as an intensity ratio and in dB.

(b) For a 1,500 Hz tone at 40 dB SPL incident on the hearing aid, what is the intensity of the tone that is transmitted to the tympanic membrane by the hearing aid?

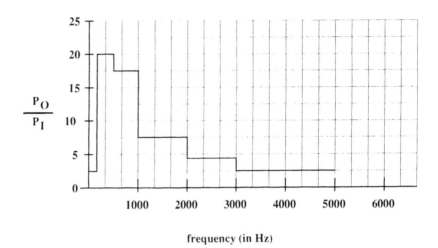

FIG. VII.3   The pressure amplification of a hypothetical hearing aid as a function of frequency.

9. (a) Give the names of the various structures identified by letters in Figure VII.4.

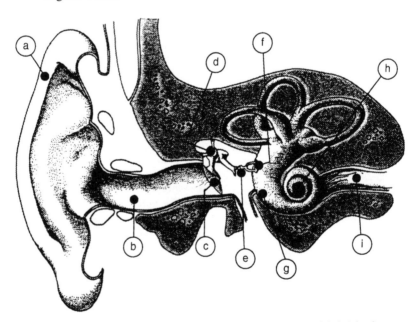

FIG. VII.4   A cross-section of the ear with various structures labeled by letters. Adapted from *Human Information Processing: An Introduction to Psychology* (p. 66) by P. H. Lindsay and D. A. Norman, 1972, New York: Academic Press. Copyright 1972 by Academic Press, Inc. Reprinted by permission.

(b) For each location where there is an energy transduction (c, f, and h), state what the change is (e.g., a loudspeaker is electrical-to-acoustical).

10. The movement of the basilar membrane encodes both intensity and frequency information about a pure tone signal.
   (a) Which aspect(s) of the motion correspond to intensity?
   (b) Which correspond to frequency?

11. Complete the following sentences to make them true:
   (a) A tone of frequency 2,500 Hz has a period of _____ seconds, and
   (b) so it has a period of _____ ms.
   (c) A tone with period 100 ms has frequency _____ Hz.
   (d) A change of _____ dB is equivalent to a 2 to 1 ratio of intensities.
   (e) A high pass filter blocks the passage of _____ frequencies.
   (f) In a mammal, the _____ is a transducer that converts sound pressure in either air or water into pressure in a different fluid.
   (g) One organ of the ear amounts to a collection of fairly narrow band pass filters; it is the _____ .
   (h) The ratio of outer to inner hair cells in the human and the cat is

   _____ .
   (i) If the hair cells near the helicotrema are destroyed, the person suffers from hearing loss in the _____ frequencies.
   (j) Suppose Reissner's membrane is ruptured, so that the fluids in the scala media and scala vestibuli mix freely, but the ear is otherwise normal. The consequence to hearing in that ear is _____

12. Frequency has to do with the repetition pattern of a wave in time. One way it can be converted into a spatial measure is through wavelength. This is not the way the basilar membrane encodes frequency as a spatial measure.
   (a) Why does it not use wavelength?
   (b) Could wavelength have been used for any of the audible frequencies? Explain your answer.
   (c) On what principle does the conversion from frequency to distance take place?

Neural

13. (a) Explain what is meant by saying that the basilar membrane is equivalent to a series of moderately sharply tuned frequency filters.
   (b) What is the connection between the idea of the basilar membrane being a series of tuned frequency filters and the tuning curves that are used to describe the overall activity pattern of individual auditory neurons?

14. Outline the major features and differences between the place and temporal theories for the coding of frequency and intensity at the peripheral auditory system. Discuss the neurophysiological evidence that is relevant to the two theories. Include, where appropriate, the functioning of the basilar membrane and the relevance of the poststimulus and interval histograms, tuning curves, and input–output functions for single neurons.

15. Hearing loss can take various forms. For each of the instances described here, give a plausible account of the cause of the observed hearing loss in terms of a structure in the ear and that structure's function:
    (a) The person shows a roughly 30 dB loss in the minimum audible intensity for frequencies throughout the normal audible frequency range.
    (b) The person is effectively deaf to frequencies greater than about 3,000 Hz, but shows nearly normal hearing for frequencies below that level.

16. Suppose that a microelectrode is imbedded in the auditory nerve of an animal and that a 500 Hz pure tone stimulus causes an increase in the firing rate that is measured on the electrode.
    (a) Describe what you would do experimentally and how you would process the data in order to develop both a poststimulus histogram and an interval histogram.
    (b) On the assumption that the firing rate is well below the maximum firing rate, sketch the typical pattern found for each type of histogram.
    (c) Suppose that you increase the stimulus intensity by 5 dB and hold the frequency fixed. Sketch (approximately) how each histogram in (b) will change.
    (d) Suppose you decrease the frequency from 500 Hz to 400 Hz and hold the intensity fixed. Assuming that the firing rate continues to fall between the spontaneous and the maximum firing rates for the fiber, sketch (approximately) how each of the histograms in (b) changes.

17. Figure VII.5 depicts the neural tuning curves for three auditory nerve fibers, designated #1, #2, and #3. Each tuning curve was obtained using a criterion firing rate of the spontaneous rate plus 10% of the difference between the maximum firing rate and the spontaneous rate. At their characteristic frequencies, each of these fibers has a dynamic range of 25 dB, measured from the intensity that produces the criterion firing rate for the tuning curve.
    (a) What is the characteristic frequency (CF) of each fiber?

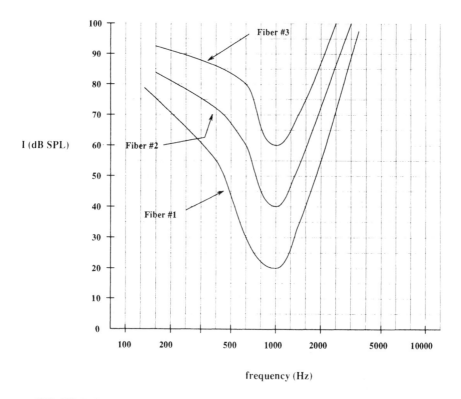

FIG. VII.5   Neural tuning curves for three different auditory nerve fibers.

(b) What is the overall dynamic range of the three fibers taken together when a tone of the frequency of the CF of fiber #1 is presented?

(c) For a 75 dB, 500 Hz tone, sketch the expected interval histograms for fibers #1 and #2. Be sure to label your axes carefully and show relevant numerical values wherever possible. Your sketches should show clearly which features of the two interval histograms will be the same and which will be different. (Give as much detail as possible.)

18. Fill in the 15 missing items (some may be a pair of words or a number) in the following passage:

In the middle ear, bones called (a) _____ form a lever system that is attached to a membrane on the surface of the cochlea called the (b) _____ . They transmit sound induced vibrations of the (c) _____ , which is the boundary between the outer and middle ears, to traveling waves on the (d) _____ , which partitions the cochlea into two main chambers. Despite their separation, the fluid in these two

chambers is connected by means of a small hole, called the (e) _____ .
Pressure in this fluid is relieved by a second membrane, the (f) _____ ,
also on the surface of the cochlea. The effect of the sound-induced
pressure changes in the cochlea is, as was remarked earlier, to cause the
partition (item d above) to vibrate, which in turn induces a sheering
motion of some of the (g) _____ , the number of which is approximately
(h) _____ in human beings. On the basis of their anatomical properties,
these are grouped into two types, called (i) _____ and _____ . The result
of such sheering motion is the creation of neural (j) _____ . There are
various ways that physiologists describe such neural activity. One is to
plot the proportion of interspike durations for each of a number of time
intervals; such plots are called (k) _____ histograms. A second is to
record the durations from signal onset to the occurrence of a spike and
to plot the proportion of such durations lying in each of a number of
time intervals; this is called a (l) _____ histogram. And a third is to plot
the locus of *(I, f)* pairs that all have the same firing rate on a single
neuron; this is called a (m) _____ . Activity on individual neurons codes
signal (n) _____ as rate of firing. The time between two successive
neural spikes is an integral multiple of the (o) _____ of the signal.

19. Suppose that an auditory neuron has firing rate contours shown in Fig.
    VII.6 where the three curves correspond to 10%, 50%, and 90% of the
    distance between spontaneous firing and maximum firing for that neu-
    ron. (The 10% curve is the one usually called the tuning curve.)
    (a) Sketch the type of interval histograms that would be expected to be
        found for the intensity-frequency pairs labeled a, b, and c. Be sure

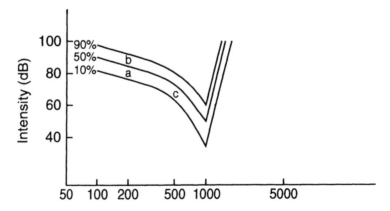

FIG. VII.6   Firing rate contours of a single neural fiber. They correspond to firing
rates at 10%, 50%, and 90% of the difference in rates between the resting (spontaneous) and maximum rates for that fiber.

to label your axes carefully and show relevant numerical values. Include quantitative detail in so far as possible.

(b) For the same three points, sketch the form of the poststimulus histogram for a signal of duration 500 ms. Again, label the axes clearly.

20. Suppose that a pure tone stimulus produces a spiking rate of 100 sps in a group of fibers all of whose CF is that of the input tone. Assume that (a) the organism is going to generate the equivalent of an interval histogram in order to estimate the period of the tone, (b) no more than 30 ms is to be devoted to acquiring all the information that goes into the histogram, and (c) it has the accuracy that is guaranteed by having on average a total 1,500 observations in the histogram. How many distinct neurons are needed?

21. In the simple geometric-distribution model for the interval histogram that is outlined in Section III.4.36, suppose that the spiking probability is $Q = \frac{2}{3}$. If a total of 2,700 observations are made, how many are expected to occur in the mode at $3T$, where T is the period of the input signal?

22. Suppose that tones (I, f) and (I', f') cause a particular neuron to spike at rates r and r', respectively. Consider the spiking when both signals are on at the same time. Explain why one does not in general expect pure additivity to hold, that is, the neuron does not in general spike at the rate $r + r'$. When might additivity hold?

23. Indicate each statement as True or False.

(a) If a medium can sustain both longitudinal and transverse waves, then both types have the same speed of propagation.

(b) The distance along the basilar membrane from the basal (oval window) end to the point of the peak amplitude of the traveling wave is greater the lower the frequency of the sound source.

(c) There are approximately three times as many outer hair cells as inner ones, and so roughly 75% of the activity in the auditory nerve is attributable to the outer hair cells.

(d) The hair cells are, in effect, simple resonators (i.e., very narrow band filters) that are tuned to resonate at different sound frequencies, and when they resonate there is an electrochemical process that generates pulses on the afferent nerve fibers that synapse on the cell.

(e) A major role for the middle ear is to increase the pressure applied to the oval window to overcome the impedance mismatch between air and water.

(f) A sound source that is approaching a fixed observer at velocity v and an observer that is approaching a fixed sound source at velocity v are auditorily equivalent situations, and in particular the apparent frequency increase for the observer (the Doppler effect) is the same in the two cases.

(g) Suppose that a sound wave in air approaches a water surface at an angle. Most of the energy will be reflected, but some will be refracted. The angle of reflection is equal to the angle of refraction, both angles being measured from a perpendicular to the surface of the water.

(h) Sound propagation is very efficient in a vacuum because the density is zero and so there is no acoustic impedance.

(i) In general, more sound intensity is lost when a sound passes from a low density medium to a high density medium than vice versa.

(j) 0 dB SPL means there is no sound intensity.

(k) Assume that a sound source is emitting a sound of a constant frequency. Then the further away the sound source is from an observer, the lower the apparent frequency.

PART IV. PSYCHOPHYSICS OF PURE TONES

Local Psychophysics

1. For a Yes–No design, some have plotted $P(Y|s)$ as a function of signal intensity in dB and then defined a jnd in terms of this plot. In terms of the ROC curve, discuss why this may not be a very satisfactory way to determine the detection threshold.

2. Suppose that Weber's law, Equation IV.1, holds and that $\Delta I/I = 0.05$. What is the Weber fraction in dB?

3. In Fig. IV.4, what is the value of $\Delta I/I$ for large I? What does it correspond to in terms of the generalized Weber's law of Equation IV.2.?

4. Suppose that in the generalized Weber's law, Equation IV.3, the Weber fraction has the value d at the absolute threshold I_0. Express b/a in terms of d/a and I_0.

5. Describe a two-alternative, forced-choice (2AFC) procedure used to measure the jnd for intensity. Be sure to include the following:

    (a) The stimulus or stimuli used on each trial — specify which stimulus parameters are varied from trial to trial and which are held constant.

    (b) Sketch a typical psychometric function that illustrates the type of data that would be obtained from an experiment using this procedure (label the axes!).

    (c) Show the intensity jnd on the graph of part (b).

Global Psychophysics

6. Prepare reasonably accurate sketches of the following functions, carefully labeling the axes you are using:

(a) The near-miss to Weber's law.

(b) The tuning curve of a peripheral auditory neuron.

(c) The psychometric function obtained in a two-alternative, forced-choice discrimination experiment.

(d) Equal-loudness contours for pure tones.

(e) The magnitude estimation function for the loudness of a pure tone.

7. In Fechner's law, Equation IV.7, suppose that the absolute threshold is at I_0, and so $L(I_0) = 0$. Evaluate the constant B and rewrite Equation IV.7 more compactly in terms of b/a and I_0. Using the result from Exercise 4, rewrite it in terms of d/a. Simplify these expressions as much as you can.

8. Using Fig. IV.12, find all the equal loudness solutions to the following equivalences:

(a) (60 dB, 200 Hz) ~ (? dB, 4,000 Hz).

(b) (10 dB, 1,000 Hz) ~ (? dB, 100 Hz).

(c) (80 dB, 1,000 Hz) ~ (80 dB, ?).

9. Calculate the exponent of Stevens' law, Equation IV.10, for Fig. IV.13. Show how you get this number.

10. Suppose that loudness is given by Stevens' law, Equation IV.10, with $\beta = 0.3$. What dB change corresponds to reducing the loudness by a factor of two?

11. In a two-interval design, suppose the signal in the first interval is the presentation to *each* ear of a tone of frequency f and intensity I, and the signal in the second interval is a tone of frequency f and intensity I' presented to *just one* ear. Suppose the intensity I' is adjusted until the subject says that the signals in the two intervals are equal in loudness. Suppose that the data for equal loudness are such that for every intensity I above 35 dB the value of I' must be 9 dB larger than I for an equal loudness judgment. Draw a sketch of this equal loudness contour. Label axes carefully.

12. Suppose that subjective loudness L and intensity in dB have the following corresponding values:

L	dB
10	10
20	20
?	30

What is the value for ? if

(a) Fechner's law describes the relation; or if

(b) Stevens' law describes the relation.

13. Give brief definitions of the following seven terms:
    (a) jnd
    (b) Weber's law
    (c) Stevens' law
    (d) equal loudness contour
    (e) magnitude estimation
    (f) two-alternative, forced-choice design
    (g) psychometric function

14. In Fig. IV.16, suppose that a 60 dB tone is applied to the normal ear. What intensity level (in dB) of a tone of the same frequency must be applied to the deaf ear to sound equally loud in the case of (a) neural loss and (b) conductive loss?

15. The plot of magnitude estimation of loudness as a function of duration with signal intensity in dB as a parameter is shown (idealized) in Fig. VII.7. Construct and sketch the intensity-duration trade-off function for the loudness level corresponding to 50 dB at 1 s duration.

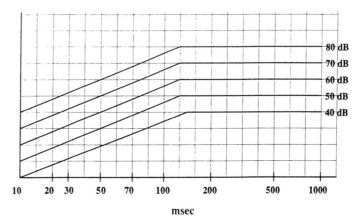

FIG. VII.7   An idealized plot of magnitude estimates, on a logarithmic scale, versus signal duration for five intensity levels.

16. The following questions concern Fig. VII.8:
    (a) What do these data tell us about the effect of signal duration on the subject's ability to detect a signal?
    (b) Are the low frequency (below 1,000 Hz) signals more or less affected than the high frequency (above 1,000 Hz) signals by signal duration? Explain your answer briefly.

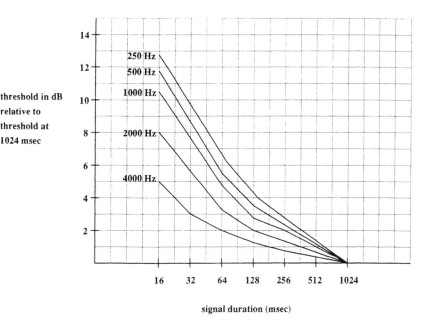

FIG. VII.8 Detection thresholds as a function of signal duration with frequency as a parameter. The dependent variable is the threshold in dB relative to the threshold at 1,024 ms.

17. Suppose that the perceived loudness of a tone is related to its intensity by the following version of Fechner's law:

$$L = 30 \log I - 100.$$

(a) Suppose that I_2 is perceived to be 60 loudness units lower than I_1. What is the ratio I_2/I_1?

(b) What is their intensity difference in dB?

(c) What is their pressure ratio?

18. Suppose (even though it is not empirically accurate) that Weber's law $\Delta(I)/I = a$ holds for intensity discrimination of pure tones. Then, according to Stevens' law, what would be the loudness ratio of the stimulus $I + \Delta(I)$ to the stimulus I, that is, the loudness ratio of stimuli that differ by one jnd?

19. (a) Sketch the general shape of the equal loudness contours (label axes carefully).

(b) Suppose that loudness as a function of intensity is, for each frequency, described by Stevens' power law. Given the form shown in (a), what can you say about the dependence of the exponent in Stevens' law as a function of frequency? Explain.

20. Suppose that the perceived loudness of a pure tone is related to its intensity by the Stevens' law:

$$L = AI^{0.3},$$

where A is a constant. If I_1 is perceived to be four times as loud as I_2, then:

(a) What is their intensity ratio, that is, I_1/I_2?

(b) What is their intensity difference in dB?

(c) What is their pressure ratio, p_1/p_2?

21. A subject with partial hearing loss in one ear is asked to assign numbers to presentations of a 1,500 Hz tone at various intensities. The subject is instructed to assign the numbers in such a fashion that ratios of numbers capture subjective loudness ratios. The procedure is repeated twice, once to the normal ear (N) and once to the deficient ear (D). The results of the experiment are shown in Fig. VII.9.

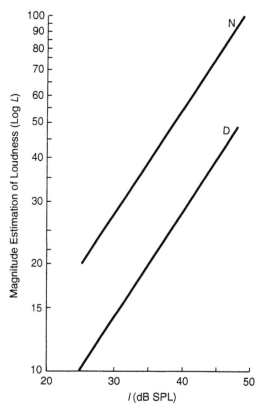

FIG. VII.9 Magnitude estimates to the normal (N) and deficient (D) ear of a hypothetical subject with hearing loss in one ear.

(a) What is this experimental procedure called?

(b) Are the reported results in the figure consistent with Stevens' law? Explain.

(c) If a 43 dB, 1,500 Hz tone is presented to the subject's deficient ear, what is the loudness estimate that you expect the subject to give?

(d) Suppose that the same 43 dB, 1,500 Hz tone is being presented to the deficient ear, and the subject adjusts the intensity of another 1,500 Hz tone presented to the normal ear so that the two tones are perceived as equally loud. What will be the intensity of the adjusted tone?

22. For each of the following descriptions, sketch as accurately as you can the empirical functions involved. In each case, be sure to label clearly the two axes of the graph, indicate the units involved, and indicate any key numerical values.

(a) Tuning curve of a peripheral auditory fiber.

(b) Absolute threshold for a pure tone.

(c) Interval histogram (from a peripheral auditory neuron) for a pure tone.

(d) Poststimulus histogram (from a peripheral auditory neuron) for a pure tone.

(e) Typical male hearing loss with age for different frequencies.

(f) Absolute identification performance when there are 10 pure tone signals equally spaced in dB.

Bridging the Local and Global

23. Discuss the absolute identification paradox that arises when comparing the data for two signals with those when there are a number of other signals that must also be identified. Describe one proposed solution to the paradox.

24. (a) An individual auditory neuron can be said to be a filter. Explain what this means.

(b) The attention mechanism proposed to account for the absolute identification paradox can also be described as being a filter. Explain what this means.

PART V. DESCRIPTIVE PHYSICS
OF COMPLEX TONES

Superposition and Standing Waves

1. (a) Distinguish among longitudinal, transverse, and standing waves.

(b) Give an example of each type.

(c) What, if any, relations hold among them with respect to speed of propagation?

2. Two musicians have tuned their instruments to produce 688 Hz tones. Suppose that, while sounding this note, one of the musicians is walking toward a stationary observer at a speed of 1 m/s while the other musician is walking away from the observer at a speed of 1 m/s. (This could happen in a parade situation.) Describe and explain in as much detail as you can what the observer will perceive.

3. Suppose a 10 cm wire is plucked to produce its fifth harmonic. The resulting sound wave causes a nearby half-open tube to resonate.
    (a) What is the length of the tube so that the resulting standing wave is its third harmonic?
    (b) Same question as (a) but under the assumption that the tube is open at both ends.

4. Consider a hypothetical auditory disease that affects the basilar membrane (BM) in the following way. It causes portions of the BM to become four times more taut (tense) than is normal, but other than that the performance of the BM remains unchanged. The progress of the disease is gradual, beginning at the oval window (basal) end of the BM and extending regularly over a year toward the helicotrema (apical) end until after a year the entire BM is affected. For present purposes we may consider the BM as composed of independent fibers, not unlike the strings of a piano, which have different resonance frequencies by virtue of their different lengths and tensions. The speed of sound on each fiber is $c = (\tau/\rho)^{1/2}$, where τ is its tension, which is increased by a factor of four, and ρ is its linear density, which is not affected by the disease.
    (a) What will happen to the resonance frequency of a given fiber (point on the BM) when the disease affects it?
    (b) Suppose that the disease has been diagnosed shortly after it has begun in a young person with previously normal hearing. Show in two figures how the absolute threshold curve appears when first discovered and at the end of a year. Be sure to label key numerical points on the axes.

Spectrum

5. Evidence from studies of sound localization using pure tones supports the Duplex Theory of sound localization. Recall that this theory states that there are two mechanisms, each drawing on different aspects of the physical stimulus, which are used in localizing the direction from which a sound is coming.
    (a) Discuss these two mechanisms briefly. Make clear the conditions under which each is useful.

(b) A sound localization experiment is done using a square wave having a period of 2.5 msec. Sketch the amplitude-frequency (i.e., Fourier) spectrum of the square wave making clear the numerical values of the frequencies and their relative amplitudes.

(c) Explain how the duplex theory can predict two different ways whereby a square wave can be localized.

6. Suppose a periodic sound has the amplitude-frequency (i.e., Fourier) spectrum shown in Fig. VII.10. Suppose that when a second signal is added to this sound the resulting spectrum is exactly the same except that the amplitude is 0 at the fundamental frequency of original sound.

(a) What word is used to describe the interaction of the two signals?

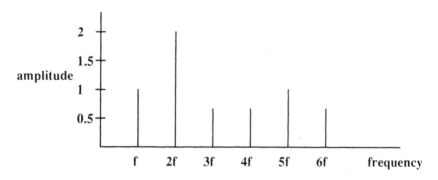

FIG. VII.10   The spectrum of a periodic sound wave.

(b) State the characteristics of the signal added in terms of its spectrum and phase relative to that of the original wave.

7. Suppose a sound signal is a square wave of period 2 ms.

(a) Sketch the amplitude-frequency (Fourier) spectrum of this signal.
    Now suppose that a second sound signal is added to the square wave, resulting in exactly the same spectrum as in (a) except that the amplitudes at each frequency are cut in half.

(b) What type of interference has occurred?

(c) What is the plot of amplitude versus time for the sum of the two signals? Provide as much detail as possible.

(d) Describe as fully as possible the second signal that was added to the first one.

8. Suppose that a periodic wave has the spectrum shown in panel a of Fig. VII.11. Another periodic wave is added to the first one and the resulting spectrum is that of panel b. Note that the two spectra differ only at 2 and 3 kHz.

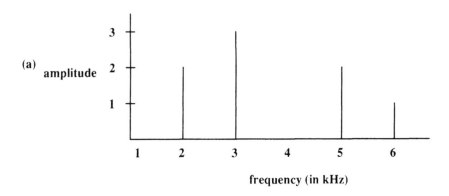

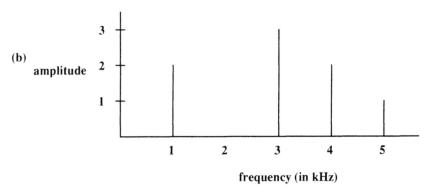

FIG. VII.11 (a) The spectrum of a periodic sound wave. (b) The resulting spectrum after a wave has been added to that of panel a.

(a) What is the spectrum of the wave that was added to the wave having the spectrum of panel a to result in the wave having the spectrum of panel b?

(b) What are the phase relations between its component sine waves and those of the original wave?

Distortion

9. (a) Sketch the relation between the output amplitude and input amplitude of a half-wave rectifier.

(b) If a square wave of pressure amplitude 0.001 dynes/cm^2 and period 1 ms is passed through this rectifier, what is the frequency spectrum of the output?

(c) What would you hear listening to this output?

10. Suppose there are two sound waves. The first is a sine wave of period T and maximum pressure amplitude P; the second is the half-wave rectified version of the first.

(a) What is the frequency of the sine wave?

(b) What is the frequency of the rectified sine wave?

(c) What are the maximum and minimum pressure amplitudes of the rectified wave?

(d) Sketch these two waves as well as the third wave that is their sum.

(e) What are the maximum and minimum pressure amplitudes of the sum of the two waves?

(f) What is the frequency of the sum wave?

11. Suppose a wave has period T and the shape shown in panel a of Fig. VII.12 where all triangles are congruent; it will be referred to as wave a. If it is rectified into the shape shown in panel b, which will be called wave b, then answer the following, giving explanations in each case.

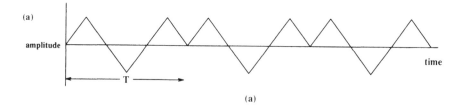

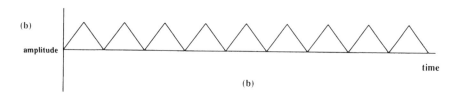

FIG. VII.12 (a) The waveform of a periodic wave. (b) The wave resulting from rectifying the wave of panel a.

(a) What is the frequency of wave b in terms of T?

(b) If the speed of propagation of wave a is 500 m/s, what is the speed of propagation of wave b in the same medium?

(c) If the wavelength of wave a is 5 m, what is that of wave b?

(d) In a Fourier (spectral) decomposition of wave b, only even harmonics are present. In terms of the frequency of wave a, state the frequencies of the first three harmonics that are present.

(e) If a pure tone is matched in pitch to wave b, what will its frequency be?

Noise

12. (a) Write $E - N_0$ as compactly as you can.
    (b) Explain what an increase in each of the terms P, D, W, and N does to the detectability of signal in noise.
13. Conversation can be difficult when there is a substantial noise background, as in a moving automobile with open windows. Are any of the three methods for noise suppression that were described in Section V.5.3 potentially suitable for improving the signal-to-noise ratio in such cases? Explain your answer.
14. For the reproduction of music on tapes, which of the three methods for noise suppression (Section V.5.3) are potentially useful? Explain your answer for including or ruling out each of the methods.

PART VI. PSYCHOPHYSICS OF COMPLEX SOUNDS

Masking and Critical Bands

1. A complex signal is composed of 600, 700, 800, 900, and 1,000 Hz components at equal intensities. It is comparatively easy to isolate the 600 Hz component by alternating in time the complex with a 600 Hz tone of the same intensity. It is far more difficult to do so for the 1,000 Hz component. Why?
2. Suppose that two tones, each 60 dB above threshold, are presented simultaneously. In case (i) the frequencies are 2,000 and 2,200 Hz and in case (ii) they are 2,000 and 3,000 Hz.
   (a) Which sound pair, (i) or (ii), will be subjectively louder?
   (b) What is the reasoning behind your answer, that is, what data and concepts lead you to this conclusion (aside from actually running the experiment itself)?
3. Describe one experiment, involving a pure tone to be detected and band pass noise to mask the tone, that has been used to establish the correctness of the critical band hypothesis. Be sure to:
   (a) State clearly the critical band hypothesis, and
   (b) Describe briefly the experimental procedure and the resulting data that are predicted by the theory.
4. Figure VII.13 idealizes the classical data on critical bands obtained by Fletcher in 1940. Shown is the ratio of signal intensity, I_{signal}, to noise masker intensity (per Hz), I_{masker}, as a function of the bandwidth of the noise in Hz. In the calculations, the masker intensity should be left as intensity per Hz.

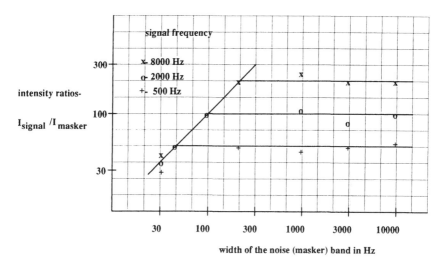

FIG. VII.13 Idealized critical band data showing the signal-to-noise intensity ratio as a function of bandwidth for tones of three frequencies, 500, 2,000, and 8,000 Hz.

(a) According to the graph what is the critical bandwidth for a 2,000 Hz tone? For a 8,000 Hz tone?

(b) For noise of bandwidth 100 Hz, what is the difference in dB between a just detectable intensity of the 500 Hz tone and the noise masker intensity?

(c) Assuming that the pressure of the masker is 0.002 dynes/cm^2, what is its level in dB SPL?

(d) Assuming the masker of part (c), what is the level of I_{signal} in dB SPL?

(e) Same question as (b) except for noise of bandwidth of 5,000 Hz.

5. Suppose two pure tones *(I, f)* and *(I', f')* have been chosen so: (i) they are in different critical bands, and (ii) they are each judged separately in a magnitude estimation experiment to have the same loudness level, 60.

(a) Suppose that both tones are presented simultaneously and their sum is magnitude estimated; what value do you expect them to be given?

(b) Suppose a pure tone of frequency *f* is matched in loudness to the sum of tones in (a), and the matching intensity is *I''*. Assuming Stevens' law is applicable with exponent 0.3, what is the ratio *I''/I*?

(c) What is the dB difference between *I''* and *I*?

6. One type of evidence favoring the critical band hypothesis has to do with the loudness of a band of white noise as the bandwidth is varied.

(a) Describe the data that are found and the interpretation that is given to these results.

(b) In terms of the auditory nerve, to what does the critical band correspond?

Missing Fundamental

7. Explain the logic of Licklider's high and low pass noise experiment aimed at deciding whether distortion is the source of the phenomenon of the missing fundamental.

8. A 1,000 Hz tone is sounded continuously. A pair of tones with frequencies 1,250 and 1,500 Hz are turned on together for 1 s, then off for 1 s, and so on. Consequently, a complex of three tones (1,000 Hz, 1,250 Hz, 1,500 Hz) alternates with a single tone (1,000 Hz). The perception is of a pitch that rises and falls repeatedly.

(a) In terms of one of the phenomenon discussed in the text, describe what is probably happening.

(b) What would one hear if high pass noise masks 1,250 Hz and above, but not 1,000 Hz?

(c) What would one hear if low pass noise masks frequencies below 1,000 Hz, but not 1,000 Hz and above?

9. Suppose a sound consists of the simultaneous presentation of three pure tones — 1,000 Hz, 1,500 Hz, and 2,500 Hz.

(a) This sound has a pitch. What pure tone frequency would be judged to have the same pitch? Why do you think this?

(b) Aside from what is perceived in (a), what will be perceived if a pure tone of 502 Hz is added to the above three pure tones? Explain.

(c) Aside from what is perceived in (a), what will be perceived if a pure tone of 1,002 Hz is added to the above three pure tones? Explain.

10. Place theorists have attempted to understand the phenomenon of the missing fundamental in terms of distortion products, among them being the difference frequencies. So, for example, when 800, 1,000, and 1,200 Hz are presented, 200 Hz is the distortion product arising from all of the successive differences. Empirically, the complex 850, 1,050, and 1,250 Hz, which is the previous sequence but with 50 Hz added to each, is matched in pitch by subjects to 204 Hz. Discuss this finding in terms of the place theory. (See Demonstration 23.)

Precedence

11. (a) Explain what the problems are in amplifying sound in a large auditorium if one tries to use a single loudspeaker system in the front of the auditorium.

    (b) Describe the nature of the solution to this problem. On what psychological phenomenon does the solution depend? Make explicit any numerical constraints that are involved.

12. If echos require a delay of about 500 ms, calculate the size of a water-filled chamber that will result in echoes for a person listening in the water.

Signal Induction

13. Suppose that some 100 ms gaps are introduced into a passage of ongoing speech. We know that this will cause some deterioration in intelligibility, but if the gaps are filled with white noise much of the intelligibility is restored.
    (a) What is the basic principle of reconstruction illustrated by this example?
    (b) Assuming that this principle is correct and using what you know about pure tone masking, what would you anticipate if:

        (i) A loud 100 Hz tone is inserted in the gaps?
        (ii) A loud 3,000 Hz tone is inserted in the gaps?

    In both cases, explain your answer in a sentence.

Speech

14. "Painted" spectrograms are used to simulate speech.
    (a) Describe what they are.
    (b) To what do the larger dark blobs of the spectogram correspond?
    (c) By what rationale is the intensity variable reduced to a binary value?
    (d) In digitally approximating a painted spectogram, what is a reasonable temporal sampling rate?
15. The perception of distinguishable speech sounds, phonemes, is said to be "categorical."
    (a) What does this mean?
    (b) Cite two empirical demonstrations of the categorical nature of phonemic perception.
    (c) Discuss the evidence that these categories are inborn and that they are subject to modification by experience.
16. Outline the resonance process whereby the vocal track molds the fundamental buzz produced by the glottis.
17. Describe how the resonances of the vocal track are numbered in terms of:
    (a) the harmonics of the fundamental buzz;
    (b) the harmonics of the vocal track, as a half-open tube;
    (c) the formants of speech.

REVIEW QUESTIONS COVERING
THE ENTIRE TEXT

1. Complete the following sentences so that they become true statements:
   (a) If I in dB, relative to some intensity I_0, is negative, then I/I_0 is
   _____ .
   (b) The standard (SPL) sound pressure reference level p_0 is _____
   dynes/cm^2.
   (c) The threshold for auditory pain is approximately _____ dB.
   (d) Consider the refraction of sound at a boundary between two media
   i and r. If the speed in medium i, c_i, is greater than that in medium
   r, c_r, then the angle of incidence is _____ than the angle of
   refraction.
   (e) Equal loudness curves are usually generated by means of a
   _____ procedure.
   (f) In intensity discrimination experiments, the observed deviations
   from Weber's law are typically such that the Weber fraction _____ as signal intensity increases.
   (g) Equal dB differences correspond to equal intensity _____ .
   (h) The fundamental frequency of a tube having one closed and one
   open end is _____ the fundamental frequency of a tube of the same
   length that is open at both ends.
   (i) Fechner's law is the assertion that a subjective scale is a _____
   function of intensity.
   (j) The fact that the directional localization of sound coming directly
   from a source is not disrupted by reflections of the same sound that
   arrives slightly later is called the _____ effect.
2. A woman traveling in an unfriendly country fears that her room will be
   bugged so that her private conversations can be overheard. She is able
   to bring with her just one pure tone sound source to try to defeat the
   bug. Her frequency options are 300, 500, 1,000, 3,000, or 5,000 Hz.
   (a) Which option should she select and why?
   Suppose that when she gets to her hotel she concludes that the
   bug is probably located in the wall phone in the room (see Fig. VII.14).
   (b) Where should she locate her sound source and where should she
   conduct her conversations? Explain your answer.

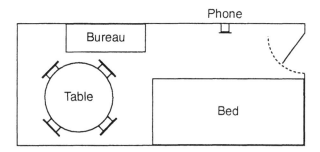

FIG. VII.14   Schematic of a room in which a sound "bug" is located in the telephone.

3. Indicate whether each of the following statements is True or False.
   (a) The vocal tract can be changed in length and shape.
   (b) Aspirin causes irreversible hearing loss.
   (c) A tuning curve shows intensity-frequency pairs for which the firing rate is constant.
   (d) The human vocal tract can, for some purposes, be modeled as a half-open tube.
   (e) The rate of firing of peripheral auditory neurons is controlled primarily by the frequency of the stimulus.
   (f) Absolute thresholds can be expressed as an equal-loudness contour.
   (g) The natural frequency of a string on a musical instrument is affected by both its length and tension.
   (h) The temporal theory of neural coding lays emphasis on the pattern of activity over the basilar membrane and over the entire set of peripheral fibers.
4. Draw graphs showing typical cases of the following functions. In each case, provide as much labeling of axes and as great detail about the function as you can:
   (a) Poststimulus histogram of a peripheral auditory neuron responding to a pure tone.
   (b) Interval histogram of a peripheral auditory neuron responding to a pure tone.
   (c) A typical tuning curve of a peripheral auditory neuron responding to a pure tone.
   (d) Spectrum of high pass, white noise.
   (e) Equal loudness contours for pure tones.
   (f) Intensity Weber function for a pure tone.
5. Explain the difference between:
   (a) Neural and psychophysical tuning curves.
   (b) Transverse and longitudinal waves.

(c) Harmonic and formant.

(d) Magnitude estimation and magnitude production.

6. Complete the following sentences so that they become true statements:
   (a) In detecting faint pure tones, the ear is most sensitive at about _____ Hz.
   (b) The dB scale converts ratios into _____ .
   (c) Stevens's law for the growth of loudness says that subjective loudness is a _____ function of pressure.
   (d) The maximum audible frequency for young people with no hearing loss is about _____ Hz.
   (e) The Weber fraction for intensity discrimination _____ with intensity and
   (f) it _____ with frequency.
   (g) The angle of refraction exceeds the angle of reflection when the velocity of propagation in the first medium _____ that of the second medium.
   (h) To reduce the transmission of sound, a wall should differ from air in _____ by as large a ratio as possible.
   (i) When a sound intensity is given in sound level (SL), the intensity is measured relative to _____ of the observer.
   (j) If an observer is driving away from a source, the perceived frequency is _____ than the actual frequency.

ANSWERS TO SELECTED EXERCISES

Part II

6. (a) 1,284 Hz, (b) 6,420 m/s, (c) aluminum.

12. (a) $T(s) = 1/f(Hz) = (1/3,000)$ s $= (1/3)$ ms.
    (b) $f_o = f_s c/(c - v_s) = 3,000 \times 344/(344 - 44) = (3,000/300)344 = 3,440$ Hz.
    (c) He must move away from a source, namely the sound arriving at the point where he is, which has frequency 3,440 Hz, at a velocity v_0 sufficient to reduce it to 3,000 Hz: $f_0/f_{s'} = (c - v_0)/c$, substituting $3,000/3,440 = (344 - v_0)/344$, and solving by inspection, $v_0 = 44$ ms, that is, exactly the speed of the police car. In fact, if he always moves to maintain the frequency unchanged, he will stay a constant distance from the police car, no matter what speed they go.

24. (a) $f = c/\lambda = 344(m/s)/.688(m) = .344 \times 10^3/.688 = \frac{1}{2} \times 10^3 = 500$ Hz.
    (b) same as (a).
    (c) $\lambda = c/f = 3.44 \times 10^5(cm/s) \times 10^{-2}(m/cm)/500(1/s) = 3.44 \times 10^3/\frac{1}{2} \times 10^3 = 6.88$ m $= 688$ cm.

(d) $4R/(1 + R)^2 \approx 4/R = 4/4{,}000 = 1/1{,}000$ (exact: $1/1{,}000.5$).

(e) It is reflected.

Part III

2. An earplug fails to attenuate sounds if it permits any substantial direct path for air to reach the tympanic membrane; therefore, it is important that it fit snugly into the ear. This either means that it should be tailored to the individual using it or that it should be of relatively soft material. Second, the attenuation is increased as the impedance mismatch between air and the substance used increases. So the acoustic impedance of the earplug should be as different as possible from that of air, either by making R as small or as large as possible.

10. (a) The intensity of the sound controls the maximum amplitude of the envelope of the traveling wave and therefore the maximum deflection of the cilia.

    (b) The frequency of the sound determines the rather sharp termination of the motion of the traveling wave along the basilar membrane and therefore determines which cilia at the apical end are not moving at all. Also, at each point along the basilar membrane where any motion occurs, the oscillation is at the frequency of the sound wave; therefore, the cilia that move do so at the frequency of the sound wave.

23. (a) F, (b) T, (c) F, (d) F, (e) T, (f) F, (g) F, (h) F, (i) F, (j) F, (k) F.

Part IV

1. The Yes–No experiment involves, for each signal intensity $I(s)$, determining both $P(Y|s)$ and $P(Y|n)$, and there are a continuum of possibilities. Thus, $P(Y|s)$ versus $I(s)$ can be almost any increasing function, depending on where the behavior lies on the ROC curve. There is no clear-cut function, and so no clear-cut concept of the detection threshold.

7. $L(I) = A \log [1 + a(I - I_0)/d]$.

10. About 10 dB.

19. (b) The exponent increases with the distance in either direction from the frequency corresponding to the most sensitive detection because the equal loudness contours become increasingly compressed in dB.

Part V

2. In addition to the basic pure tone, beating at 4 Hz will occur because of Doppler effects that can be calculated.

6. (a) Destructive interference.
   (b) The signal added must be a pure tone of the frequency of the fundamental of the given signal of the same intensity but 180° out of phase, so cancellation will occur.
   10. (a) $1/T$, (b) $2/T$, (c) P and 0, (e) $2P$ and 0, (f) $1/T$.

Part VI

2. (a) (ii).
   (b) Because those in (i) lie in the same critical band, thus interact, and have a level of activity less than the sum of the two individually; whereas those in (ii) lie in different critical bands and so additivity is to be expected.
5. (a) $L = A(2I)^{0.3} = 2^{0.3}AI^{0.3} = 1.231 \times 60 = 73.9$
   (b) $I''/I = 2$.
   (c) Approximately 3 dB.
9. (a) 500 Hz because that is the common fundamental of the given tones, and so it is the predicted pitch according to other results about the missing fundamental.
   (b) Both the illusory pitch of 500 Hz as well as the 502 Hz tone should be heard. They seem to coexist in totally different realms and they will fail to produce beats because, as we know, no energy exists at the frequency in question.
   (c) The two signals at 1,000 Hz and 1,002 Hz will interact to produce a 2 Hz beat, but at the same time the missing fundamental will continue to be present.

PART VIII

References

The references are separated into books and articles. This has been done because the books tend (although there are exceptions) to be more general and accessible than the rather technical articles. Moreover, many of the latter are included simply because they are original sources of some of the figures.

BOOKS

Anderson, N. H. (1981, 1982). *Foundations of information integration theory* (Vols. 1–2). New York: Academic Press.

Békésy, G. von (1960). *Experiments in hearing* (E. G. Wever, Trans. and ed.) New York: McGraw-Hill.

Boff, K. R., Kaufman, L., & Thomas, J. P. (Eds.). (1986). *Handbook of perception and human performance* (Vol. 1). New York: Wiley.

Bolanowski, S. J., Jr., & Gescheider, G. A. (1991). *Ratio scaling of psychological Magnitude, in honor of the memory of S. S. Stevens*. Hillsdale, NJ: Lawrence Erlbaum Associates.

Borden, G. J., & Harris, K. S. (1984). *Speech science primer*. Baltimore: Williams & Wilkins.

Boring, E. G. (1950). *A history of experimental psychology*. New York: Appleton-Century-Crofts.

Burns, W. (1968). *Noise and man*. London: John Murray.

Bregman, A. S. (1990). *Auditory scene analysis: The perceptual organization of sound*. Cambridge, MA: MIT Press.

Carterette, E. C., & Friedman, M. P. (Eds.). (1978). *Handbook of perception: Vol. IV. Hearing*. New York: Academic Press.

Cornsweet, T. M. (1970). *Visual perception*. New York: Academic Press.

Dooling, R. J., & Hulse, S. H. (Eds.). (1989). *The comparative psychology of audition, perceiving complex sounds*. Hillsdale, NJ: Lawrence Erlbaum Associates.

Dowling, W. J., & Harwood, D. L. (1986). *Music cognition.* Orlando, FL: Academic Press.

Egan, J. P. (1975). *Signal detection theory and ROC analysis.* New York: Academic Press.

Fechner, G. T. (1966). *Elemente der psychophysik.* Leipzig: Breitkopf und Hartel. Translation of Volume I by H. E. Adler, *Elements of psychophysics.* New York: Holt, Rinehart & Winston. (Original work published 1860)

Fletcher, H. (1953). *Speech and hearing in communication.* New York: Van Nostrand.

Gluck, W. L. (1971). *Hearing, physiology and psychophysics.* New York: Oxford University Press.

Gluck, W. L., Gescheider, G. A., & Frisina, R. D. (1989). *Hearing: Physiological acoustics, neural coding, and psychoacoustics.* New York: Oxford University Press.

Green, D. M. (1976). *An introduction to hearing.* Hillsdale, NJ: Lawrence Erlbaum Associates.

Green, D. M. (1988). *Profile analysis.* New York: Oxford University Press.

Green, D. M., & Swets, J. (1974). *Signal detection theory and psychophysics* Huntington, NY: Robert E. Krieger. (Original work published 1966)

Halliday, D., & Resnick, R. (1978). *Physics.* New York: Wiley. (Original work published 1960)

Handel, S. (1989). *Listening.* Cambridge, MA: MIT Press.

Harnad, S. (Ed.). (1987). *Categorical perception, the groundwork of cognition.* Cambridge; New York: Cambridge University Press.

Helmholtz, H. L. F. von (1954). *Die Lehre von den Tonempfindungen als physiologiche Grundlage für die Theorie der Musik.* Braunschweig: Verlag von Fr. Vieweg u. Sohn. Translation of the fourth and last German edition of 1877 by A. J. Ellis, *On the sensations of tone as a physiological basis for the theory of music.* New York: Dover. (Original work published 1863)

Hirsh, I. J. (1952). *The measurement of hearing.* New York: McGraw-Hill.

Johnson, K. W., Walker, W. B., & Cutnell, J. D. (1981). *The science of hi-fidelity.* Dubuque, Iowa: Kendall/Hunt.

Kiang, N. Y.-S., Watanabe, T., Thomas, E. C., & Clark, L. F. (1965). *Discharge patterns of single fibers in the cat's auditory nerve.* Cambridge, MA: MIT Press.

Krumhansl, C. L. (1990). *Cognitive foundations of musical pitch.* New York: Oxford University Press.

Kryter, K. D. (1970). *The effects of noise on man.* New York: Academic Press.

Kubovy, M., & Pomerantz, J. R. (Eds.). (1981). *Perceptual organization.* Hillsdale, NJ: Lawrence Erlbaum Associates.

Laming, D. (1986). *Sensory analysis.* New York: Academic Press.

Levine, M. W., & Shefner, J. M. (1991). *Fundamentals of sensation and perception.* 2nd Ed. Pacific Grove, CA: Brooks/Cole.

Lieberman, P., & Blumstein, S. A. (1988). Speech physiology, speech perception, and acoustic phonetics. Cambridge: Cambridge University Press.

Lindsay, P. H., & Norman, D. A. (1972). *Human information processing: An introduction to psychology.* New York: Academic Press.

Link, S. W. (1992). *The wave theory of difference and similarity.* Hillsdale, NJ: Lawrence Erlbaum Associates.

Macmillan, N. A., & Creelman, C. D. (1991). *Detection theory: A user's guide.* New York: Cambridge University Press.

Massaro, D. W. (1987). *Speech perception by ear and eye: A paradigm for psychological inquiry.* Hillsdale, NJ: Lawrence Erlbaum Associates.

Miller, G. A. (1981). *Language and speech.* San Francisco: W. H. Freeman.

Moore, B. C. J. (1982). *An introduction to the psychology of hearing* (2nd ed.). New York: Academic Press.

Morrison, P., & Morrison, P. (1982). *Powers of ten.* New York: Scientific American Books.

Pickles, J. O. (1988). *An introduction to the physiology of hearing* (2nd ed.). New York: Academic Press.

Pierce, J. R. (1974). *Almost all about waves.* Cambridge, MA: MIT Press.

Pierce, J. R. (1983). *The science of musical sound.* San Francisco: W. H. Freeman.

Potter, R. K., Kupp, G. A., & Kupp, H. G. (1966). *Visible Speech.* New York: Dover Publications.

Roederer, J. G. (1975). *Introduction to the physics and psychophysics of music* (2nd ed.). New York: Springer-Verlag.

Rossing, T. D. (1982). *The science of sound.* Reading, MA: Addison-Wesley.

Schiffman, H. R. (1982). *Sensation and perception* (2nd ed.). New York: Wiley.

Stevens, S. S. (1975). *Psychophysics.* New York: Wiley.

Stevens, S. S., Warshofsky, F., & Editors of *Life.* (1965). *Sound and hearing.* New York: Time Inc.

Stuhlman, O. (1943). *An introduction to biophysics.* New York: Wiley.

Tobias, J. V. (Ed.). (1970, 1972). *Foundations of modern auditory theory* (Vols. 1-2). New York: Academic Press.

Warren, R. M. (1982). *Auditory perception: A new synthesis.* New York: Pergamon Press.

Weast, R. C., & Astle, M. J. (Eds.). (1980). *CRC handbook of chemistry and physics.* Boca Raton, FL: CRC Press.

Wever, E. G. (1970). *Theory of hearing.* New York: Dover. (Original work published 1949).

Yost, W. A., & Nielsen, D. W. (1985). *Fundamentals of hearing* (2nd ed.). Orlando: Holt, Rinehart & Winston.

ARTICLES AND CHAPTERS

Alper, J. (1991). Antinoise creates the sounds of silence. *Science, 252,* 508-509.

Berg, B. G. (1989). Analysis of weights in multiple observation tasks. *Journal of the Acoustical Society of America, 86,* 1743-1746.

Berg, B. G., & Green, D. M. (1990). Spectral weights in profile listening. *Journal of the Acoustical Society of America, 88,* 758-766.

Braida, L. D., & Durlach, N. I. (1972). Intensity perception II: Resolution in one-interval paradigms. *Journal of the Acoustical Society of America, 51,* 483-502.

Brugge, J. F., & Merzenich, M. M. (1973). Patterns of activity of single neurons of the auditory cortex in monkeys. In A. G. Moller (Ed), *Basic mechanisms in hearing* (pp. 745-766). New York: Academic Press.

Davis, H. (1983). An active process in cochlear mechanics. *Hearing Research, 9,* 79-90.

Delattre, P. C., Liberman, A. M., & Cooper, F. S. (1955). Acoustic loci and transitional cues for consonants. *Journal of the Acoustical Society of America, 27,* 769-773.

Durlach, N. I., Braida, L. D., & Ito, Y. (1986). Toward a model for discrimination of broadband signals. *Journal of the Acoustical Society of America, 80,* 63-72.

Fedderson, W. E., Sandel, T. T., Teas, D. C., & Jeffress, L. A. (1957). Localization of high-frequency tones. *Journal of the Acoustical Society of America, 29,* 988-991.

Green, D. M., & Luce, R. D. (1976). Variability of magnitude estimates: A timing theory analysis. *Perception & Psychophysics, 15,* 291-300.

Green, D. M., & Yost, W. A. (1976). Binaural analysis. In W. Keidel & D. Neff (Eds.), *Handbook of sensory physiology: Vol. V: Auditory system* (pp. 461-480). Berlin: Hiedelberg, and New York: Springer-Verlag.

Hall, J. W. (1987). Experiments on comodulation masking release. In W. A. Yost & C. S. Watson (Eds.), *Auditory processing of complex sounds.* Hillsdale, NJ: Lawrence Erlbaum Associates.

Hawkins, J. E., Jr., & Johnson, L.-G. (1976). Pattern of sensorineural degeneration in human ears exposed to noise. In D. Henderson, R. P. Hamernik, D. S. Dosanih, & J. H. Mills (Eds.), *Effects of noise on hearing* (pp. 91-110). New York: Raven Press.

Hawkins, J. E., & Stevens, S. S. (1950). The masking of pure tones and of speech by white noise. *Journal of the Acoustical Society of America, 22,* 6-13.

Iverson, G. J., & Pavel, M. (1981). Invariant properties of masking phenomena in psychoacoustics and their theoretical consequences. *SIAM-AMS Proceedings, 13,* 17-24.

Jesteadt, W., Wier, C. C., & Green D. M. (1977). Intensity discrimination as a function of frequency and sensation level. *Journal of the Acoustical Society of America, 61,* 169-171.

Kiang, N. Y.-S. (1968). A survey of recent developments in the study of auditory physiology. *Annals of Otology, Rhinology and Laryngology, 77,* 656-675.

Kiang, N. Y.-S., & Moxon, E. C. (1972). Physiological considerations in artificial stimulation of the inner ear. *Annals of Otology, Rhinology and Laryngology, 81,* 714-730.

Klein, M., Coles, M. G. H., & Donchin, E. (1984). People with absolute pitch process tones without producing a P300. *Science, 223,* 1306-1309.

Kreuger, L. E. (1989). Reconciling Fechner and Stevens: Toward a unified psychophysical law. *Behavior and Brain Sciences, 12,* 251-320.

Liberman, A. M. (1957). Some results of research on speech perception. *Journal of the Acoustical Society of America, 29,* 117-123.

Liberman, A. M. (1982). On finding that speech is special. *American Psychologist, 37,* 148-167.

Liberman, A. M., Delattre, P. C., & Cooper, F. S. (1952). The role of selected stimulus-variables in the perception of the unvoiced stop consonants. *American Journal of Psychology, 65,* 497-516.

Liberman, A. M., Delattre, P. C., Gerstman, L. J., & Cooper, F. S. (1956). Tempo of frequency change as a cue for distinguishing classes of speech sounds. *Journal of Experimental Psychology, 52,* 127-137.

Liberman, A. M., & Mattingly, I. G. (1985). The motor theory of speech revisited. *Cognition, 21,* 1-36.

Licklider, J. C. R. (1954). Periodicity pitch and place pitch. *Journal of the Acoustical Society of America, 26,* 945 (A).

Lockhead, G. (1992). The repeal of psychophysical scaling laws. *Behavior and Brain Sciences, 15,* 543-601.

Luce, R. D., & Green, D. M. (1974). Neural coding and psychophysical discrimination data. *Journal of the Acoustical Society of America, 56,* 1554-1564.

Luce, R. D., & Green, D. M. (1978). Two tests of a neural attention hypothesis for auditory psychophysics. *Perception & Psychophysics, 23,* 363-371.

Luce, R. D., & Nosofsky, R. M. (1984). Attention, stimulus range, and identification of loudness. In S. Kornblum & J. Requin (Eds.), *Preparatory states & processes* (pp. 3-25). Hillsdale, NJ: Lawrence Erlbaum Associates.

Marley, A. A. J., & Cook, V. T. (1984). A fixed rehearsal capacity interpretation of limits on absolute identification performance. *British Journal of Mathematical and Statistical Psychology, 37,* 136-151.

Marley, A. A. J., & Cook, V. T. (1986). A limited capacity rehearsal capacity for psychophysical judgments applied to magnitude estimation. *Journal of Mathematical Psychology, 30,* 339-390.

Miller, G. A. (1947). Sensitivity to changes in the intensity of white noise and its relation to masking and loudness. *Journal of the Acoustical Society of America, 19,* 609-619.

Miller, G. A. (1956). The magical number seven plus or minus two: Some limits on our capacity for processing information. *Psychological Review, 63,* 81-97.

Miller, J. L. (1990). Speech perception. In D. Osherson & H. Lasnik (Eds.), *Language. An introduction to cognitive science* (Vol. 1, pp. 69-93). Cambridge, MA: MIT Press.

Mills, A. W. (1972). Auditory localization. In J. V. Tobias (Ed.), *Foundations of modern auditory theory* (Vol. 2, pp. 303-348). New York: Academic Press.

Patterson, R. D., & Green, D. M. (1978). Auditory masking. In E. C. Carterette & M. P. Friedman (Eds.), *Handbook of perception: Vol. IV. Hearing* (pp. 337-361). New York: Academic Press.

Reynolds, G. S., & Stevens, S. S. (1960). Binaural summation of loudness. *Journal of the Acoustical Society of America, 32,* 1337-1344.

Rose, J. E., Brugge, J. F., Anderson, D. J., & Hind, J. E. (1967). Phase-locked response to low-frequency tones in single auditory nerve fibers of the squirrel monkey. *Journal of Neurophysiology, 30,* 769-793.

Rose, J. E., Hind, J. E., Anderson, D. J., & Brugge, J. F. (1971). Some effects of stimulus intensity on response of auditory nerve fibers in the squirrel monkey. *Journal of Neurophysiology, 34,* 685-689.

Sachs, M. B., & Abbas, P. J. (1974). Rate versus level functions for auditory-nerve fibers in cats: Tone-burst stimuli. *Journal of the Acoustical Society of America, 56,* 1835-1847.

Scharf, B. (1970). Critical bands. In J. V. Tobias (Ed.), *Foundations of modern auditory theory* (Vol. I, pp. 159-202). New York: Academic Press.

Schouten, J. F., Ritsma, R. J., & Cardoza, B. L. (1962). Pitch of the residue. *Journal of the Acoustical Society of America, 34,* 1418-1424.

Seebeck, A. (1841). Beobachtungen über einige Bedingungen der Enstehung von Tönen. *Annalen der Physik und Chemie, 53,* 417-437.

Seebeck, A. (1843). Über die Sirene. *Annalen der Physik und Chemie, 60,* 449-481.

Shaw, E. A. G. (1966). Earcanal pressure generated by a free sound field. *Journal of the Acoustical Society of America, 39,* 465-470.

Sivian, L. J., & White, S. D. (1933). On minimum audible sound fields. *Journal of the Acoustical Society of America, 4,* 288-321.

Spoendlin, H. (1970). Structural basis of peripheral frequency analysis. In R. Plomp & G. F. Smoorenburg (Eds.), *Frequency analysis and periodicity detection in hearing* (pp. 2-36). Leiden, the Netherlands: A. W. Sijthoff.

Stevens, J. C., & Hall, J. W. (1966). Brightness and loudness as functions of stimulus duration. *Perception & Psychophysics, 1,* 319-327.

Stevens, S. S., & Greenbaum, H. B. (1966). Regression effect in psychophysical judgment. *Perception & Psychophysics, 1,* 439-446.

Teas, D. C., Konishi, T., & Nielsen, D. W. (1972). Electrophysiological studies on the spatial distribution of the crossed olivocochlear bundle along the guinea pig cochlea. *Journal of the Acoustical Society of America, 51,* 1256-1264.

Teghtsoonian, R. (1971). On the exponents in Stevens' law and the constant in Ekman's law. *Psychological Review, 78,* 71-80.

Treisman, M. (1985). The magical number seven and some other features of category scaling: Properties of a model for absolute judgment. *Journal of Mathematical Psychology, 29,* 175-230.

Treisman, M., & Williams, T. C. (1984). A theory of criterion setting with an application to sequential dependencies. *Psychological Review, 91,* 68-111.

Vogten, L. L. M. (1974). Pure tone masking; a new result from a new method. In E. Zwicker & E. Terhardt (Eds.), *Facts and models in hearing* (pp. 142-155). Berlin: Springer-Verlag.

Warren, R. M., Obusek, C. J., & Ackroff, J. M. (1972). Auditory induction: Perceptual synthesis of absent sounds. *Science, 176,* 1149-1151.

Weber, D. L., Green, D. M., & Luce, R. D. (1977). Effects of practice and distribution of auditory signals on absolute identification. *Perception & Psychophysics, 22,* 223-231.

Wegel, R. L., & Lane, C. E. (1924). The auditory masking of one pure tone by another and its probable relation to the dynamics of the inner ear. *Physical Review, 23,* 266-285.

Weir, C., Jesteadt, W., & Green, D. M. (1977). Frequency discrimination as a function of frequency and sensation level. *Journal of the Acoustical Society of America, 61,* 178–184.

Yost, W. A., & Sheft, S. (1989). Across-critical-band processing of amplitude-modulated tones. *Journal of the Acoustical Society of America, 85,* 848–857.

Zwicker, E. (1974). On a psychoacoustical equivalent of tuning curves. In E. Zwicker & E. Terhardt (Eds.), *Facts and models in hearing* (pp. 132–141). Berlin: Springer-Verlag.

Zwislocki, J. (1960). Theory of temporal auditory summation. *Journal of the Acoustical Society of America, 32,* 1046–1060.

Name Index

Bold face numbers indicate references whereas ordinary type identifies citations in the text itself.

Subject Index

APPENDIX:
THE DEMONSTRATION DISC

These demonstrations are drawn from three sources. Many of them are from or adapted from the original set of demonstration tapes that Dr. David M. Green, then of Harvard University, had prepared under a grant from the National Science Foundation. These sets of tapes, which came to be called the "Harvard tapes," were very rapidly exhausted and for a period were unavailable except by making copies of the cassette tapes, which were not of the best quality. In 1984, at the request of the Acoustical Society of America's Committee on Education in Acoustics, Drs. T.D. Rossing and W.D. Ward looked into the possibility of re-issuing the Green tapes in a higher quality medium. This was done in 1987 by Drs. A.J.M. Houtsma and W.M. Wagenaars of the Institute for Perception Research (IPO), Eindhoven, The Netherlands and T.D. Rossing of Northern Illinois University, with sponsorship of the Acoustical Society of America and the technical assistance of IPO and the Phillips Company. The product was a compact disc *Auditory Demonstrations* (Phillips 1126-061) that consisted of many, but not all, of the Harvard tapes either digitally re-mastered or redone plus some new demonstrations made especially for this purpose. Independently of that project, Drs. A. Bregman, M. Kubovy, and R.S. Shepard prepared a tape of demonstrations to accompany the 1981 book *Perceptual Organization* by M. Kubovy and J.R. Pomerantz, published by Lawrence Erlbaum Associates.

In developing the present text, I found myself using some of the demonstrations from the Phillips disc, two of the Harvard tapes that had not been placed on that CD, plus a few from the Bregman, Kubovy, and Shepard tape. It was clear to me that many instructors would find access to all three sources difficult, so it seemed reasonable to prepare a new CD that includes just the demonstrations referred to in the text. I am grateful for the permission to reproduce the following materials on the demonstration disc:

Demonstrations 1, 2, 3, 4, 5, 6, 7, 8, 9, 10, 11, 12, 13, 17, 20, and 23, courtesy of the copyright holders A.J.M. Houtsma, T.D. Rossing, and W.M. Wagenaars; Demonstrations 14, 15, 16, 18, and 19, courtesy of the copyright holder, Albert S. Bregman; and Demonstrations 21 and 22, courtesy of the copyright holder, David M. Green.

CONTENTS

[1]In many of the writeups from the Phillips CD, it is made clear which of Harvard tapes was the original source.

[2]The demonstrations requiring the use of ear phones are in italics.

Credits: The following material is taken verbatim from the manual accompanying the Phillips CD:

Many people in the United States and Europe have contributed to the realization of this project. A preliminary scenario by T.D. Rossing was developed through frequent discussions with A.J.M. Houtsma and W.M. Wagenaars, who composed and synthesized the audio material with 16-bit digital techniques. Th. de Jong of IPO provided invaluable technical assistance. The narration by Prof. Ira J. Hirsh was recorded at the Central

Institute for the Deaf in Saint Louis. Speech samples in Demonstrations 4 and 35 were provided by, respective, J. 't Hart and Dr. Sanford Fidell. The instrumental scales of Demonstration 30 were played by bassoonist B. van den Brink of the Brabant Orchestra. The text booklet ("libretto") was written by T.D. Rossing and A.J.M. Houtsma. A trial version of the demonstrations was field-tested and critically reviewed by D.E. hall, W.M. Hartmann and W.D. Ward, which led to substantial improvements. Special thanks go to the IPO director H. Bouma, to G. van Hoeyen of Philips Polygram, and to A. Rehnberg and G.J.A. Vogelaar of PDO for their enthusiastic administrative and technical support.

In addition, Dr. Houtsma has provided us with high quality tapes of the two Green demonstration that were not included on the Phillips disc.

Dr. Bregman has recreated in higher quality, digital format the several demonstrations from his, Kubovy, and Shepard's tape that I use. I wish to thank him for doing so.

The following descriptions of the demonstration are taken from the manual accompanying the Phillips CD and from the original Green manual for those not on that CD. Those for the Bregman demonstrations were prepared by Dr. Bregman, and I thank him.

DEMONSTRATION 1. EFFECT OF ECHOES (1:47)

This so-called "ghoulies and ghosties" demonstration (No. 2 on the "Harvard tapes") has become somewhat of a classic, and so it is reproduced here exactly as it was presented there. The reader is Dr. Sanford Fidell.

An important property of sound in practically all enclosed space is that reflections occur from the walls, ceiling, and floor. For a typical living space, 50 to 90 percent of the energy is reflected at the borders. These reflections are heard as echoes if sufficient time elapses between the initial sound and the reflected sound. Since sound travels about a foot per millisecond, delays between the initial and secondary sound will be of the order of 10 to 20 ms for a modest room. Practically no one reports hearing echoes in typical small classrooms when a transient sound is initiated by a snap of the fingers. The echoes are not heard, although the reflected sound may arrive as much as 30 to 50 ms later. This demonstration is designed to make the point that these echoes do exist and are appreciable in size. Our hearing mechanism somehow manages to suppress the later-arriving reflections, and they are simply not noticed.

The demonstration makes these reflections evident, however, by playing the recorded sound backward in time. The transient sound is the blow of a hammer on a brick, the more sustained sound is the narration of an old Scottish prayer. Three different acoustic environments are used, an anechoic (echoless) room, a typical conference room, similar acoustically to many living rooms, and finally a highly reverberant room with cement floor, hard plaster walls and ceiling. Little reverberation is apparent in any of the rooms when the recording is played forward, but the reversed playback makes the echoes evident in the environment where they do occur.

Note that changes in the quality of the voice are evident as one changes rooms even when the recording is played forward. These changes in quality are caused by differences in amount and duration of the reflections occurring in these different environments. The reflections are not heard as echoes, however, but as subtle, and difficult to describe, changes in voice quality. All recordings were made with the speaker's mouth about 0.3 meters from the microphone.

Commentary

"First in an anechoic room, then in a conference room, and finally in a very reverberant space, you will hear a hammer striking a brick followed by an old Scottish prayer. Playing these sounds backwards focuses our attention on the echoes that occur."

References

L. Cremer, H.A. Müller, and T.J. Schultz (1982), *Principles and Applications of Room Acoustics,* Vol. 1 (Applied Science, London).

H. Kutruff (1979), *Room Acoustics,* 2nd ed. (Applied Science, London).

V.M.A. Peutz (1971), "Articulatory loss of constants as a criterion for speech transmission in a room," J. Audio Eng. Soc. *19,* 915–19.

M.R. Schroeder (1980), "Acoustics in human communication: room acoustics, music, and speech," J. Acoust. Soc. Am. *68,* 22–28.

DEMONSTRATION 2. BINAURAL LATERALIZATION (3:14)

The most important benefit we derive from binaural hearing is the sense of localization of the sound source. Although some degree of localization is possible in monaural listening, binaural listening greatly enhances our ability to sense the direction of the sound source.

Although localization also includes up-down and front-back discrimination, most attention is focused on side-to-side discrimination or *lateralization*. When we listen with headphones, we lose front-back information, so that lateralization becomes exaggerated; the image of the source appears to switch from one side of the head to the other by moving "through the head", or the sound source appears to be "in the head."

Lord Rayleigh (1907) was one of the first to recognize the importance of time and intensity cues at low frequency and high frequency, respectively.

Low-frequency sounds are lateralized mainly on the basis of interaural time difference, whereas high-frequency sounds are localized mainly on the basis of interaural intensity differences.

In the first example, tones of 500 Hz and then 2000 Hz are heard with alternating interaural phases of plus and minus 45 degrees. At 500 Hz, the image switches from side to side as the phase changes. At 2000 Hz, on the other hand, no such movement is perceived. (The interaural time difference varies from $\Delta t = \Delta\phi/2\pi f = 250$ to -250 μs in the first case, but only 62.5 to -62.5 μs at 200 Hz).

In the second example, a 100-μs pulse (heard as a "click") is presented with an interaural time difference that cycles from 5 ms to -5 ms, so that the source of the click appears to move between left and right.

The third example uses tones of 250 and 4000 Hz to illustrate the effects of interaural intensity difference at low and high frequency. The interaural intensity changes (in 1.25 s) from 32 dB to -32 dB. In both cases, the image moves from side to side. Although the auditory system processes interaural intensity cues at both low and high frequency, the head does not cast much of an acoustic shadow at low frequency (due to diffraction), and hence there is little intensity difference even when the source is located to one side of the head.

Commentary

"Tones of 500 and 2000 Hz are heard with alternating interaural phases of plus and minus 45 degrees."
"Next the interaural arrival time of a click is varied. The apparent location of the click appears to move."
"Finally, the interaural intensity differences of 250-Hz and a 4000-Hz tone are varied."

References

J. Blauert (1983), *Spatial Hearing* (MIT Press, Cambridge, MA).

W.M. Hartmann (1983), "Localization of sound in rooms," J. Acoust. Soc. Am. *74*, 1380–91.

E.R. Hafter and R.H. Dye (1983), "Detection of interaural differences of time in trains of high-frequency clicks as a function of interclick interval and number," J. Acoust. Soc. Am. *73*, 644–51.

Lord Rayleigh (J.W. Strutt) (1907), "On our perception of sound direction," Phil. Mag. *13*, 214–32.

H. Wallach, E.B. Newman and M.R. Rosenweig (1949), "The precedence effect in sound localization," Am. J. Psych. *62*, 315–36.

DEMONSTRATION 3. FREQUENCY RESPONSE OF THE EAR (2:07)

Although sounds with a greater sound pressure level usually sound louder, this is not always the case. The sensitivity of the ear varies with the frequency and the quality of the sound. Many years ago Fletcher and Munson (1933) determined curves of equal loudness for pure tones (that is, tones of a single frequency). The curves shown below, recommended by the International Standards Organization, are similar to those of Fletcher and Munson. These curves demonstrate the relative insensitivity of the ear to sounds of low frequency at moderate to low intensity levels. Hearing sensitivity reaches a maximum around 4000 Hz, which is near the first resonance frequency of the outer ear canal, and again peaks around 13 kHz, the frequency of the second resonance.

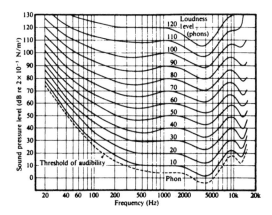

Equal-loudness curves for pure tones (frontal incidence). The loudness levels are expressed in phons.

(from Rossing, 1982)

The contours of equal loudness are labeled in units called *phons,* the level in phons being numerically equal to the sound pressure level in decibels at $f = 1000$ Hz. The phon is a rather arbitrary unit, however, and it is not widely used in measuring sound.

In this demonstration, we compare the thresholds of audibility (in a room) of tones having frequencies of 125, 250, 500, 1000, 2000, 4000, and 8000 Hz. The tones are 100 ms in length and decreases in 10 steps of -5 dB each.

Naturally, the threshold of audibility in a room depends very much on the character of the background noise. Nevertheless, in most rooms the threshold should increase measurably at low frequency. The listener should be reminded that pure tones cause standing waves in a room, especially at the higher frequencies, in which the maximum and minimum levels may differ by 10 dB or more.

Commentary

"First adjust the level of the following calibration tone so that it is just audible."
"You will now hear tones at several frequencies, presented in 10 decreasing steps of 5 decibels. Count the number of steps you hear at each frequency. Frequency staircases are presented twice."

References

H. Fletcher and W.A. Munson (1933), "Loudness, its definition, measurement and calculation," J. Acoust. Soc. Am. *5*, 82–108.

ISO R226 (1961), "Normal equal-loudness contours for pure tones and normal threshold of hearing under free-field listening conditions," (International Standards Organization, Geneva, Switzerland).

DEMONSTRATION 4. PRIMARY AND SECONDARY BEATS (1:32)

If two pure tones have slightly different frequencies f_1 and $f_2 = f_1 + \Delta f$, the phase difference $\phi_2 - \phi_1$ changes continuously with time. The amplitude of the resultant tone varies between $A + A_2$ and $A_1 - A_2$, where A_1 and A_2 are the individual amplitudes. These slow periodic variations in amplitude at frequency Δf are called *beats,* or perhaps we should say *primary beats,* to distinguish them from second-order beats, that will be described in the next paragraph. Beats are easily heard when Δf is less than 10 Hz, and may be perceived up to about 15 Hz.

A sensation of beats also occurs when the frequencies of two tones f_1 and f_2 are nearly, but not quite, in a simple ratio. If $f_2 = 2f_1 + \delta$ (mistuned octave), beats are heard at a frequency δ. In general, when $f_2 = (n/m)f_1 + \delta$, $m\delta$ beats occur each second. These are called *second-order beats* or *beats of mistuned consonances,* because the relationship $f_2 = (n/m)f_1$, where n and m are integers, defines consonant musical intervals, such as a perfect fifth (3/2), a perfect fourth (4/3), and a major third (5/4), etc.

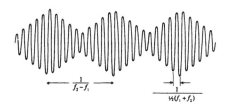

Waveform with beats due to pure tones with frequencies f_1 and $f_2 = f_1 + \Delta f$.

(from Rossing, 1982)

Primary beats can be easily understood as an example of linear superposition in the ear. Second-order beats between pure tones are not quite so easy to explain, however. Helmholtz (1877) adopted an explanation based on combination tones (Demonstration 34 of the Phillips CD), but an explanation by means of aural harmonics was favored by others, including Wegel and Lane (1924). This theory, which explains second-order beats as resulting from primary beats between aural harmonics of f_1 and f_2, predicts the correct frequency $mf_2 - nf_1$, but cannot explain why the aural harmonics themselves are not heard (Lawrence and Yantis, 1957).

An explanation which does not require nonlinear distortion in the ear is favored by Plomp (1966) and others. According to this theory, the ear recognizes periodic variations in waveform, probably as a periodicity in nerve impulses evoked when the displacement of the basilar membrane exceeds a critical value. This implies that simple tones can interfere over much larger frequency differences than the critical bandwidth, and also that the ear can detect changing phase (even though it is a poor detector of phase in the steady state).

Beats of mistuned consonances have long been used by piano tuners, for example, to tune fifths, fourths, and even octaves on the piano. Violinists also make use of them in tuning their instruments. In the case of musical tones, however, primary beats between harmonics occur at the same rate as second-order beats, and two types of beats cannot be distinguished.

In the first example, pure tones having frequencies of 1000 and 1004 Hz are presented together, giving rise to primary beats at a 4-Hz rate.

In the next example, tones with frequencies of 2004 Hz, 1502 Hz, and 1334.67 Hz are combined with a 1000-Hz tone to give secondary beats at a 4-Hz rate (n/m = 2/1, 3/2, and 4/3, respectively).

It is instructive to compare the apparent strengths of the beats in each case.

Commentary

"Two tones having frequencies of 1000 and 1004 Hz are presented separately and then together. The sequence is presented twice."

DEMONSTRATION 5. CANCELLED HARMONICS (1:33)

This demonstration illustrates Fourier analysis of a complex tone consisting of 20 harmonics of a 200-Hz fundamental. The demonstration also illustrates how our auditory system, like our other senses, has the ability to listen to complex sounds in different modes. When we listen *analytically,* we hear the different components separately; when we listen *holistically,* we focus on the whole sound and pay little or no attention to the components.

When the relative amplitudes of all 20 harmonics remain steady (even if the total intensity changes), we tend to hear them holistically. However, when one of the harmonics is turned off and on, it stands out clearly. The same is true if one of the harmonics is given a "vibrato" (i.e., its frequency, its amplitude, or its phase is modulated at a slow rate).

Commentary

"A complex tone is presented, followed by several cancellations and restorations of a particular harmonic. This is done for harmonics 1 through 10."

References

R. Plomp (1964), "The ear as a frequency analyzer," J. Acoust. Soc. Am. *36,* 1628-367.

H. Duifhuis (1970), "Audibility of high harmonics in a periodic pulse," J. Acoust. Soc. Am. *48,* 888-93.

DEMONSTRATION 6. DISTORTION (2:17)

This demonstration illustrates some audible effects of distortion external to the auditory system. These effects are of interest, not only because distortion commonly occurs in sound recording and reproducing systems, but because distortion is an important topic in auditory theory. This demonstration replicates one presented by W.M. Hartmann in the "Harvard tapes" (Auditory Demonstration Tapes, Harvard University, 1978). Both harmonic and intermodulation distortion are illustrated.

Our first example presents a 440-Hz sinewave tone, distorted by a symmetrical compressor.

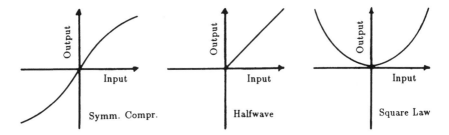

A symmetrical compressor has an input-output relation such as that shown at the left. The important property is that the function describing the relation between input and output is an odd function—that is, f(x) is equal to −f(−x). Because of the symmetry, only odd harmonics of the original sinewave are present in the output. A simple example of a symmetrical compressor would be a limiter. In this demonstration, the distorted tone alternates with its 3rd harmonic (which serves as a "pointer").

Next the 440-Hz tone is distorted asymmetrically by a half-wave rectifier, which generates strong even-numbered harmonics. The distorted tone alternates with its 2nd harmonic.

When two pure tones (sinusoids) are present simultaneously, distortion produces not only harmonics of each tone but also tones with frequencies $nf_1 - mf_2$, where m and n are integers. The prominent cubic difference tone $(2f_1 - f_2)$ which occurs when tones of 700 and 1000 Hz are distorted by a symmetrical compressor alternates with a 400-Hz pointer in the third example.

As a general rule the ear is rather insensitive to the relative phase angles between low-order harmonics of a complex tone. Distortion, however, especially if present in the right amount, can produce noticeable changes in the perceived quality of a complex tone when phase angles are changes. This is shown in the last demonstration in which the phase angle between a 440-Hz fundamental and its 880-Hz second harmonic is varied, first without distortion and with the complex fed through a square-law device.

Commentary

"First you hear a 440-Hz sinusoidal tone distorted by a symmetrical compressor. It alternates with its 3rd harmonic."

"Next the 440-Hz tone is distorted asymmetrically by a half-wave rectifier. The distorted tone alternates with its 2nd harmonic."

"Now two tones of 700 and 1000 Hz distorted by a symmetrical compressor. These tones alternate with a 400-Hz pointer to the cubic difference tone."

"You will hear a 440-Hz pure tone plus its second harmonic added with a phase varying from minus 90 to plus 90 degrees. This is followed by the same tones, distorted through a square-law device."

References

J.L. Goldstein (1967), "Auditory nonlinearity," J. Acoust. Soc. Am. *41*, 676–89.

J.L. Hall (1972), "Monaural phase effect: Cancellation and reinforcement of distortion products $f_2 - f_1$ and $2f_1 - f_2$," J. Acoust. Soc. Am. *51*, 1872–81.

DEMONSTRATION 7. FILTERED NOISE (1:50)

This demonstration shows the effects of filtering broadband white noise with low-pass, high-pass, and band-pass filters, and also a filter with a 3 dB/octave rolloff.

First, we hear a sample of white noise. Then it is passed through a low-pass filter with the cutoff frequency set at 10,000, 4000, 2000, 1000, and 500 Hz. Next it is passed through a high-pass filter with cutoff frequencies of 500, 1000, 2000, 4000, and 10,000 Hz, then through a band-pass filter to give 1/3-octave bands with center frequencies of 500, 1000, 2000, 4000, and 8000 Hz.

The last part of the demonstration compares samples of white and pink noise having the same power. The spectral difference can be seen in the graphs below. White noise has a constant spectrum level N_0 (same power in every $\Delta f = 1$ Hz band), and thus appears "flat" in a graph of sound level versus frequency (left). Pink noise, on the other hand, has the same amount of power in frequency bands whose widths are proportional to frequency (a so-called "constant-Q system where $\Delta f = Kf$), so that its spectrum level is inversely proportional to the frequency f. Spectrum levels N_0 are shown in the graph on the left for white and pink noise. The graph on the right shows plots of the power in proportional bands, $N_0\Delta f = KN_0 f$, as a function of $\log f$. This yields a "flat" function for pink noise, and a "ramp" function with 3 dB/octave slope for white noise. In the demonstration, the samples of white and pink noise have been adjusted to have the same power in the frequency range 50–10,000 Hz.

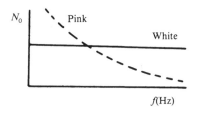

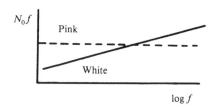

Commentary

"This is a sample of white noise."
"Now this same noise is passed through a low-pass filter with decreasing cutoff frequencies."
"Now the noise is passed through a high-pass filter with increasing cutoff frequencies."
"Next you will hear 1/3-octave noise bands with increasing center frequencies."
"Finally you will hear samples of white and pink noise having the same sound power."

References

R. Plomp (1970), "Timbre as a multidimensional attribute of complex tones," in *Frequency Analysis and Periodicity Detection in Hearing,* ed. R. Plomp and G. Smoorenburg (Sijthoff, Leiden).

D.M. Green (1983), "Profile analysis: a different view of auditory intensity discrimination," Am. Psychol. *38,* 133–42.

N.I. Durlach, L.D. Braida and Y. Ito (1986), "Towards a model for discrimination of broadband signals," J. Acoust. Soc. Am. *80,* 63–72.

DEMONSTRATION 8. BINAURAL BEATS (0:42)

An important issue in the study of sound localization concerns the ear's ability to process phase differences at the two ears. One way to study this phenomenon is to present two sinusoids of slightly different frequencies, one to each ear. At low frequencies the sound may appear to fluctuate or beat slowly at a rate equal to the frequency difference between the two tones.

Note that these *binaural beats* are quite unlike the physical beats that can be heard by a single ear (Demonstration 42). There, the small difference in the two frequencies caused the physical stimulus to wax and wane in intensity; if this fluctuation was slow enough, it was experienced as a beating sensation. With binaural beats, however, the interaction between the two tones occurs because of some kind of interaction in the nervous system of the inputs from each ear.

One might expect that these binaural beats would occur only at low frequencies, since at higher frequencies it is difficult to imagine that the nervous system can preserve the temporal structure of the waveform at each ear — a condition that must be met for their interaction to be noticeable. This conjecture is supported by quantitative measurements (Licklider, Webster, and Hedlun, 1950). They found that the best binural beats occurred at frequency separations of about 30 Hz near 400 Hz and much smaller frequency separations at the higher frequencies. No binaural beats are evident above about 1500 Hz. Tobias (1965) found that men appear to perceive binaural beats at a higher frequency than women, but this needs more exploration.

Commentary

"A 250-Hz tone is presented to the left ear while a 251-Hz tone is presented to the right ear."

References

J.C.R. Licklider, J.C. Webster, and J.M. Hedlun (1950), "On the frequency limits of binaural beats," J. Acoust. Soc. Am. *22*, 468–73.

D.R. Perrott and M.A. Nelson (1969), "Limits for the detection of binaural beats," J. Acoust. Soc. Am. *46*, 1477–81.

J.V. Tobias (1965), "Consistency of sex differences in binaural-beat perception," Intl. Audiology *4*, 179–82.

DEMONSTRATION 9. ASYMMETRY OF MASKING BY PULSED TONES (1:31)

A pure tone masks tones of higher frequency more effectively than tones of lower frequency. This may be explained by reference to the simplified response of the basilar membrane for two pure tones A and B shown in the figure below. In (a), the excitations barely overlap; little masking occurs. In (b) there is appreciable overlap; tone B masks tone A more than A masks B. In (c) the more intense tone B almost completely masks the higher-frequency tone A. In (d) the more intense tone A does not mask the lower-frequency tone B.

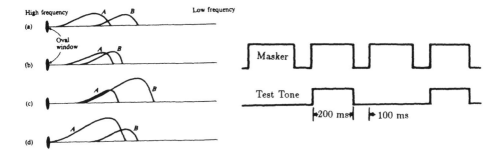

This demonstration uses tones of 1200 and 2000 Hz, presented as 200-ms tone bursts separated by 100 ms (see figure above). The test tone, which appears every other pulse, decreases in 10 steps of 5 dB each, except the first step which is 15 dB.

Commentary

"A masking tone alternates with the combination of masking tone plus a stepwise-decreasing test tone. First the masker is 1200 Hz and the test tone is 2000 Hz, then the masker is 2000 Hz and the test tone is 1200 Hz. Count how many steps of the test tone can be heard in each case."

References

G. von Bekesy (1970), "Traveling waves as frequency analyzers in the cochlea," Nature *225*, 1207–09.

J.P. Egan and H.W. Hake (1950), "On the masking pattern of a simple auditory stimulus," J. Acoust. Soc. Am. *22*, 622–30.

R. Patterson and D. Green (1978), "Auditory masking," in *Handbook of Perception,* Vol. 4: *Hearing,* ed. E. Carterette and M. Friedman (Academic Press, New York) pp. 337–62.

T.D. Rossing (1982), *The Science of Sound* (Addison-Wesley, Reading, MA). Chap. 6.

J.J. Zwislocki (1978), "Masking: Experimental and theoretical aspects of simultaneous, forward, backward, and central masking," in *Handbook of Perception,* Vol. 4: *Hearing,* ed. E. Carterette and M. Friedman (Academic Press, New York) pp. 283–336.

DEMONSTRATION 10. CRITICAL BANDS BY MASKING (1:50)

This demonstration of the masking of a single 2000-Hz tone by spectrally flat (white) noise of different bandwidths is based on the experiments of Fletcher (1940). First, we use broadband noise and the noise with bandwidths of 1000, 250, and 10 Hz.

In order to determine the level of the tone that can just be heard in the presence of the noise, in each case, we present the 2000-Hz tone in 10 decreasing steps of 5 decibels each.

Since the critical bandwidth at 2000 Hz is about 280 Hz, you would expect to hear more steps in the 2000-Hz tone staircase when the noise bandwidth is reduced below this value.

Since the spectrum level of the noise is kept constant, its intensity (and its subjective loudness) will decrease markedly as the bandwidth is decreased.

Commentary

"You will hear a 2000-Hz tone in 10 decreasing steps of 5 decibels. Count how many steps you can hear. Series are presented twice."
"Now the signal is masked with broadband noise."
"Next the noise has a bandwidth of 1000 Hz."
"Next noise with a bandwidth of 250 Hz is used."
"Finally, the bandwidth is reduced to only 10 Hz."

References

H. Fletcher (1940), "Auditory patterns," Rev. Mod. Phys. *12*, 47–65.
B,. Scharf (1970), "Critical bands," in *Foundations of Modern Auditory Theory,* Vol. 1, ed. J.V. Tobias (Academic Press, New York), pp. 157–202.
E. Zwicker, G. Flottorp, and S.S. Stevens (1957), "Critical bandwidth in loudness summation," J. Acoust. Soc. Am. *29*, 548–57.

DEMONSTRATION 11. MASKING LEVEL DIFFERENCES (2:03)

Besides enabling us to localize sound sources, binaural hearing helps us to receive auditory signals in noisy environments. Licklider (1948) discovered the phenomenon called "masking level difference" for speech; Hirsh (1948) demonstrated it for sinusoidal signals, as in this demonstration.

The first example in the demonstration begins by playing a 500-Hz signal of 100 ms duration in the left ear. Then this signal is masked by noise. The staircase procedure is used, so that you can count the level at which the signal becomes inaudible. The staircase contains 10 steps; the first step is -10 dB, and the remaining 9 steps are -3 dB each.

In the third example, noise is added to the other ear. The noise now appears to have a different spatial location (albeit inside the head) from the signal, and the signal is much easier to hear. In the fourth example, the signal is again made difficult to hear by adding a signal to the noise in the right ear, so that the auditory images of signal and noise again coincide.

The fifth example demonstrates that inverting the signal at one of the ears places the noise and signal in different auditory locations. In this configuration, the signal is easy to hear.

The signal, which is similar to No. 11 in the "Harvard tapes" can be summarized as follows: 1) S_L; 2) $S_L N_L$; 3) $S_L N_{LR}$; 4) $S_{LR} N_{LR}$; 5) $S_L S_R N_{LR}$, where S = signal, S = signal of reversed phase, N = noise, L = left, R = right. The signal is more easily heard in examples 1, 3, and 5. In the original Harvard tapes, the demonstration is repeated at 2000 Hz, where the effect has faded, thus demonstrating the strong frequency dependence of masking level difference (Hirsh, 1948).

Commentary

"A stepwise decreasing 500-Hz tone is applied to the left ear. Staircases are presented twice. Count the number of steps you can hear."
"Now the signal is masked with noise."
"Next the same masking noise is applied to both ears."
"Now both signal and noise appear in both ears."
"Finally signal and noise appear in both ears, but the signal phase is reversed in one of the ears."

References

J.L. Flanagan and B.J. Watson (1966), "Binaural unmasking of complex signals," J. Acoust. Soc. Am. 40, 456–68.

I.J. Hirsh (1948), "The influence of interaural phase on interaural summation and inhibition," J. Acoust. Soc. Am. 20, 536–44.

L.A. Jeffress, H.C. Blodgett, T.T. Sandel, and C.L. Wood (1956), "Masking of tonal signals," J. Acoust. Soc. Am. 28, 416–26.

T. Houtgast (1974), Lateral Suppression in Hearing (Acad. Pers. BV, Amsterdam).

H. Levitt and L.R. Rabiner (1967), "Binaural release from masking for speech and gain in intelligibility," J. Acoust. Soc. Am. 42, 601–08.

J.C.R. Licklider (1948), "The influence of interaural phase relations upon the masking of speech by white noise," J. Acoust. Soc. Am. 20, 150–59.

D. McFadden (1975), "Masking and the binaural system," in Human Communication and its Disorders, ed. E. Eagles (Raven Press, New York).

D.E. Robinson and L.A. Jeffress (1963), "Effect of varying the interaural noise correlation on the detectability of tonal signals," J. Acoust. Soc. Am. 35, 1947–52.

DEMONSTRATION 12. VIRTUAL PITCH (0:41)

A complex tone consisting of 10 harmonics of 200 Hz having equal amplitude is presented, first with all harmonics, then without the fundamental, then without the two lowest harmonics, etc. Low-frequency noise (300-Hz lowpass, −10 dB) is included to mask a 200-Hz difference tone that might be generated due to distortion in playback equipment.

Commentary

"You will hear a complex tone with 10 harmonics, first complete and then with the lower harmonics successively removed. Does the pitch of the complex change? The demonstrations is repeated once."

References

A.J.M. Houtsma and J.L. Goldstein (1972), "The central origin of the pitch of complex tones: evidence from musical interval recognition," J. Acoust. Soc. Am. *51,* 520–529.

J.F. Schouten (1940), "The perception of subjective tones," Proc. Kon. Ned. Akad. Wetenschap *41,* 1086–1093.

A. Seebeck (1841), "Beobachtungen über einige Bedingungen der Entstehung von Tönen," Ann. Phys. Chem. *53,* 417–436.

DEMONSTRATION 13. MASKING SPECTRAL AND VIRTUAL PITCH (1:28)

This demonstration uses masking noise of high and low frequency to mask out, alternately, a melody carried by single pure tones of low frequency and the same melody resulting from virtual pitch from groups of three tones of high frequency (4th, 5th, and 6th harmonics). The inability of the low-frequency noise to mask the virtual pitch in the same range points out the inadequacy of the place theory of pitch.

Commentary

"You will hear the familiar Westminster chime melody played with pairs of tones. The first tone of each pair is a sinusoid, the second a complex tone of the same pitch."

"Now the pure-tones notes are masked with low-pass noise. You will still hear the pitches of the complex tone."

"Finally the complex tone is masked by high-pass noise. The pure-tone melody is still heard."

References

J.C.R. Licklider (1955), "Influence of phase coherence upon the pitch of complex tones," J. Acoust. Soc. Am. *27,* 996 (A).

R.J. Ritsma and B.L. Cardozo (1963/64), "The perception of pitch," Philips Techn. Review *25,* 37–43.

DEMONSTRATION 14. TONE GLIDES WITH GAPS (2:32)

Part 1: A tone repetitively glides up and down in frequency. The instants of reversal from ascending to descending glide and from descending to ascending glide have been spliced out and replaced by silence. The gaps are easily heard.

Part 2: The gaps at the peaks and valleys have been replaced by loud bursts of white noise. The tone sounds continuous and seems to glide through the noise burst. The gliding tone goes from 1464 Hz to 2297 Hz and back again in 2 sec. The glides are exponential (equal pitch change per unit time). The noise is white and its peak amplitude is 10.6 times that of the tone, i.e., 20.5 dB larger.

References

Bregman, A.S. (1990). Auditory Scene Analysis: The Perceptual Organization of Sound. Cambridge, Mass.: Bradford Books, MIT Press. pp. 28, 363, 367, 420–428.
Dannenbring, G.L. (1976). Perceived auditory continuity with alternately rising and falling frequency transitions. Canadian Journal of Psychology, *30,* 99–114.

DEMONSTRATION 15. PITCH STREAMING AND PITCH GLIDES (2:07)

Bregman and Campbell's (1971) loop of three high tones alternating with three low tones, producing streaming. The frequencies of the six tones, in the order in which they occur in the loop, are 2500, 350, 2000, 430, 1600, and 550 Hz. All tones are sinusoidal, of equal intensity, and are 0.1 s in duration, exclusive of the decay. The start of the decay of each tone is synchronous with the start of the onset of the next. The onsets are 10 ms in duration following a quarter-sine wave function, and the decays are exponential with a time constant (50 percent decay) of 0.004 s.

Bergman's and Dannenbring (1973) illustration of the effects of continuity in streaming.
Part 1: Loop of alternating high and low tones connected by pitch glides, which tends to resist streaming.
Part 2: The same loop of tones without the pitch-glides (i.e., with disconnected tones) is more likely to produce streaming. In the connected condition, the steady states are 100 ms, and the pitch glides are also 100 ms.
In the disconnected condition, the 100 ms steady states are preceded by a 10 ms rise and followed by a 10 ms fall in intensity which are linear in amplitude. However, each tone is unchanging in frequency. The timing of the loop is the same as in the connected condition. The frequency transitions are exponential. Intensities of the steady-state parts are the same as the pitch glides and are the same for all frequencies. The frequencies of the tones are 2000, 1600, 614, and 400, as in Bregman & Dannenbring (1973).

References

Bregman, A.S. (1990). Auditory Scene Analysis: The Perceptual Organization of Sound. Cambridge, Mass.: Bradford Books, MIT Press. pp. 50, 133-136, 139, 147.

Bregman, A.S., & Campbell, J. (1971). Primary auditory stream segregation and perception of order in rapid sequences of tones. Journal of Experimental Psychology, *89*, 244-249.

Bregman, A.S., & Dannenbring, G. (1973). The effect of continuity on auditory stream segregation. Perception and Psychophysics, *13*, 308-312.

DEMONSTRATION 16. FUSING, STREAMING, AND PITCH GLIDES (2:01)

A pure tone (A) alternates with a complex tone having two pure tone components (B and C).

The durations of all tones are 200 msec and the silence between A and B is always 100 msec. The cycle length is 600 ms. All the pure tone components are of equal amplitude.

Part 1: The components, B and C, of the complex tone are synchronous in onset, and neither is near the frequency of the preceding pure tone A. The components of the complex tone are heard as fused, producing a rich timbre, and the complex tone is perceptually isolated from the single pure tone. The frequencies of A, B, and C are 1800, 650 and 300 Hz, respectively.

Part 2: The components of the complex tone are not synchronous in onset, and the preceding pure tone, A, is near in frequency to upper component, B, of the complex tone BC. This causes B to be pulled into a sequential stream with A. The result is the isolation of the lower component C of the complex tone as a separate stream. The rich timbre of the complex tone (AB) is lost and only pure tones are heard. The frequencies of A, B, and C are 700, 650 and 300 Hz, respectively. The onset of C precedes that of B by 60 ms.

References

Bregman, A.S. (1990). Auditory Scene Analysis: The Perceptual Organization of Sound. Cambridge, Mass.: Bradford Books, MIT Press. pp. 29, 216-221.

Bregman, A.S., & Pinker, S. (1978). Auditory streaming and the building of timbre. Canadian Journal of Psychology, *32*, 19-31.

DEMONSTRATION 17. PITCH STREAMING (1:22)

It is clear in listening to melodies that sequences of tones can form coherent patterns. This is called *temporal coherence*. When tones do not form patterns, but seem isolated, that is called *fission*.

Temporal coherence and fission are illustrated in a demonstration first presented by van Noorden (1975) and included in the "Harvard tapes" (1978). Van Noorden describes it as a "galloping rhythm."

We present tones A and B in the sequence ABA ABA. Tone A has a frequency of 2000 Hz, tone B varies from 1000 to 4000 Hz and back again to 1000 Hz. Near the crossover points, the tones appear to form a coherent pattern, characterized by a galloping rhythm, but at large intervals the tones seem isolated, illustrating fission.

Commentary

"In this experiment a fixed tone A and a variable tone B alternate in a fast sequence ABA ABA. At some places you may hear a "galloping rhythm," while at other places the sequences of tone A and B seem isolated."

References

A.S. Bregman (1978), "Auditory streaming: competition among alternative organizations," Percept. Psychophys. *23*, 391–98.

L.P.A.S. van Noorden (1975), *Temporal Coherence in the Perception of Tone Sequences*. Doctoral dissertation with phonograph record (Institute for Perception Research, Eindhoven, The Netherlands).

Harvard University Laboratory of psychophysics (1978), "Auditory demonstration tapes," No. 18.

DEMONSTRATION 18. FUSING, STREAMING, AND TEMPORAL PATTERNING (1:52)

Three pure tones glide up and down together in frequency, maintaining the frequency ratios 3:4:5. These fuse into a complex sound. A fourth tone, which glides up and down in frequency in a different pattern, is thereby isolated and is heard as a second sound.

The slow gliding of the three components is imposed by a 0.4 Hz frequency modulation (period = 2.5 s). The faster gliding of the isolated fourth tone is imposed by a 2 Hz frequency modulation (period = 0.5 s).

Reference

Bregman, A.S. (1990). Auditory Scene Analysis: The Perceptual Organization of Sound. Cambridge, Mass.: Bradford Books, MIT Press. pp. 101–102, 257–260.

DEMONSTRATION 19. EFFECT OF DISTRACTORS ON STREAMING (1:19)

Part 1: A pair of target tones is played once, then played again, bracketed by two lower distractor tones. The frequencies of the target tones are 2200 and 2400 Hz, and that of both of the distractor tones is 1460 Hz. All tones are of equal intensity. Each tone has a 7 ms linear rise in amplitude, a 45-ms steady state and a 5 ms linear decay. There is a warning click (10 ms white noise burst) 1 s before each demonstration.

In Part 1, the order of the target tones is hard to judge. A warning click is followed 1.5 s later by a sequence of the two target tones, with no silence between them. Then the sequence of the two targets bracketed before and after by the distractor tones is played. This presentation occurs twice. Onset-to-onset time for the tones in this sequence is 65 ms).

Part 2: The addition of a stream of tones at the same frequency as the distractor tones "strips off" the distractor tones, isolating the target tones in their own stream. The order of the target tones is easier to judge. The onset-to-onset time of the tones in the capturing stream is set to be equal to that for the two distractor tones taken alone (i.e., without regard to the target tones that they bracket). This means the distractors fall into an isochronous stream (onset-to-onset time = 195 ms) with the capturing tones.

References

Bregman, A.S. (1990). Auditory Scene Analysis: The Perceptual Organization of Sound. Cambridge, Mass.: Bradford Books, MIT Press. pp. 14–15, 132–133, 140, 165–166, 192–193, 444–445.

Bregman, S.A. & Rudnicky, A. (1975). Auditory segregation: stream or streams? Journal of Experimental Psychology: Human Perception and Performance, 1, 263–267.

DEMONSTRATION 20. AN AUDITORY ILLUSION (0:38)

Presenting certain tone sequences to both ears produces some interesting auditory illusions, including the one in this demonstration, described by Deutsch (1975).

Tones of 400 and 800 Hz alternate in both ears in opposite phase; that is, when the left ear receives 400 Hz, the right ear receives 800 Hz. About 99% of listeners hear a single low-frequency tone in one ear and a high-frequency tone in the other ear. Quite remarkably, when the headphones are reversed, most listeners hear the high tone and the low tone in the same ears as before (Deutsch, 1974).

Right-handed subjects usually hear the high tone in their right ear and the low tone in their left ear, regardless of how the headphones are oriented. Left-handed subjects, on the other hand, are just as likely to hear the high tone in the right ear as in the left. This is because in right-handed people, the left hemisphere is dominant (and is primary auditory input is from the right ear), whereas in left-handed people, either hemisphere may be dominant. High tones apparently are perceived as being heard at the ear that feeds the dominant hemisphere (Deutsch, 1975).

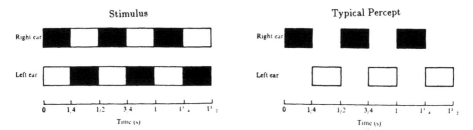

Commentary

"Try to guess the signal you are listening to in each ear."

References

D. Deutsch (1974), "An auditory illusion," Nature *251*, 307–09.
D. Deutsch (1975), "Musical Illusions," Sci. Am. *223*(4), 92–104.

DEMONSTRATION 21. SPEECH TRANSFORMATION (3:43)

One of the remarkable properties of speech is the fact that the information conveyed by the wave form is invariant under extreme transformations. A homely example of such transformations occurs when one hears speech in an ordinary room, for the acoustics of the room produce various delays and changes in the power spectrum. The room is, after all, a spatial filter. In one demonstration (#2) of this series we attempt to illustrate some of those transformations via a consideration of echoes. The study of various transformations of the waveform, especially those that leave the speech information intact, has been of major interest to the Bell Telephone Laboratories. The demonstrations presented here are all prepared by the speech group at BTL.

The first example simply illustrates that digitizing the amplitude of the speech waveform does not produce a very serious change in the intelligibility of the speech waveform. The sampling rate is 10 kHz, that is, a sample of the pressure waveform is quantized and represented by either 12, 9, 4, 2, or 1 bits. In the last case, 1 bit, the quantization consists of making the speech amplitude have a "1" or "0" value. Thus the speech waveform is essentially a square wave of variable duty cycle. For 2 bits, four values of amplitude are used, for 4 bits sixteen values of amplitude are used, etc. Notice at even at the 1 bit quantization the intelligibility is high and one can in fact tell whether the speaker is a man or a woman.

In the second example, the amplitude quantization is held at 12 bits so that the error is representing the pressure amplitude is very small, but the sampling rate is changed from 10 kHz to 5 kHz to 1.25 kHz. Notice that changing the sampling rate, that is, the duration of each sample, has a profound effect upon the intelligibility.

The reason for the differences in these two demonstrations is easy to see if one looks at the power spectrum of the speech waveform. Amplitude quantization has a relatively small effect on the power spectrum, it essentially introduces some high frequency noise. This was illustrated in some spectrograms from the chapter by Licklider and Miller (1951), in S.S. Stevens' handbook article. Changing the sampling rate, however, severely disturbs the power spectrum, especially as it introduces new components in the speech band.

The third example is self-explanatory, and represents a computer simulation of speech, that is, the generation of speech waveforms according to rules stored in the computer. For more details on this very interesting demonstration, the article by Coker, Umeda, and Browman (1973) is recommended.

The fourth example illustrates vocoder speech. This is a bandwidth compression scheme, first suggested by Homer Dudley (1939) in his classic article. Basically, Dudley's approach is to maintain the power spectrum of speech as a function of time, but to ignore the fine variation in the speech waveform. The engineering consequence of these manipulations is to reduce the bandwidth of speech by nearly a factor of ten. Since the cost of a large scale communication system is nearly proportional with bandwidth, the economic advantage of these manipulations is apparent. The vocoder has never been used as a device in telephone communications in the United States, although it is widely used in military applications, especially because it allows one to scramble the various channels of the waveform and thus provide a private communication channel.

Many modern-day vocoders are of the linear predictive type. This type of vocoder is illustrated in the final band of this tape. For more information concerning linear prediction vocoders, Atal and Hanauer (1971) is recommended.

References

Coker, C.H., Umeda, N., and Browman, C.P. Automatic synthesis from ordinary English text, IEEE Transactions on Audio Electroacoustics, 1973, AU-21, 293–298.

Atal, B.S. and Hanauer, S.L. Speech analysis and synthesis by linear prediction of the speech wave, *Journal of the Acoustical Society of America,* 1971, *50,* 637–655.

Licklider, J.C.R., and Miller, G. The perception of speech, *Handbook of Experimental Psychology,* S.S. Stevens (ed.), New York: J. Wiley & Sons, Inc., 1951.

Dudley, H. Remaking Speech, *Journal of the Acoustical Society of America,* 1939, *11,* 169–177.

CONTENTS

DEMONSTRATION 22. CATEGORICAL SPEECH PERCEPTION (5:17)

The following demonstrations were constructed at the Haskins Laboratories and illustrate the categorical nature of speech perception. "Categorical" refers to the fact that although speech sounds may differ along a continuum, such as the starting frequency of the second format, we perceive such variations in terms of only one or two categories. These categories divide the stimulus continuum into two or three distinctive sounds or phonemes. Within the categories, discrimination tends to be difficult; across the categories, discrimination is easy. The following demonstrations do not concern themselves with discrimination per se, but do illustrate the rather dramatic change in perception of the speech sound as we move along the stimulus continuum. The first demonstration illustrates the place continuum (so called because the variation pertains to the locus of the tongue as the sound is initiated). Physically, the tapes were constructed by varying the onset frequency of the second formant in twelves steps of approximately 135 Hz. The figure shows that the starting frequency for the second formant was changed systematically, while the first formant remained the same. The figure illustrates samples 1, 6, and 13 as they would be represented in a stylized spectrographic display of the utterances.

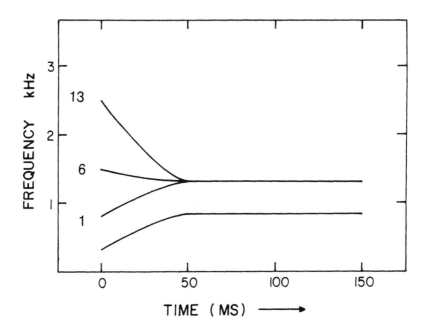

The second demonstration presents the second formant transition cues in isolation. No abrupt changes in the sound is encountered as we systematically vary the stimulus. The same set of sounds, when coupled with the first formant frequency, produces the BA DA GA sequence that was heard in the first demonstration.

The third demonstration is an example of the effect of the duration of a silent interval inserted between a voiceless fricative, S, and a voiced vowel, A. This illustrates a "manner continuum", referring to the presence or absence between fricative and vowel of a voiceless obstruent or stop (such as P, T, K). Here continuous variations in the duration of the silent interval give rise to the perceived categories, SA and STA. Again, thirteen utterances occur in succession, and the gap is zero for the first utterance, 120 ms for the last, in steps of 10 ms. The second figure shows an oscillographic representation of a typical utterance with the gap labeled.

The final continuum illustrated is a "voicing continuum" and illustrates a change from GA to KA. The abrupt perceptual switch is induced by varying the duration of the interval between the beginning of the utterance, that is, the release of the initial stop, signaled by a brief burst of noise, and the onset of voicing, signaled by periodic excitation of the vocal tract. In the eight utterances, each lasting roughly 300 ms the delay in "voice onset" is varied from zero to 70 ms in 10 ms steps.

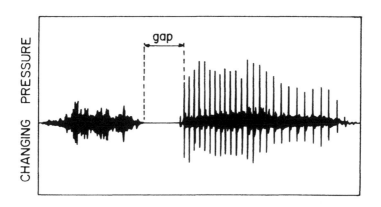

References

Cutting, J.E., Rosner, B.S., and Ford, C.F. Perceptual categories for musiclike sounds: Implications for theories of speech perception. *Quarterly Journal of Experimental Psychology,* 1976, *28,* 361–378.

Liberman, A.M., Cooper, F. S., Shankweiler, D.S., and Studdert-Kennedy, M. Perception of the Speech Code," *Psychological Review,* 1967, *74,* 431–661.

Studdert-Kennedy, M. Speech perception. Chapter 8 in: *Contemporary Issues in Experimental Phonetics,* N.J. Lass (ed.) New York: Academic Press, 1976.

CONTENTS

DEMONSTRATION 23: SHIFT OF VIRTUAL PITCH (1:08)

A tone having strong partials with frequencies of 800, 1000, and 1200 Hz will have a virtual pitch corresponding to the 200-Hz missing fundamental, as in Demonstration 12. If each of these partials is shifted upward by 20 Hz, however, they are no longer exact harmonics of any fundamental frequency around 200 Hz. The auditory system will accept them as being "nearly harmonic" and identify a virtual pitch slightly above 200 Hz (approximately $\frac{1}{3}(\frac{820}{4} + \frac{1020}{5} + \frac{1220}{6}) = 204$ Hz in this case). The auditory system appears to search for a "nearly common factor" in the frequencies of the partials.

Note that if the virtual pitch were created by some kind of distortion, the resulting difference tone would remain at 200 Hz when the partials were shifted upward by the same amount.

In this demonstration, the three partials in a complex tone, 0.5 s in duration, are shifted upward in ten 20-Hz steps while maintaining a 200-Hz spacing between partials. You will almost certainly hear a virtual pitch that rises from 200 to about $\frac{1}{3}(\frac{1000}{4} + \frac{1200}{5} + \frac{1400}{6}) = 241$ Hz. At the same time, you may have noticed a second rising virtual pitch that ends up at $\frac{1}{3}(\frac{1000}{5} + \frac{1200}{6} + \frac{1400}{7}) = 200$ Hz and possibly even a third one, as shown in Fig. 2 in Schouten et al. (1962).

In the second part of the demonstration it is shown that virtual pitches of a complex tone having partials of 800, 1000, and 1200 Hz and one having partials of 850, 1050, and 1250 Hz can be matched to harmonic complex tones with fundamentals of 200 and 210 Hz, respectively.

Commentary

"You will hear a three-tone harmonic complex with its partials shifted upward in equal steps until the complex is harmonic again. The sequence is repeated once."

"Now you hear a three-tone complex of 800, 1000, and 1200 Hz, followed by a complex of 850, 1050 and 1250 Hz. As you can hear, their virtual pitches are well matched by the regular harmonic tones with fundamentals of 200 and 210 Hz. The sequence is repeated once."

References

J.F. Schouten, R.L. Ritsma and B.L. Cardozo (1962), "Pitch of the residue," J. Acoust. Soc. Am. *34*, 1418–1424.

G.F. Smoorenburg (1970), "Pitch perception of two-frequency stimuli," J. Acoust. Soc. Am. *48*, 926–942.

Printed and bound by CPI Group (UK) Ltd, Croydon, CR0 4YY

22/10/2024

01777623-0010